ALLEZEIT WACH
1842

Fetal Heart Rate Monitoring

Clinical Practice and Pathophysiology

Edited by W. Künzel

With 157 Figures

Springer-Verlag
Berlin Heidelberg New York Tokyo

Professor Dr. Wolfgang Künzel
Universitäts-Frauenklinik
Klinikstr. 28, D-6300 Gießen

Library of Congress Cataloging in Publication Data. Main entry under title: Fetal heart rate monitoring. Includes bibliographies and index. 1. Fetal heart rate monitoring. I. Künzel, W. (Wolfgang), 1936– . [DNLM: 1. Fetal Heart—physiology. 2. Fetal Heart—physiopathology. 3. Fetal Monitoring. WQ 210.5.F4195] RG 628.3.H42F45 1985 618.3′2 85-2811

ISBN 978-3-642-70360-7 ISBN 978-3-642-70358-4 (eBook)
DOI 10.1007/978-3-642-70358-4

Softcover reprint of the hardcover 1st edition 1985

2123/3130-543210

Preface

In the past decade fetal heart rate monitoring has become a generally accepted method for fetal surveillance during pregnancy and labor. Although its importance has been doubted recently, I personally feel that this method has become an important obstetric tool. It has not only improved our knowledge about fetal behavior and fetal condition throughout gestation, but it has especially improved fetal surveillance during labor; the most dangerous period of human life has never been as safe as nowadays. The only people who can question the advantage of fetal heart rate monitoring are those who did not experience the period before fetal heart rate monitoring was generally introduced.

The first paper on the history of fetal heart rate monitoring takes us back to the beginning of fetal surveillance and provides an introduction to the different aspects of fetal observation which are covered later in this volume. Common practices of fetal surveillance in different countries are discussed, and the paths that future developments will take are suggested. An outline of the physiological aspects of fetal heart rate regulation is followed by discussion of the pathophysiology with which the obstetrician is very often confronted.

Although there is no doubt that fetal heart rate deviations combined with an increase in baseline fetal heart rate and a loss of oscillations signify fetal deterioration, there is still controversy over the interpretation of the different heart rate patterns. We know that decelerations express fetal hypoxia, but it remains unclear to what extent these heart rate alterations affect the acid-base status of the fetus. We know that a loss of oscillations is often followed by fetal compromise, but essentially we know nothing about the cause and regulations of these heart rate patterns. We know that during fetal hypoxia the chemo- and pressoreceptors are stimulated, but we do not know the preference of these receptors during hypoxia.

In looking over the fetal heart rate charts available in delivery rooms, one sometimes feels like an individual doing research with tunnel vision or the keyhole syndrome in one's own microcosm, as Longo pointed out at the symposium *Respiratory Gas Exchange and Blood Flow in the Placenta* [edited by L. D. Longo and H. Bartels, U.S. Department of Health, Education, and Welfare publication no. (NIH) 73-361] 12 years ago in Hannover. He emphasized this situation by citing the allegory of The Blind Men and the Elephant by John Godfrey Saxe. At that time I was a young investigator working in the department of physiology with Bartels and Moll in Hannover. I was very impressed by his talk and I cannot resist presenting this poem again here.

The Blind Men and the Elephant

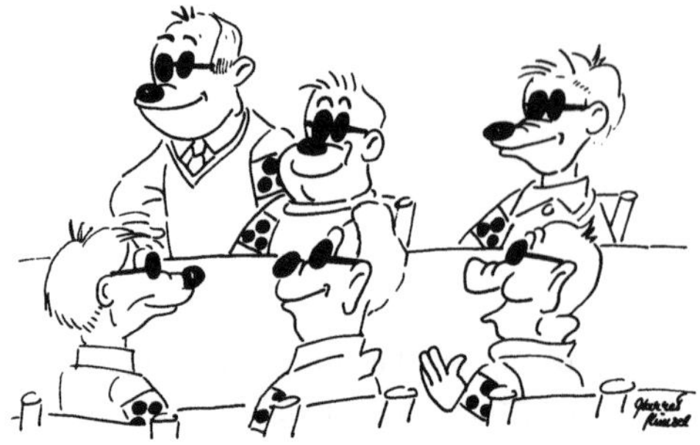

It was six men of Indostan
To learning much inclined,
Who went to see the Elephant
(Though all of them were blind),
That each by observation
Might satisfy his mind.

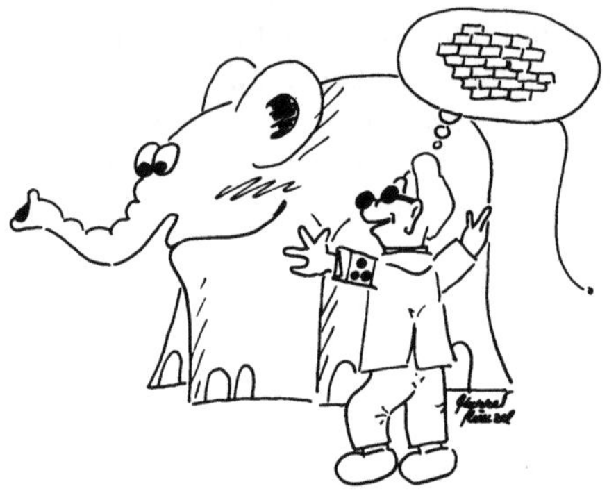

The First approached the Elephant,
And happening to fall
Against his broad and sturdy side,
At once began to bawl:
"God bless me! but the Elephant
Is very like a wall!"

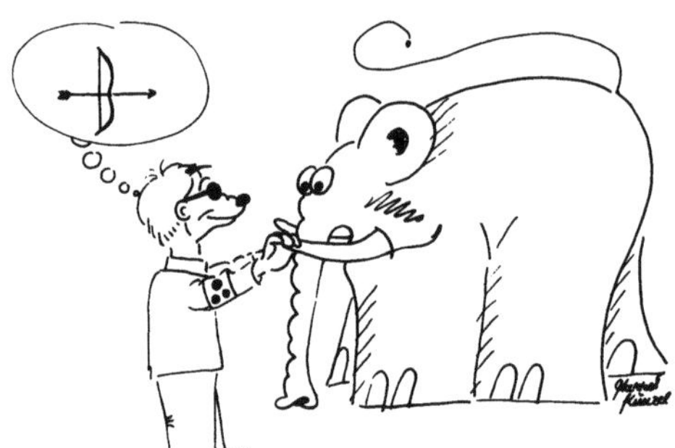

The Second, feeling of the tusk,
Cried, "Ho! what have we here.
So very round and smooth and sharp?
To me 'tis mighty clear
This wonder of an Elephant
Is very like a spear!"

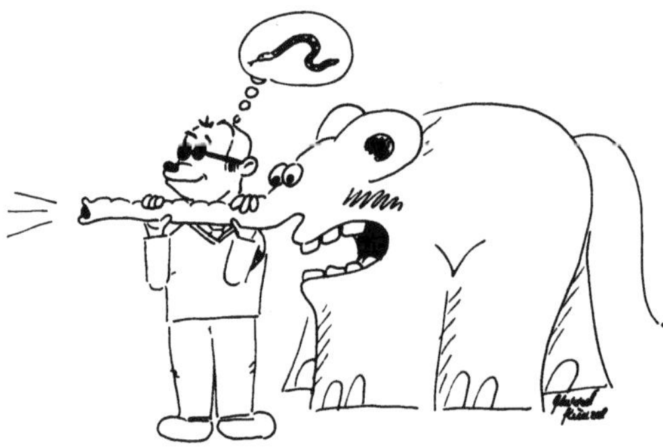

The Third approached the animal,
And happening to take
The squirming trunk within his hands,
Thus boldly up and spake:
"I see," quoth he, "the Elephant
Is very like a snake."

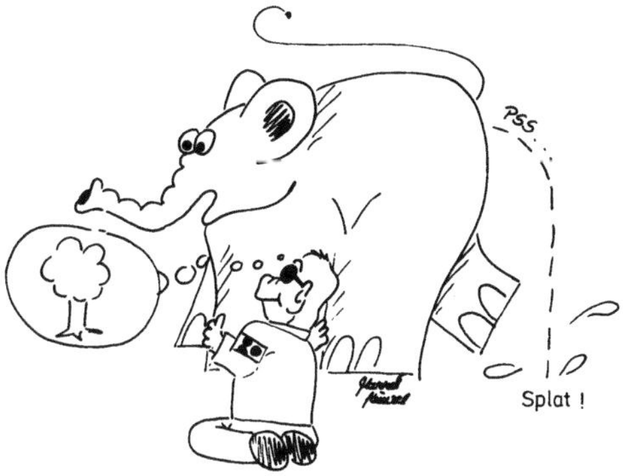

The Fourth reached out an eager hand,
And felt about the knee,
"What most this wonderous beast is like
Is mighty plain," said he;
"Tis clear enough the Elephant
Is very like a tree!"

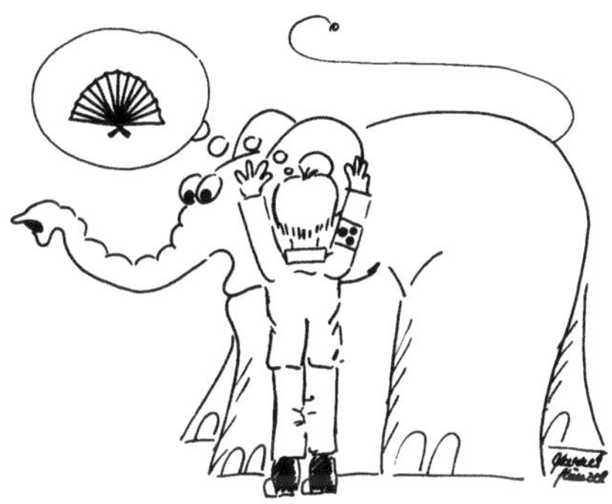

The Fifth, who chanced to touch the ear,
Said: "E'en the blindest man
Can tell what this resembles most;
Deny the fact who can,
This marvel of an Elephant
Is very like a fan!"

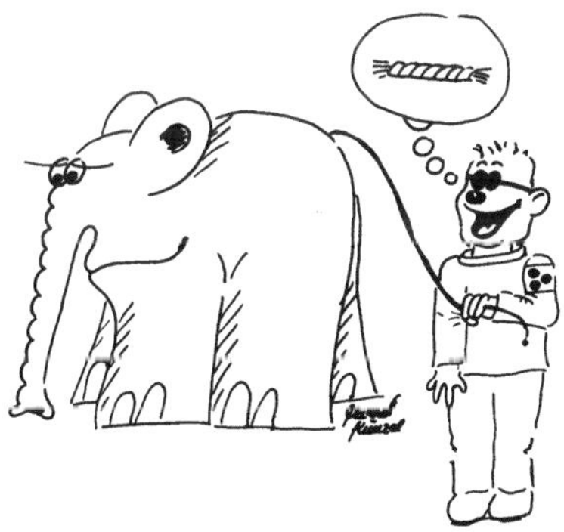

The Sixth no sooner had begun
About the beast to grope,
Than, seizing on the swinging tail
That fell within his scope,
"I see," quoth he, "the Elephant
Is very like a rope!"

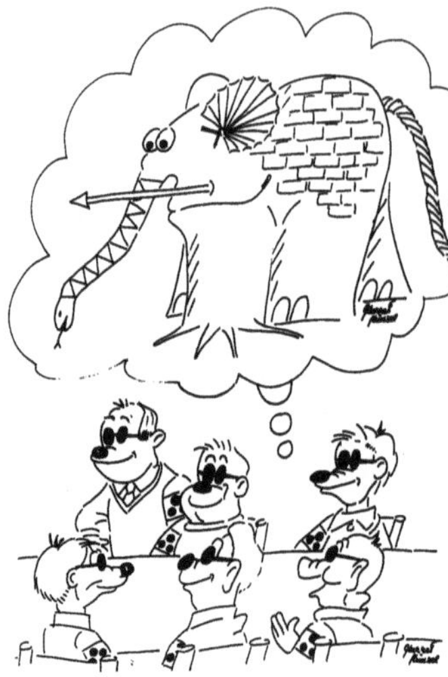

And so these men of Indostan
Disputed loud and long,
Each in his own opinion
Exceeding stiff and strong,
Though each was partly in the right,
And all were in the wrong!

Moral

So oft in scientific wars
The disputants, I ween,
Rail on in utter ignorance
Of what each other mean,
And prate about an elephant
Not one of them has seen!

John Godfrey Saxe

I hope in this volume that we do not adhere to a "keyhole meaning"; that we are not "blind men"; and that the papers presented here will stimulate discussion, clear up misunderstandings, and provide us with knowledge that helps us to proceed in our research.

Gießen

W. Künzel

Table of Contents

Clinical Application and Validity

History of Fetal Heart Rate Monitoring
K.-H. Wulf (With 10 Figures) 3

Necessity of Fetal Heart Rate Monitoring
from a Dutch Point of View
T. K. A. B. Eskes (With 3 Figures) 16

Changing Trends of Fetal Heart Rate Monitoring
in the United States
S. Y. Yeh (With 2 Figures) 22

The Dublin Randomised Controlled Trial
of Intrapartum Electronic Fetal Heart Rate Monitoring
P. Boylan, D. MacDonald, A. Grant, M. Pereira, and I. Chalmers
(With 3 Figures) 34

The Use of Fetal Surveillance During Labor
in the Federal Republic of Germany
V. M. Roemer, K. Bühler, and D. G. Kieback (With 13 Figures) . . . 40

Present and Future Technical Advances
in Fetal Heart Rate Monitoring
H. D. Junge (With 5 Figures) 53

Physiology of Fetal Heart Rate During Intrauterine Life

Antenatal Heart Rate Analysis at the Bedside
Using a Microprocessor
G. S. Dawes and C. W. G. Redman 63

Fetal Hemodynamic Alterations During Advancing Gestation
M. A. Heymann (With 1 Figure) 66

Pathophysiology of Fetal Heart Rate Deceleration

Incidence and Pattern of Fetal Heart Rate Alterations During Labor
J. Melchior and N. Bernard (With 6 Figures) 73

Fetal Hemodynamic Responses to Reduced Uterine Blood Flow in the Sheep Fetus
J. T. PARER (With 10 Figures) 82

Variability of Fetal Heart Rate Deceleration, Blood Pressure, and Acid Base Alterations During Defined Repetitive Hypoxic Stress
E. KASTENDIECK, W. KÜNZEL, and A. JENSEN (With 7 Figures) 94

Fetal Heart Rate Response to Hypoxia in the Subhuman Primate
E. MUELLER-HEUBACH (With 6 Figures) 104

Fetal Heart Rate Alterations in Partial and Total Cord Occlusion
W. KÜNZEL (With 10 Figures) 114

Neurohumoral and Metabolic Response of the Fetus to Hypoxia

Adrenal-Medullary Activity and Cardiovascular Control in the Fetal Sheep
C. T. JONES and G. WEI (With 6 Figures) 127

The Dip Area: A Measure of Acid Base Alterations?
W. KÜNZEL, E. KASTENDIECK, M. HOHMANN, and A. JENSEN (With 8 Figures) 136

Fetal Heart Rate and Fetal Deterioration: Clinical and Experimental Observations
A. JENSEN, W. KÜNZEL, and M. HOHMANN (With 19 Figures) 144

Kinetics of Lactic Acid Accumulation and Removal in the Fetus
W. MOLL and E. KASTENDIECK (With 8 Figures) 161

Pharmacological Aspects of Fetal Heart Rate Regulation During Hypoxia
C. B. MARTIN, JR. (With 8 Figures) 170

Pathophysiology of Fetal Heart Rate Variability and Base Line Fetal Heart Rate

The Control of Fetal Heart Rate and Its Variability in Lambs
G. S. DAWES 187

Short- and Long-Term Variability in Fetal Heart Rate Pattern and Its Relation to Basal Heart Frequency
J. DE HAAN (With 7 Figures) 191

Long-Term Observation of Fetal Heart Rate Irregularities
H. D. JUNGE (With 6 Figures) 201

Fetal Heart Rate Patterns in Experimental Intrauterine Growth Retardation
J. F. CLAPP, III, N. S. PERESS, P. M. CATALANO, and L. I. MANN (With 7 Figures) 212

Chemoreceptor and Baroreceptor Function
with Respect to Fetal Heart Rate Variability
H. Acker (With 10 Figures) 223

Blood Flow Measurements in the Human Fetus
J. W. Wladimiroff, H. M. Tonge, and P. C. Struijk (With 2 Figures) . 234

Subject Index 240

List of Contributors

You will find the addresses at the beginning of the respective contribution

Acker, H. 223
Bernard, N. 73
Boylan, P. 34
Bühler, K. 40
Catalano, P.M. 212
Chalmers, I. 34
Clapp, J.F., III 212
Dawes, G.S. 63, 187
Eskes, T.K.A.B. 16
Grant, A. 34
deHaan, J. 191
Heymann, M.A. 66
Hohmann, M. 136, 145
Jensen, A. 94, 136, 145
Jones, C.T. 127
Junge, H.D. 53, 201
Kastendieck, E. 94, 136, 161
Kieback, D.G. 40
Künzel, W. 94, 114, 136, 145
MacDonald, D. 34
Mann, L.I. 212
Martin, C.B., Jr. 170
Melchior, J. 73
Moll, W. 161
Mueller-Heubach, E. 104
Parer, J.T. 82
Pereira, M. 34
Peress, N.S. 212
Redman, C.W.G. 63
Roemer, V.M. 40
Struijk, P.C. 234
Tonge, H.M. 234
Wei, G. 127
Wladimiroff, J.W. 234
Wulf, K.-H. 3
Yeh, S. 22

Clinical Application and Validity

History of Fetal Heart Rate Monitoring

K.-H. Wulf[1]

The history of fetal heart rate monitoring is a combination of progress in both biomedical technique and obstetrics at the same time. Technical developments range from the first obstetric stethoscopes of around 1800 via the second generation cardiotocographs to the modern computer-operated cardiotocograph evaluation systems of our, as it were, third-generation obstetric monitoring equipment. The importance of fetal heart monitoring for obstetrics has increased with technical progress.

Obstetric auscultation was reported as early as the eighteenth century. Interest then centered primarily on the acoustic recognition of fetal movement and the splashing sounds of the amniotic fluid. Fetal heartbeat was not mentioned at that time. Auscultation of fetal heartbeats began in the early nineteenth century. In 1818 the Swiss surgeon Mayor described the characteristic double tone and frequency of the acoustic activity of the fetal heart, but the exact details of his findings are not known. No publication by Mayor himself exists; only a reference in the annals of the University Library of Geneva has come down to us. The Parisian doctor and nobleman Jean-Alexandre Le Jumeau, Vicomte de Kergaradec (1822) (Fig. 1), is rightly considered the real pioneer and founder of fetal heartbeat auscultation. On 26 December 1821 before the Royal Academy of Medicine in Paris, Kergaradec reported hearing fetal heartbeats in eight pregnant women. Among his audience was his teacher Laennec, the founder of auscultation of the thoracic organs, who later confirmed his observations. Kergaradec himself was not an obstetrician, but he nevertheless immediately recognized the importance of fetal heart monitoring for practical obstetrics. He summarized its possible applications in seven points (Table 1).

News of the revolutionary technique spread quickly throughout Europe. Its acceptance by established obstetricians was, however, a slow process, hindered by a great deal of prejudice. In Germany Kergaradec's discovery was taken up particularly by the schools of obstetrics in Berlin under Kluge and in Würzburg under de Outrepont. In 1823 detailed findings by Lau (1823) in Berlin and Haus (1823) and Ulsamer (1828) in Würzburg appeared. But there was no shortage of doubting voices among renowned obstetricians: Duges (Paris; 1822) considered it for theoretical reasons impossible to hear the fetal heart through the abdominal wall of the mother and von Siebold warned: "Let the obstetricians not neglect the perfecting of their sense of touch because they want to hear." There were numerous disputes over the technique of listening. Many obstetricians favored direct auscultation with the naked ear. Others demanded the use of a stethoscope for reasons of decency and nothing else. The best position for the pregnant woman and the obstetrician was also a controversial question. Normally at that time pregnant women were examined through their clothing in a standing position. It was regarded as indecent to expose

[1] Univ.-Frauenklinik und Hebammenschule, Josef-Schneider-Str. 4, D-8700 Würzburg

Fetal Heart Rate Monitoring
Ed. by W. Künzel

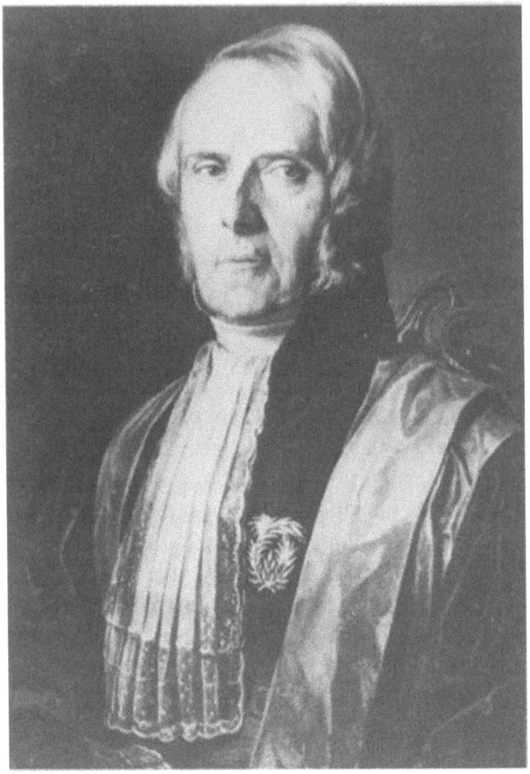

Fig. 1. Jean Alexandre Le Jumeau, Vicomte de Kergaradec, Paris (1787–1877)

the body. This respect for the sense of shame and modesty of the woman must undoubtedly have inhibited the spread of obstetric auscultation. In addition there was a fixed obstetric ritual which gave pride of place to the sense of touch. Even in 1830 the great Osiander wrote in his textbook: "The obstetrician must carry out all his duties right up to the birth of the child by touch, like a blind man."

It is therefore understandable that the first systematic and extensive studies were not published until 10–20 years after the discovery of the fetal heartbeat. Here I would mention the work of:

Evory Kennedy	(Dublin)	1833
Anton Hohl	(Dresden)	1833
Jean Anne Henri Depaul	(Paris)	1847

There now followed exact reports on the average rates of fetal heartbeat and its variations (Table 2). The increase in frequency with fetal movement or fever in the mother was noted. A temperature rise of 0.1 of a degree was said to lead to an increase in heart rate of 3 beats/min. The decrease in rate as pregnancy progresses was also often mentioned. There is a negative correlation between gestational age, weight, length, and diameter of the fetus. If the average heartbeat rate is 144/min, the birth weight can be expected to be less than about 3000 g. When the weight is

Table 1. Applications of fetal heart rate monitoring. (Kergaradec 1822)

No. 1	A certain sign of pregnancy
No. 2	A sign of fetal health (strength and frequency of heart tones)
No. 3	Diagnosis of multiple pregnancy
No. 4	Diagnosis of fetal position
No. 5	Diagnosis of placenta localization
No. 6	Diagnosis of extrauterine pregnancy
No. 7	Detection of placental or uterine souffle

Table 2. Early reports of fetal heart rate

		Beats/min
Normal frequency		
Dubois	(1831)	144
Hohl	(1833)	140
Von Höfft	(1838)	140
Nägele	(1838)	135
Frankenhäuser	(1859)	136
Hüter	(1862)	132
Fetal weight—gestational age		
< 2900 g		144
> 2900 g		128
(Bolzoni 1884)		
Differences in sex		
Female		144
Male		124
(Frankenhäuser 1860)		

greater the rate is on average 128/min. The findings on sex difference are interesting. Frankenhäuser (1860) in particular points out that with girls one can expect a higher average rate of about 144/min compared with 124/min in boys. These figures are confirmed in principle by others, though they emphasize that the differences are too small to permit a reliable prediction of sex in individual cases. The influence of the contractions on heart rate and rhythm was also discovered, as were the effects of head and umbilical cord compression.

The essential pathomechanisms of heart rate alterations, which are central to our diagnostic procedures today, were known in principle 100 years ago. Several theories about the cause of alterations in heart rate *sub partu* were developed, based above all on extensive and very careful clinical observations. But experimental approaches were also under way. Important contributions to the mechanism of alterations in heart rate were made by Schwartz (Kiel), Schultze (Jena), and Seitz (Munich). Schwartz (1858) was probably the first to investigate fetal breathing activity (Fig. 2). He developed the concept of asphyxia in connection with the first breath and considers the reason for the bradycardial reactions of the fetus to the contractions in the

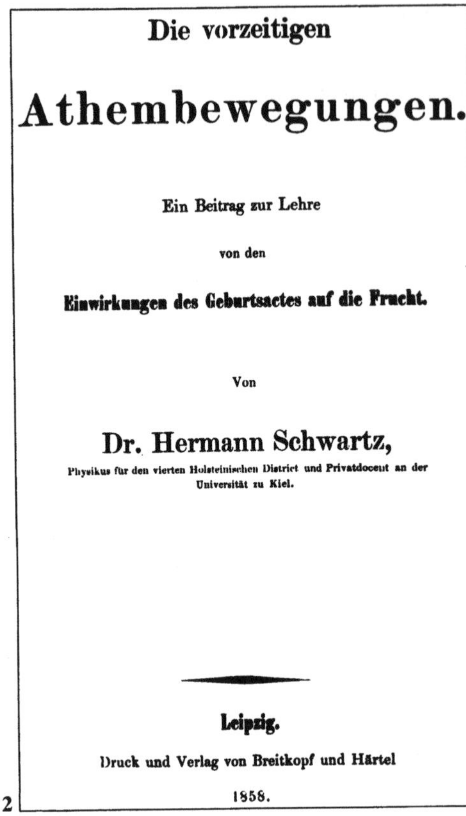

Die vorzeitigen

Athembewegungen.

Ein Beitrag zur Lehre

von den

Einwirkungen des Geburtsactes auf die Frucht.

Von

Dr. Hermann Schwartz,

Physikus für den vierten Holsteinischen District und Privatdocent an der Universität zu Kiel.

Leipzig.

Druck und Verlag von Breitkopf und Härtel

1858.

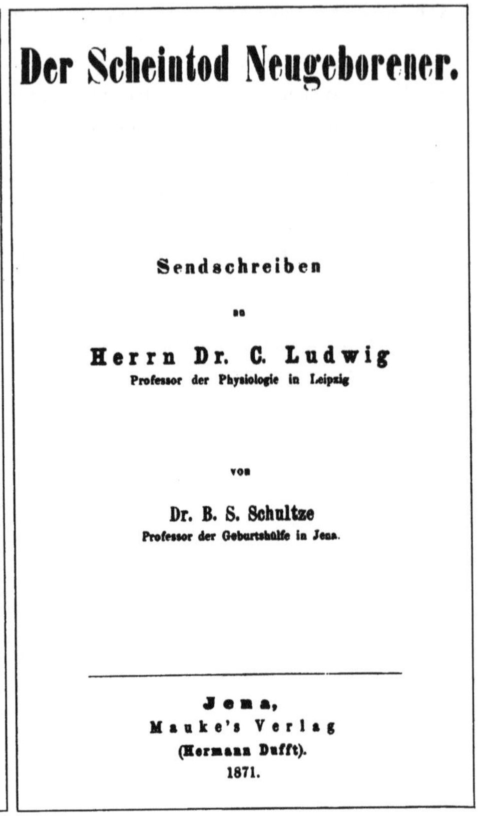

Der Scheintod Neugeborener.

Sendschreiben

an

Herrn Dr. C. Ludwig

Professor der Physiologie in Leipzig

von

Dr. B. S. Schultze

Professor der Geburtshülfe in Jena.

Jena,

Mauke's Verlag

(Hermann Dufft).

1871.

Fig. 2. Title page from textbook by Hermann Schwartz, Kiel (1858): fetal breathing movements

Fig. 3. Title page from textbook by Bernhard Sigismund Schultze, Jena (1871): apparent death of newborn babies

impairment of the placental respiration to be reduction of the uterine blood flow in the course of labor. He postulated a stagnation hypoxia in the fetoplacental circulation.

Schultze (1871) made intensive studies of the "apparent death" of newborn babies (Fig. 3). He stressed the importance of CO_2 intoxication in his pathogenetic investigations, suggesting that an accumulation of CO_2 led to vagal irritation, with consequent bradycardia. Seitz (1903) investigated above all the phenomenon of pressure. He clarified the mechanism of head compression and emphasized the importance of pressoreceptors for the regulation of heart rate (Fig. 4). Basically, however, Seitz continued to believe in Schwartz's theory of asphyxia. He gives the proportion of bradycardial reaction *sub partu* as 5%–22% during the first stage of labor, increasing to 62%, 87%, and 95% during the second stage. He says that tachycardia can be expected in 8% of all births at the beginning and in 2% at the end of a single contraction. This is an early indication of a biphasic course of heart rate curves during labor.

The inclusion of obstetric auscultation in the textbooks and the change of opinion in medical schools is also interesting. We find the first indications in the *Theoretical/*

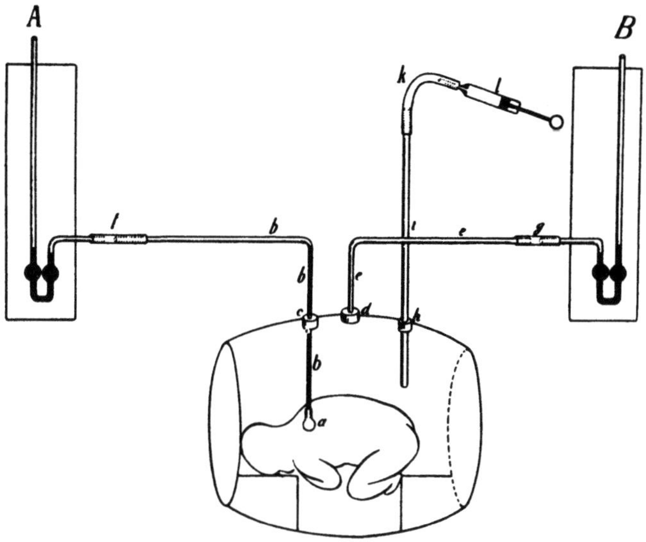

Fig. 4. Ludwig Seitz, Munich (1903): experimental equipment for pressure recordings

Practical Handbook of Obstetrics by Froriep. In his Weimar *Notes on Natural History and Medicine* in 1822, Froriep had already reported Kergaradec's discovery, and provided a translation of the French papers in the same year. Busch (Marburg/ Berlin 1840) and Carus (Dresden 1828) also refer quite early on to the demonstration of heartbeat as a sound indication of pregnancy in their textbooks. The significance of heart rate monitoring during labor was not yet recognized, however. Guidelines for monitoring the fetus by auscultation during birth are not found in the textbooks until the end of the last century.

The chief proponent of fetal indication for surgical intervention in the delivery is von Winkel in his textbook of obstetrics of 1889, even in the Anglo-American literature on the subject. These rules determined obstetric procedures for generations, up to the 1960s. During the same period a decisive change took place in surgical obstetrics. With decreasing maternal mortality the range of indications for surgical procedures was extended, also in the interest of the fetus.

At the turn of the century the first attempts were made to understand the processes of fetal heart activity, not only by intermittent auscultation but by recording and documenting it continuously. At the same time efforts were made to amplify fetal heartbeats so that they could be made accessible to a larger number of listeners for demonstration purposes. The pioneer of phonocardiography was Ernesto Pestalozza (1891) of Pavia. He was able to demonstrate the first recordings of the sound of fetal heartbeats on the occasion of the 10th International Medical Congress in Berlin with the aid of Dugeon's sphygmograph. No pictures are available. There is only the congress report to go by. The phonocardiograms of Hofbauer and Weiss in 1907 with the phonoscope developed by Weiss are documented. To transmit the pulse a soap bubble was used. The sound was conducted by a flexible elastic resonance-free tube. The vibrations of the membrane were portrayed photographically by means of a thin

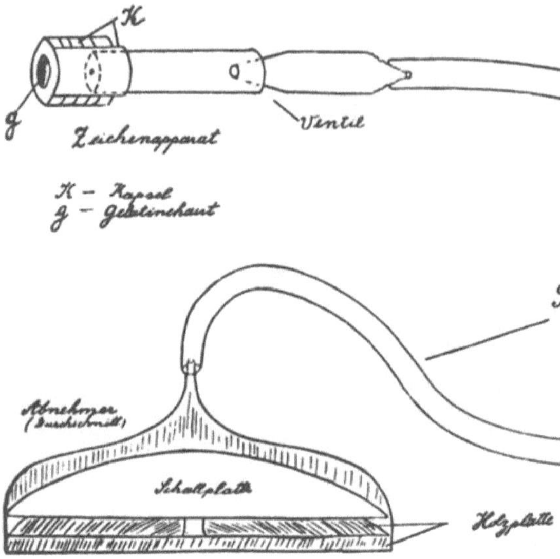

Fig. 5. Ohm's heart-sound capsule (1917)

piece of glass. None of these purely mechanical processes really established themselves.

A considerable improvement in phonocardiography began with the development of radio technology. For some recording the sound capsule of Ohm (1917) was used at first, then later electromagnetic telephonic microphones. Valve amplifiers were used to make the heartbeats audible (Fig. 5).

In 1923 Schäffer and Fleischer were able to demonstrate clearly for all to hear in the large auditorium of the Gynecological Clinic of the University of Breslau the heartbeats of the child of an 8-months pregnant woman. The sound waves were picked up by a stethoscope and then transmitted by means of a rubber tube to a so-called Waetzmann sound detector. This used sensitive microphones which had served during World War I to locate sea mines. The electrical impulses from the microphone circuit were amplified and transmitted to a high-ohm loudspeaker telephone.

Benatt (1926) also made a semimechanical experimental arrangement. The recording of the impulses was made by means of an Ohm sound-capsule. The sound waves were transmitted by a rubber tube over a fine gelatine membrane and the vibrations projected onto a light-sensitive strip of paper by means of a mirror.

Schwarz in 1926 went a step further. He transformed the sound vibrations of the Ohm capsule into electrical impulses, amplified them, and recorded them on a galvanometer. The distinct oscillations had almost the character of sound pictures (Fig. 6).

It was the investigations of Beruti (Buenos Aires) and Rech (of Heidelberg and Munich) which brought about the decisive breakthrough on the path to modern phonocardiography. Beruti (1927) and his colleagues devoted themselves intensively to the regeneration and amplification of fetal heartbeats. Their apparatus consisted first of a telephone microphone, an acoustic and electromagnetic relay, and a kymograph. The process only permitted a quantitative recording of the heartbeat. They

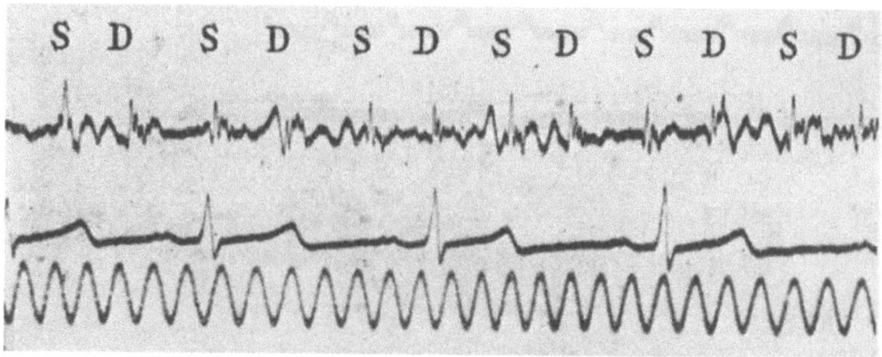

Fig. 6. G. Schwarz, Königsberg (1926): phonocardiogram of a 9-month fetus showing the two cardiac phases. *S*, systole; *D*, diastole

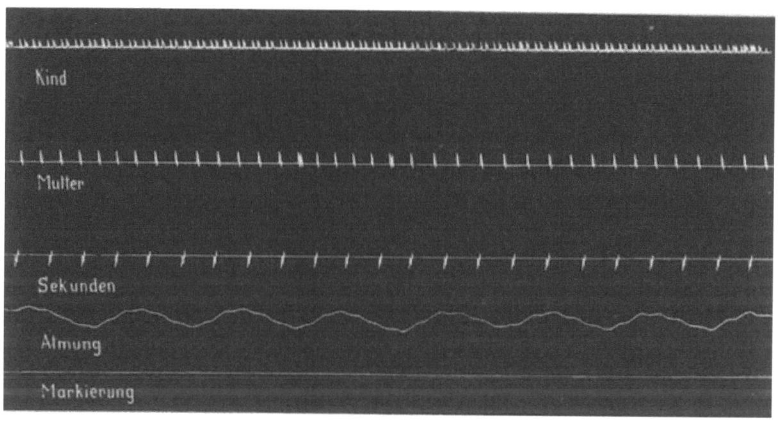

Fig. 7. W. Rech, Munich (1933): phonocardiogram of the mother and fetus. Note the fetal double tone

called it cardiotelephony and phonocardiography. It was possible to improve greatly the reproduction by constructing a contact microphone and doing without an acoustic relay. This new system made it possible to carry out auscultation from a distance and to record the heartbeats on phonographic disks. Looking ahead, Beruti prophesied "... that the doctor would soon be able to listen to the intrauterine heartbeats in his own home, transmitted from the labor ward ..." and "... that the existence of archives of records of reproductions of fetal heart activity was hardly an impossible dream." Obstetricians have had to dream for almost another 50 years.

The experimental phonocardiograms of Rech (1931) in the same period (Fig. 7) correspond to these of Beruti. The machine consisted of a mechanically coupled electromagnetic microphone with pre- and main amplifiers and an electromagnetic kymograph. This very large apparatus was housed in two separate soundproof rooms mainly to avoid feedback effects. Communication was by telephone. With the aid of frequency filters and electrical and acoustic isolation a mobile unit was later developed which could be set up in the delivery room. The size of the sound receiver

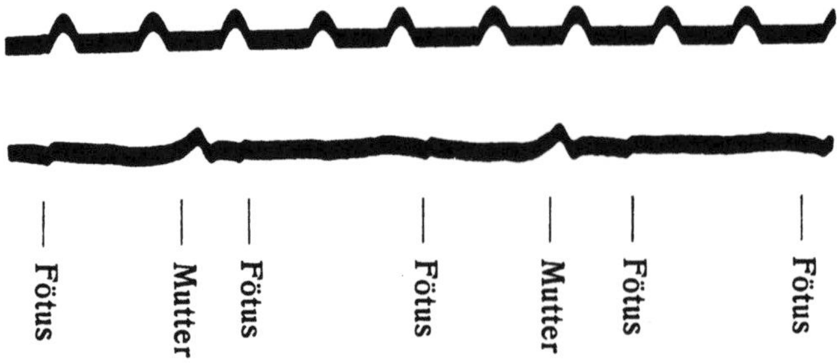

Fig. 8. Max Cremer, Munich (1906): first documented fetal electrocardiogram

remained remarkably large. It ruled out long-term supervision from the start. Nevertheless, important discoveries were made with the machine about the fetal heart rate during pregnancy and birth. Rech was able to demonstrate the influence of head compression on heart rate by experiments.

The development of phonocardiography came to a temporary halt with the studies of Palmrich (1951) and Tosetti (1958). By restriction of the frequency ranges in the recording microphones and selective amplification of the sound impulses, curves were recorded during pregnancy which could almost always be used. By means of transformation it was also possible to change the sound pictures into clear-cut trigger impulses, which is a prerequisite for frequency integration. However, these machines were not suitable for routine use in practical obstetrics with long-term monitoring of the heartbeat. There was no clear presentation of the rate. Moreover, the susceptibility to interference increased as the contractions progressed. The great breakthrough in phonocardiography was not achieved until the middle of this century.

The same applies to experiences with electrocardiography of the fetus. The first documentation of fetal ECGs was published by Cremer (1906) in the Munich medical weekly magazine (Fig. 8). The electrical impulses were recorded by an abdominal electrode over the uterus and a vaginal electrode and registered with the help of a string galvanometer developed a few years before by Einthoven. The patient was in the last month of pregnancy. As a cardiologist Cremer was primarily interested in conducting ECGs near the heart in case of heart disease. He experimented with a professional sword-swallower who was capable of swallowing silver electrodes up to 10 cm long and 1.5 cm in diameter and placing them at will in the esophagus and stomach. His success with the sword-swallower encouraged Cremer to use the same method with pregnant women in order to carry out an ECG of the fetus. He wrote: "Meanwhile I have not found a single experimental subject in whom this method of introducing the electrode was easily possible or who was prepared to volunteer for the experiment." Cremer's observation was a stroke of luck. Apart from him only Foa in 1911 succeeded in demonstrating a fetal ECG in three cases. After that there was almost 20 year's silence on the subject of fetal electrocardiography. Only some reports on more or less unsuccessful experiments appeared, e.g., Sachs in 1922. The main reason for the failure lies in the low voltage of the electrical impulses of the fetal heart which can be conducted from the abdominal wall of the mother. They have only 5–50 μV. This method did not regain importance until the develop-

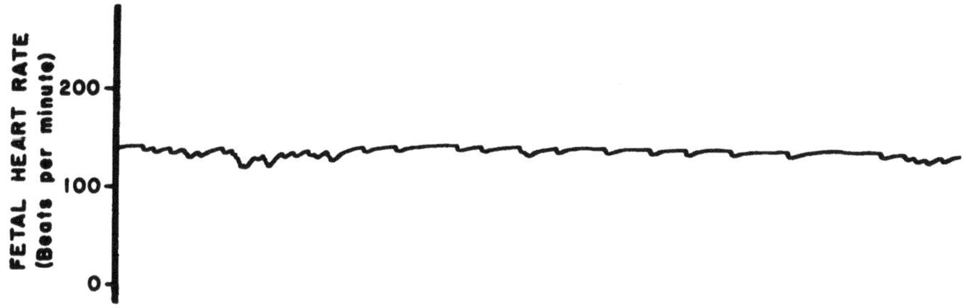

Fig. 9. Corner and Stran (1957): first documented cardiotachogram (ratemeter). *Arrows,* contraction

ment of better electronic amplifiers like those used in electroencephalograms. Enthusiastic reports from this period come particularly from Larks (1961). He was able to record fetal ECGs as early as the 10th–12th week. He summarized his findings in a monograph in 1961. In Germany it was chiefly Bolte who was working on electrocardiography, in France Sureau, and in England Southern, to mention but a few names as representative of many others. Our own investigations also go back to the 1960s.

Both systems of recording fetal heart activity, phonocardiography and electrocardiography, were so far developed by around 1960 that perfect signals were provided which could serve as trigger impulses for an integration system. The construction of usable ratemeters then followed in a few years, simultaneously in America and Germany.

The first report appeared in 1957 from the Johns Hopkins University in Baltimore by Corner and Stran. They used a crystal microphone for sound recording, and a multivibrator served as a ratemeter with a time constant of 0.2 s to suppress the second heartbeat. Only one cardiotachogram is documented (Fig. 9); no further information is known.

Hellmann and his colleagues (Hellmann et al. 1958) in Brooklyn (New York) were certainly more successful. Their prototype ratemeter was demonstrated in 1958, but detailed technical data were not given. Recording was successful in about 50% of all pregnant women before the contractions began. Long-term monitoring was difficult. About 100 cardiotachograms were available. Hellmann himself dampened his enthusiasm in view of the technical difficulties, saying: "It is a small wonder that this machine records as well as it does." Three years later in 1961, Hellmann and his team introduced an improved machine. Its method was borrowed from radar technology on the "track while scan" principle. With this apparatus the influence of various exogenous factors on the fetal heart rate were studied and the possibility of functional testing and loading systems discussed.

At the same time we built a phonocardiograph in the gynecological clinic of Kiel University. My present co-worker Herr Junge (1967), who was at that time studying for his thesis, did most of the work of developing it (Fig. 10). We were supported by Dr. Benthe as physicist. The ratemeter, a multivibrator, worked according to Lullies' method of ordinate recording; a kymograph did the recording. The first usable long-term tachograms were introduced in 1961. Our machine never went into production; in any case it lacked any kind of technical finish. Another disadvantage

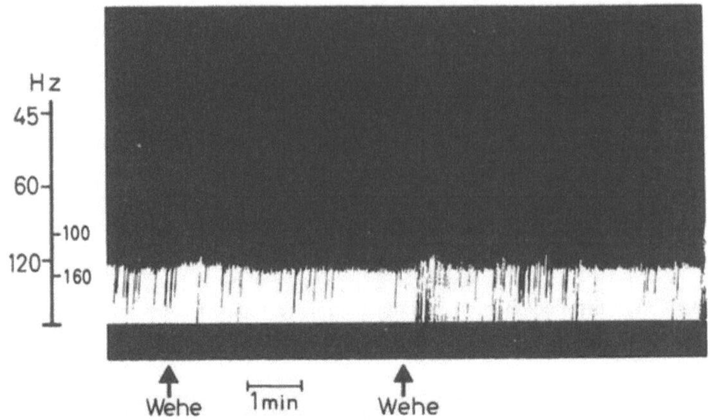

Fig. 10. Heinz-Dieter Junge, Kiel (1962): phonocardiographic ratemeter

was the liability to interference from movement of the mother and child and from uterine contractions.

The solution of this phonocardiographic problem was left to Hammacher in 1962, with his method of comparing the time of the duration and interval between the mechanical heart activity phases and the interference impulses. This brought about the breakthrough in phonotachography, which is now called cardiotocography and connected with the recording of contractions.

The first efficient ratemeter system on an electrocardiographic basis was demonstrated in 1960 by Hon and his team. The simultaneous recording of the mean curve, gained by auscultation and counting, shows the clear superiority of a continuous monitoring of the heart rate. With this prototype, Hon had already developed his concept of the physiological and pathological bradycardias dependent on uterine contractions. The technical problems of the indirect abdominal electrocardiography of the fetus lie in suppressing potential interference and above all eliminating the simultaneously recorded maternal ECG complexes. Hon tried to deal with these difficulties by making counter-poles for various maternal recordings, which was not always successful. Sureau (Paris) developed an analogue cancellation-technique, also working on the principle of subtraction. His results were not satisfactory either. Only with the introduction of computerized systems of comparison using a fade-out technique could decisive improvements be achieved, like those published by van Bemmel and his team (Nijmegen; van Bemmel et al. 1968). This development made abdominal electrocardiography competitive again as a noninvasive system of registering fetal heart rate *sub partu*.

Most of the technical problems of electrocardiography of the fetus can of course be avoided by direct internal recording. More than 30 years previously Rech (1931) had been able to show by animal experiments that excellent electrocardiograms could be obtained by the use of transabdominal needle electrodes. Caldeyro-Barcia and his team also used this method in humans in 1966. They fixed an electrode wire in the shape of a fishing hook to the fetus, introducing it into the uterus by means of an amniocenthesis needle. A "floating electrode" was introduced into the amniotic fluid in the same way by Vasicka (Vasicka and Hutchinson 1963) and remained without firm contact with the fetus. In human obstetrics such invasive methods are seldom necessary. Here risk and advantage are out of proportion to each other.

On the other hand, transcervical direct electrocardiography of the fetus has proved to be of great advantage. It can now be regarded as standard practice in heart rate monitoring during delivery. Prerequisites and disadvantages at the same time are ruptured membranes and accessibility of the leading part of the child. A whole arsenal of recording electrodes has been developed: sucking clip and screw and needle electrodes. Most widely used nowadays are probably the clip electrode of Hon and the spiral electrode of Junge/Rüttgers.

A further means of understanding fetal heart activity is offered by ultrasonography. On the basis of the Doppler effect fetal heart actions were visibly and audibly demonstrated in the middle sixties by, e.g., Callagan and his team and Bishop and Bernstein. Machines for external cardiotachometry on the basis of ultrasound were developed simultaneously by the teams of Caldeyro-Barcia in Montevideo and Mosler in Würzburg. In 1968 Mosler reported successful long-term monitoring of the fetal heart during delivery. The ultrasound Doppler signal is complex. Its main fault lies in the absence of a strictly defined parameter like, e.g., the R-peak in an ECG. This can lead to falsification of the rate curves and prevent a true beat-to-beat recording. In the meantime Mosler has succeeded by isolating a specific signal frequency in obtaining ultrasound trigger impulses, which facilitate a beat-to-beat registration which is adequate for the needs of practical obstetrics. The ultrasound Doppler signal can be improved in its stability and periodicity by the use of autocorrelation techniques. Further development of these techniques may perhaps in the future enable us to manage without invasive monitoring methods altogether.

The continuous recording of fetal heart rate during pregnancy and delivery, along with tocography, provides an abundance of data. The form and time analysis of the progress of the curves has become a special science. For practical obstetrics the differentiation of only a few typical examples of alterations in heart frequency has proved valuable. The customary schemes of gradation are based essentially on the original findings of Caldeyro-Barcia, Hon, and Hammacher. They judge the baseline heart rate according to level and oscillation characteristic and also the alterations in frequency in the form of acceleration or deceleration.

The visual analysis of cardiotocograms is subjective, at best a semiquantative process. More objectivity is certainly desirable. The construction of suitable on-line computer monitoring systems with warning indicators is technically possible. This is dealt with in later chapters. But for all our enthusiasm it must not be forgotten that although the heart rate of the fetus is undoubtedly a vital parameter it is only one of many.

From the recording of exact trigger impulses of the fetal heart for cardiotocography to wireless signal transmission by means of telemetry was at first merely a mental leap. In practice it proved more difficult than expected. Telemetric systems that were fit for use on the basis of ECGs were developed by Sureau, and from then on the basis of phonocardiography by Sokol. In Paris fetal heartbeat impulses from Los Angeles were received perfectly via Telstar. Distances are immaterial. Telemetry does not offer direct obstetrical advantages. At best it can be useful in harmonizing what is medically necessary with the wishes of the patient.

The technical possibilities for central cardiographic monitoring systems are already available. Such systems consist of bedside cardiotocographs connected to a central monitoring unit with screen and memory display and some daughter monitors. The system can be perfected by centrally operated television equipment and two-way intercom. For all the fascination of the technically possible the obstetrician who seeks personal contact with his patients feels somewhat ambivalent toward these developments. From the medical point of view the midwife belongs at the bedside of the women in labor and the place for the obstetrician is the delivery room. Technical perfection can lead to anonymity. It also encourages in our field the depersonalization of the doctor-patient relationship.

Modern obstetrics is already increasingly in the area of conflict between biomedical technology on the one hand and socio- and psychoprophylaxis on the other. It is one of our principal duties as obstetricians to mediate in this conflict. Our dilemma consists in the fact that we are simultaneously and in one person bound to the idea of medical progress and yet have a mandate to plead for the human needs of our pregnant patients. In all our present and future conduct we should remain masters of our technology and not degenerate into its slaves.

References

Benatt A (1928) Über Herztonschreibung und Embryokardie. Klin Wochenschr 7:752

Beruti JA (1927) Fernauskultation und Registrierung der fetalen Herztöne. Arch Gynakol 132:52

Busch DWH, Moser (1840) Handbuch der Geburtskunde in alphabetischer Ordnung, Vol 1. Berlin

Corner GW, Stran HM (1957) A fetal heart ratemeter. Am J Obstet Gynecol 73:191

Cremer M (1906) Über die direkte Ableitung der Aktionsströme des menschlichen Herzens vom Oesophagus und über das Elektrokardiogramm des Fötus. Münch Med Wochenschr 53:811

Depaul JH (1847) Traité théorique et pratique d'auscultation obstétricale. Paris

Duges A (1822) Mémoire sur l'auscultation appliqueé a l'etude de la grossesse, etc, par MAJ Lejunean de Kergaradec. Rev Med 8:220

Fankenhäuser F (1860) Über Nabelschnurgeräusch, Nabelschnurdruck und Hirndruck. Monatsschr Geburtsh 15:356

Goodlin RC (1973) History of fetal monitoring. Am J Obstet Gynecol 1:323

Gültekin-Zootzmann B (1975) The history of monitoring the human fetus. J Perinat Med 3:135

Hammacher K (1962) Neue Methoden zur selektiven Registrierung der fetalen Herzschlagfrequenz. Geburtshilfe Frauenheilkd 22:1542

Haus CJ (1823) Die Auskultation in Bezug auf Schwangerschaft. Würzburg

Hellmann LM, Schiffer MA, Kohl SG, Tolles WE (1958) Studies in fetal wellbeing: variations in fetal heart rate. Am J Obst Gynecol 76:998

Hofbauer JJ, Weiss O (1908) Photographische Registrierung der fötalen Herztöne. Zentralbl Gynakol 13:429

Hohl AF (1833) Die Geburtshülfliche Exploration. 1. Theil: Das Hören. Halle

Hon EH (1960) The diagnosis of fetal distress. Clin Obstet Gynecol 3:860

Junge HD (1967) Über die kontinuierliche Kontrolle der fetalen Herztätigkeit durch Aufzeichnung des fetalen Herzfrequenzdiagramms. Z Geburtshilfe Gynakol 166:159

Kennedy E (1833) Observations on obstetric auscultation, with an analysis of the evidences of pregnancy and an inquiry into the proofs of the life and death of the foetus in utero. Dublin

Kergaradec MJAL de (1822) Mémoires sur l'auscultation appliquée à l'etude de la grossesse on recherches sur deux nonveaux signes propres à faire reconnaitre plusieurs circonstances d'l'etat de gestation; lu à l'Académie royale de médecine, dans sa séance générale du 26 décembre 1821. Paris. German translation (1822) in: Frorieps Notizen aus dem Gebiete der Natur- und Heilkunde no. 35, 38

Larks SD (1961) Fetal electrocardiography. Thomas, Ill, USA
Lau CA (1823) De tubi acustici ad asiscitandam graviditatem efficacia. Dissertation, Berlin
Ohm R (1917) Über die praktische Verwertung der Registrierung des Herzschalls. Z Exp Pathol 19:299
Palmrich AH (1951) Die Variabilität des physiologischen foetalen Phonocardiogramms und dessen Abgrenzung vom pathologischen Herztonbild. Zentralbl Gynakol 73:1699
Pestalozza E (1891) Graphische Darstellung des foetalen Herzimpulses. Arch Gynakol 39:137
Rech W (1931) Untersuchungen über die Herztätigkeit des Fetus, I. Theil. Arch Gynakol 145:714
Schäffer H (1923) Die Verstärkung und Hörbarmachung der fötalen Herztöne mittels Kethodenröhren. Klin Wochenschr 2:2058
Schultze BS (1871) Der Scheintod Neugeborener. Sendschreiben an Dr C Ludwig. Jena 1871
Schwartz H (1858) Die vorzeitigen Athembewegungen. Breitkopf und Härtel, Leipzig
Schwarz G (1926) Die graphische Darstellung fetaler Herztöne. Klin Wochenschr 5:451
Seitz L (1903) Die fötalen Herztöne während der Geburt. Habilitation, München
Tosetti K (1960) Die fetale Elektrophonocardiographie beim Menschen. Bull Soc R Belge Gynécol Obstét 30:153
Ulsamer A (1828) Auscultation bei Schwangeren, als ein wichtiges Mittel zur Vervollkommnung der äußerlichen Untersuchung während der Schwangerschaft und bei der Geburt. In: Harless CF (Hrsg) Rheinische Jahrbücher für Medizin und Chirurgie. Elberfeld
van Bemmel H, Peeters L, Hengeveld SJ (1968) Influence of the maternal ECG on the abdominal fetal ECG complex. Am J Obstet Gynecol 2
Vasicka A, Hutchinson HT (1963) Simultaneous monitoring of the uterine contractility and fetal heart rate using an intraamniotic platinum electrode. Obstet Gynecol 22:271
von Winkel F (1889) Lehrbuch der Geburtshilfe.

Necessity of Fetal Heart Rate Monitoring from a Dutch Point of View

T. K. A. B. Eskes[1]

The title of this paper is somewhat intriguing. Why is it that the Netherlands should be in an exceptional position with regard to fetal heart rate (FHR) monitoring? I think that this is because of the low perinatal mortality and because 30%–35% of deliveries take place at home in the Netherlands (Table 1). It is, however, interesting to note that the obstetric referral or selection system is not that perfect if one considers the number of breech births, twin births, low-birth weights, primiparae, and intrauterine deaths which occur at home (Table 2). Compared with the years 1973–1974 these figures have halved, a promising trend. So far it has been clear that these cases cannot be electronically monitored at all! Also their outcome is not known.

Table 1. Place of delivery (percentage of total number of children born)

	1970	1980
Hospital	42.7	64.6
Home	57.3	35.4

Table 2. Data on home deliveries (absolute figures). (Government figures)[a]

	1981		1980	
	MD	Midwife	MD	Midwife
Breech	107	66	112	54
Twins	69	62	103	74
< 2501 g	518	768	569	819
Primiparae > 35 years	23	21	23	17
IUD	21	29	29	26
Total born	179 615		182 499	

[a] Obstetrical conditions like breech presentation, twins, low birth weight, primiparae older than 35 years, and intrauterine deaths are considered as indications for delivery in hospital but are nevertheless delivered at home

[1] Department of Obstetrics and Gynecology, St Radboud Hospital, P.O. Box 9101, NL-6500 HB, Nijmegen

Fetal Heart Rate Monitoring
Ed. by W. Künzel

Perinatal Mortality

With regard to perinatal mortality we have already made critical remarks in the past. The basis for this criticism was a study performed by Smits (1981) in the area of Enschede, where perinatal mortality was 25% underreported.

For years, however, low figures for perinatal mortality have been used as an argument for maintaining the obstetrical selection system as it is. In particular, a perinatal mortality rate of 2.5–3/1000 for home deliveries was thought to be sufficient to guarantee the Dutch system. It was never asked how reliable this figure was.

Van Alten (1978) later reported on a survey in the Wormerveer area. In this obstetrical center prenatal care was performed and deliveries conducted by midwives without FHR monitoring.

The conclusions could be summarized as follows:

1. Indications for hospital admissions, 15%
2. Transfer during labor, 6%
3. Neonatal clinical morbidity and transfer, 3%
4. More referrals in primigravidae than in multigravidae

Here again one can ask question whether the percentages of referrals especially during labor and postpartum are acceptable.

Perinatal Morbidity

Two recent studies are discussed because these studies touch upon the adequacy or inadequacy of the Dutch referral system of obstetric care by measuring perinatal morbidity in pregnancies and deliveries with modern perinatal tools.

1. A prospective study was carried out on cord blood gases in home deliveries by Eskes et al. (1981). The main question in this study was: what gas values are found in umbilical cord blood in so-called optimal (home) deliveries? This study was planned and performed with midwives in the Nijmegen area. Midwives operate totally freely and independently and select women for home delivery, i.e., absence of a so-called medical indication for hospital delivery.

Pregnancy surveillance consists of history taking, abdominal examination, determination of body weight and proteinuria, measurement of blood pressure, and blood investigation (blood group, lues and rubella reactions, hemoglobin). During delivery midwives perform vaginal examinations and listen to fetal heart sounds with a monoauricular stethoscope. Midwives are not permitted to administer oxytocin, but they are allowed to infiltrate the perineum with local anesthetics and to perform episiotomies.

For our study a student was allowed to take an isolated piece of the umbilical cord, to aspirate blood into syringes, and to rush to the hospital to determine gas values of umbilical cord blood stored on ice.

The time interval between birth and cord clamping was noted, 85% of cords being clamped within 3 min. The same criteria as for home deliveries were applied to a group of women who for all reasons except medical ones wanted to deliver in our university hospital unit. These women were matched for age, parity, criteria for home delivery , no drug usage, and duration of second phase. They were under the care of a resident midwife or obstetrician. During labor one of these, together with a nurse and intern, were present.

FHR monitoring was carried out in all cases. Microblood investigation was performed when indicated on the FHR record. In the final evaluation 12 cases were excluded: four because of incomplete arterial and venous values, four because of recognized artifacts of the gas values, one because of too long a delay between the sampling and the determination, and three because of lack of adequately matched controls. The final report consisted of 28 primiparous and 57 multiparous women and their matched controls. One of them delivered prematurely (37th week) and six were small for date.

Tested with the Mann-Whitney U test there was a marked significant difference in favor of the hospital group for pH, base excess (BE), and PCO_2 (Fig. 1).

For primiparous women this difference was marked for pH (*P*, 0.07) but not for the BE (*P*, 0.17). For multiparous women both parameters differed significantly ($P<10^{-4}$ and *P*, 0.0007, respectively). After presentation of this study before the Dutch Society of Obstetrics and Gynecology the main criticism was the exclusion of instrumental deliveries in the hospital group and the absence of standardization of the clamping time.

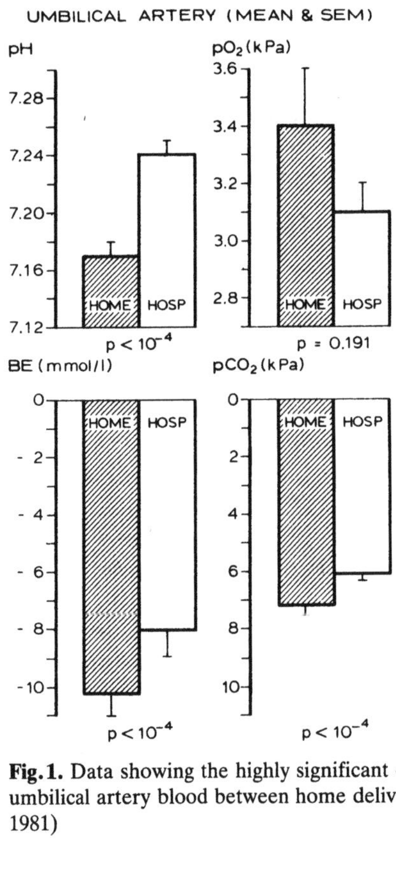

Fig. 1. Data showing the highly significant difference between pH, base excess *(BE)*, and PCO_2 in umbilical artery blood between home deliveries and matched controls in the hospital. (Eskes et al. 1981)

We argued that instrumental deliveries had to be excluded to fulfill the criteria for home delivery and that delay in clamping of the umbilical cord and/or determination of gases of blood stored at 4°C could affect arterial levels but far less venous values.

2. Discussion of a second study is worthwhile. Lievaart and De Jong (1982) conducted a prospective study comparing the outcomes of two groups of supposedly normal first pregnancies and deliveries that were solely cared for by midwives (*n*, 85) or by gynecologists (*n*, 27). The outcome was measured by arterial cord blood gases (early morbidity) and by neurological examination with the method of Heinz Prechtl (late morbidity). In the "midwife group" 19 cases, and in the "gynecologist group" 18 cases, all women with primary infertility, were excluded. The gynecologist group was electronically monitored for fetal heart rate patterns, with microblood investigation when indicated.

The acid-base values were less favourable in the midwife group than in the gynecologist group for pH (*P*, 0.011) and BE (*P*, 0.008).

Ten neurologically nonoptimal infants were found in the midwife group but none were found in the gynecologist group (*P*, 0.055). The authors concluded that these findings were incompatible with the basic philosophy of the Dutch obstetric system, which is that midwives are able to select normal pregnancies out of the group of women who present for obstetric care and can assist in maintaining the normal state in these selected cases in the course of delivery. The influence of the place of birth, home or hospital-ambulatory, could virtually be ruled out.

The main criticism of this study was the nonideal matching (infertility patients), the high number of excluded women, no report to the Dutch Society of Obstetrics and Gynecology, no publication in a national journal, and the study being nonrepresentative for the Netherlands. Although we feel ourselves that these criticisms can be partially answered more investigations of this kind, hopefully also coming from the supporters of home deliveries, must be carried out.

A separate word on the frequency of instrumental delivery: In the study of Lievaart and De Jong 7 children from 27 women with primary infertility were delivered instrumentally (25.9%). Of course one must follow critically the number of instrumental deliveries over the years, especially because it is suggested in the literature that this increase is due to FHR monitoring. In the United States, for instance, the cesarean section rate increased from 5.0 per 100 infants in 1968 to 11.4 in 1976. In the Netherlands the frequency of cesarean sections increased from 2.1% in 1971 to 3.4% in 1977.

Trends in the Radboud Hospital, Nijmegen

The trends in the frequency of operative deliveries are illustrated by the rates in the Radboud Hospital, Nijmegen, the Netherlands. Figure 2 shows the cesarean section rate as well as the forceps/vacuum rate between 1969 and 1978 in our hospital. During these years the percentage of cesarean sections rose from 2.4% to 10.9%. The percentage of forceps and vacuum extractions increased from 2.5% to about 13%. Most of the increase in cesarean section rate after 1973 is related to the management of breech presentations. From 1973, the frequency of cesarean sections

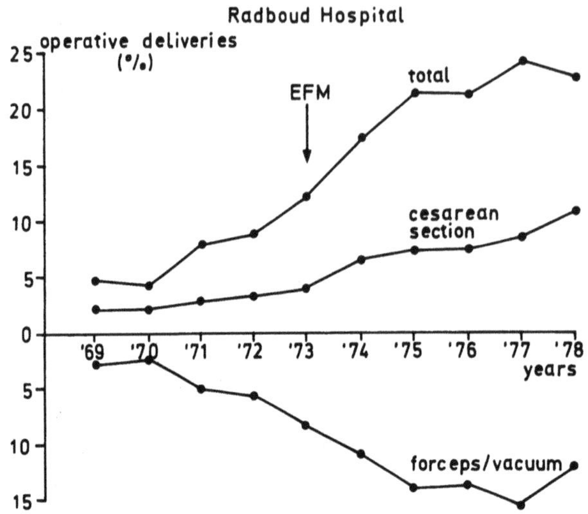

Fig. 2. Increase in operative deliveries (cesarean section and forceps/vacuum) at the Department of Obstetrics and Gynecology of the University of Nijmegen, the Netherlands. Electronic fetal monitoring *(EFM)* was applied on a routine basis in 1973. (Van Geijn 1979)

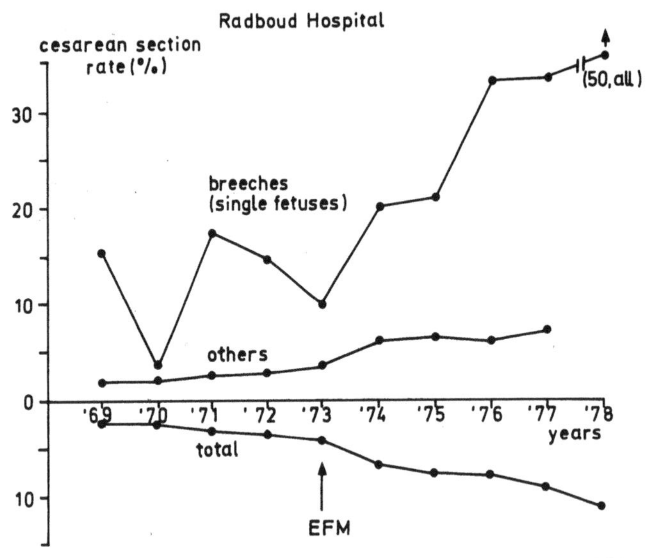

Fig. 3. Increase in the cesarean section rate at the Department of Obstetrics and Gynecology of the University of Nijmegen, the Netherlands, mainly due to a different policy toward breech presentation. *EFM,* electronic fetal monitoring. (Van Geijn 1979)

for breeches rose from 20% to 50%, which is shown in Fig. 3. The number of cesarean sections carried out for other reasons stayed at around 6%–7% during these years. Furthermore, it is evident from these figures that the cesarean section rate was already increasing before electronic fetal monitoring was introduced on a routine basis.

The effect of electronic fetal monitoring (EFM) upon the incidence of cesarean sections may vary with the manner in which EFM data are interpreted. Three of four randomized clinical trials (Haverkamp et al. 1976, 1979; Renou et al. 1976; Kelso et al. 1978) in teaching hospital settings have demonstrated significantly increased rates of primary cesarean sections in monitored women. The increase in cesarean section for fetal distress was statistically significant in two of the four trials.

Several large retrospective studies in teaching hospitals have found this increase in cesarean section rate for fetal distress to be independent of the use of EFM. The effect of EFM upon cesarean delivery rate in any particular hospital may depend upon the clinical use and norms of practice in that hospital. There is evidence that the simultaneous use of fetal scalp blood sampling provides additional information and may reduce the incidence of monitoring-associated cesarean section. The ideal use of EFM in influencing more appropriate cesarean delivery has yet to be determined. The increase in cesarean section rate which has occurred in many hospitals during the past decade most probably results from the same concerns for maximal fetal safety which have led to the widespread use of electronic fetal monitoring. The increase in cesarean section rate is therefore due to a change in attitude of the obstetrician and others toward childbirth.

Nevertheless the report of Zuspan et al. (1979) describing the report of the NIH consensus development conference on fetal monitoring will have to be the guideline for obstetrical practice in the forthcoming years. It could even be that these guidelines also hold for the terms fetus and neonate, at least for primigravidae.

References

Eskes TKAB, Jongsma HW, Houx CW (1981) Umbilical cord gases in home deliveries versus hospital based deliveries. J Reprod Med 26:405

Haverkamp AD, Thompson HE, McFee JG, Cetrulo C (1976) The evaluation of continuous fetal heart rate monitoring in high-risk pregnancy. Am J Obstet Gynecol 125:310

Haverkamp AD, Orleans M, Langendoefer S, McFee J, Murphy J, Thompson H (1979) A controlled trial of the differential effects of intrapartum fetal monitoring. Am J Obstet Gynecol 134:399

Kelso IM, Parsons RJ, Lawrence GF, Arora SS, Edmonds DK, Cooke ID (1978) An assessment of continuous fetal heart rate monitoring in labor: a randomized trial. Am J Obstet Gynecol 131:526

Lievaart M, De Jong PA (1982) Neonatal morbidity by midwives and gynecologists. A study of the system of obstetric care prevailing in the Netherlands. Am J Obstet Gynecol 144:376

Renou P, Chang A, Anderson I, Wood C (1976) Controlled trial of fetal intensive care. Am J Obstet Gynecol 126:470

Smits F (1981) The efficacy of the selection system in obstetrical care. Thesis, University of Nijmegen, The Netherlands

Van Alten D (1978) Home deliveries. Ned Tijdschr Geneeskd 122:1178

Van Geijn HP (1979) Fetal monitoring current concepts and controversies. Symposium, April 17, 1980, Catholic University Nijmegen

Zuspan FP, Quilligan EJ, Iams JD, Van Geijn HP (1979) Predictors of intrapartum fetal distress: the role of electronic monitoring. Am J Obstet Gynecol 135:287

Changing Trends of Fetal Heart Rate Monitoring in the United States

SZE-YA YEH[1]

Whenever a new development occurs, the attitude of society will usually evolve through the following psychological stages: (1) excitement, because of the new development; everyone is excited to see or to participate in the new development; (2) speculation; after a trial for a certain period, people start to question the value of this new development; some may oppose it; (3) adjustment; as time goes by, trial and error will help people to readjust their attitude toward the development; and, finally, (4) acceptance. Fetal heart rate (FHR) monitoring in the United States has gone through these stages, and is now approaching the final stage of acceptance.

Changing Trends of Intrapartum FHR Monitoring

Terminology

"Dip" Versus "Deceleration". During the 1950s, there were two major studies on FHR monitoring: those of Caldeyro-Barcia in Uruguay and Hon in the United States. At that time there were different terminologies used to describe abnormal heart rate patterns and different paper speeds and scales to record FHR. Caldeyro-Barcia used the terms "type I dip" and "type II dip" (Caldeyro-Barcia et al. 1963) while Hon used the terms "early," "late", and "variable" decelerations (Hon and Quilligan 1967). After many years of debate and adjustment, an agreement was reached in 1972 at the conference in Amsterdam among the world experts in this field to standardize the nomenclature and the recording specification. In the United States today, almost all hospitals are using the terminology and the recording specification recommended by Hon.

Baseline FHR. The terms baseline "tachycardia" and "bradycardia" have been consistently used throughout the past 2 decades, but the terms describing fetal heart beat-to-beat changes have gone through some evolution. In the literature of the sixties and early seventies, there were several terms used for this description: irregularities, beat-to-beat interval differences, oscillations, and variabilities. At present, most of the people in the United States have adopted the term "variability."

Specific Patterns. From time to time, there have been different specific patterns discovered. Some have been reported in the literature while others have been mentioned only at conferences. For example, there is a sinusoidal pattern (Manseau et al. 1972), a saltatory pattern, a saw-tooth pattern, premature ventricular contractions,

[1] Dept. of Obstetrics and Gynecology, The Allentown Hospital, 1627 Chew Street, Allentown, PA 18102, USA

Fetal Heart Rate Monitoring
Ed. by W. Künzel

and premature atrial contractions (Hon and Huang 1962). Unfortunately, there are no clear definitions given to these patterns, which has resulted in more confusion today.

Interpretation

Pattern Recognition. After the FHR monitor was introduced for clinical practice, one of the most serious problems encountered was misinterpretation of FHR patterns. On numerous occasions this caused unnecessary intervention and some perinatal mortalities due to ignorance. Although there have been several attempts to utilize computer technology for the proper diagnosis of FHR patterns (Yeh et al. 1972), the results have not been satisfactory for clinical application. After several years of proper education, this problem seems to be improving.

Late Deceleration. There has been a change in the interpretation of late deceleration patterns during the past 2 decades. In 1967, Hon made a statement that all late decelerations are ominous regardless of the amplitude of FHR drops. This statement was supported by a study carried out by Kubli et al. (1969). They found that late decelerations were associated with lower fetal capillary pH. However, there was a wide range of fetal pH associated with late decelerations. Subsequently, a re-examination of these patient data (Paul et al. 1975) revealed that baseline FHR variability played an important complementary role in determining fetal condition. Figure 1 illustrates cases of late decelerations and the fetal capillary blood pH values associated with those patterns. For those patients who had the same degree of late deceleration, the ones who had good FHR variability had higher fetal pH, and the ones who had diminished FHR variability showed fetal acidosis. FHR variability has become an essential complementary observation for the interpretation of late decelerations.

Baseline FHR Variability. The presence of fetal heart rate variability has become an important observation in the interpretation of FHR monitoring. FHR variability represents the integration of autonomic nervous system control of the heartbeats, and any condition interfering with this system will result in alteration of heart rate variability (Hon and Yeh 1969). In reality, FHR variability is an indication of fetal reserve while a periodic FHR pattern represents the fetal response to various stress conditions.

In the late sixties and the early seventies, there were two major studies investigating methods of quantifying baseline FHR variability. DeHaan et al. (1971) applied the geometrical principle and developed the index STI (short-term irregularity) for the beat-to-beat variability and LTI (long-term irregularity) for the long-term heart rate changes. Yeh et al. (1973) applied the statistical principle to develop indices for FHR variabilities, viz., DI (differential index) for the short-term variability and II (interval index) for the long-term variability. Subsequently, there have been numerous different but similar methods published and reviewed (Laros et al. 1977). Unfortunately, none of these methods have physiological bases for the index computation. Although there are a few monitoring instruments equipped with variability index computations, no definite clinical advantage has been demonstrated. At

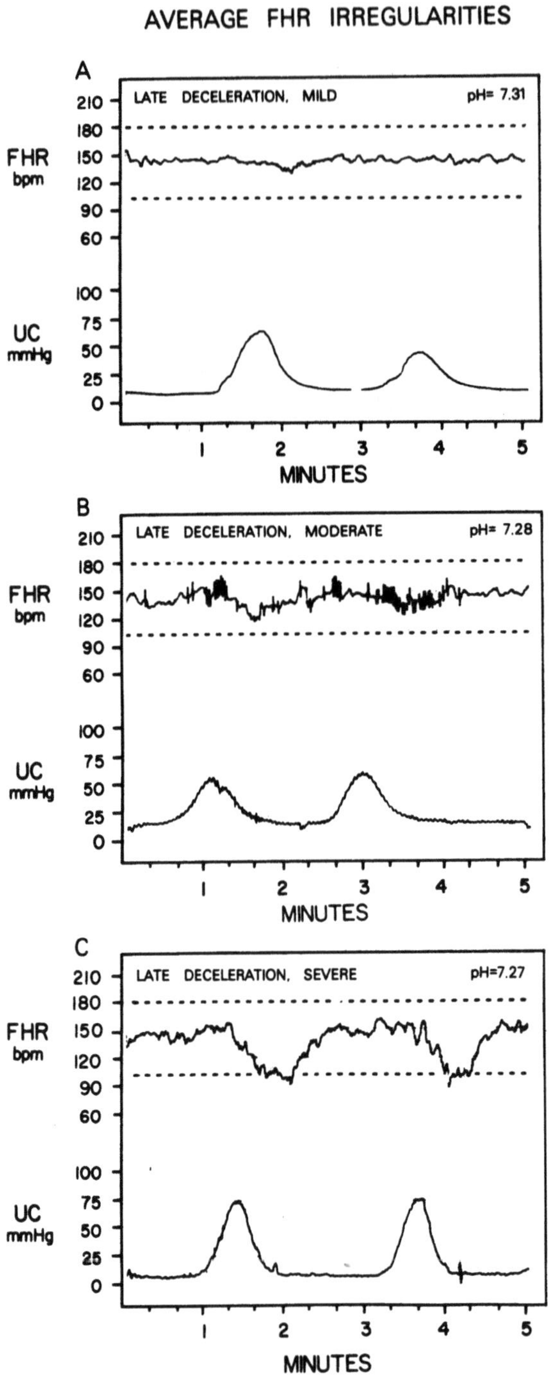

Fig. 1A–F. Fetal scalp blood pH values and late deceleration patterns. Three cases on the *left* (**A, B, C**) coincide with the three cases on the *right* (**D, E, F**) regarding the severity of the late decelerations. The former group demonstrated average FHR variability (or irregularity) while the latter

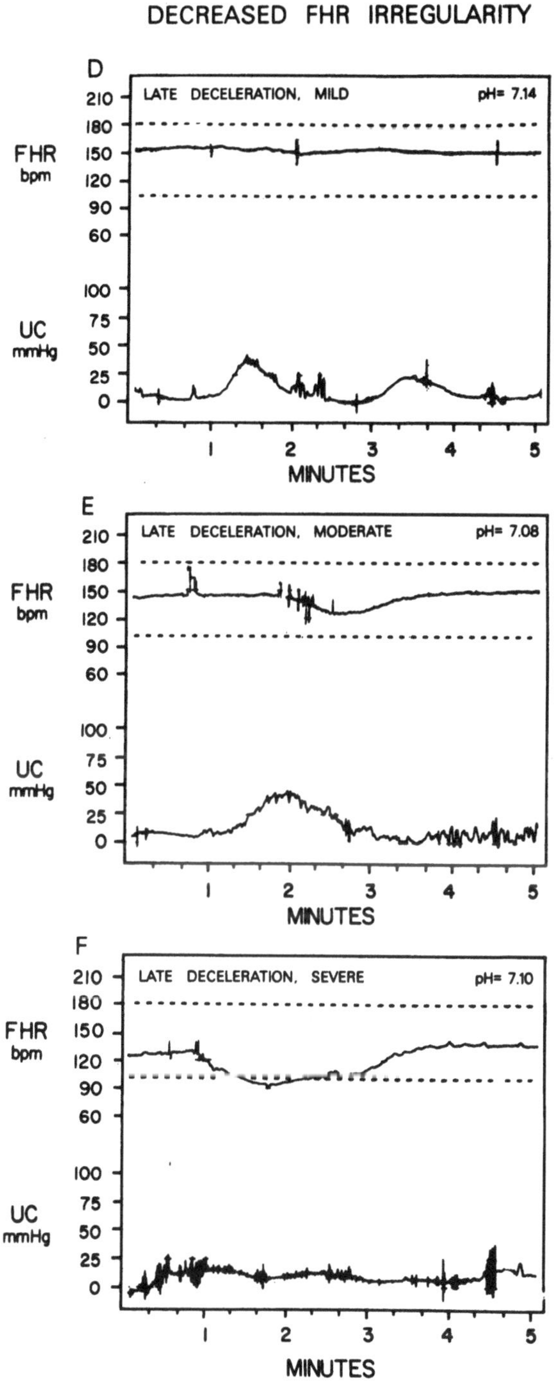

Fig. 1 (continued)
group demonstrated decreased variability. The pH values obtained within 20 min of these patterns were higher for those with average variability and lower for those with decreased variability

present, the visual observation of FHR variability is felt to be as useful as calculated indices in clinical practice.

Acceleration. In the early seventies, some investigators started to pay attention to the significance of FHR acceleration. A preliminary study on FHR acceleration by Lee et al. (1975) and the subsequent observation of FHR changes during antepartum fetal heart rate testings indicated that FHR acceleration associated with fetal movement was an indication of fetal well-being (Lee et al. 1976). Animal experiments by James et al. (1976) indicated that FHR acceleration was found when the umbilical cord was partially occluded. Goodlin stated that smooth FHR acceleration immediately following smooth variable deceleration (overshoot) may indicate severe fetal hypoxia (Goodlin and Lowe 1974). Therefore, the significance of FHR acceleration became an important issue that required a discrete interpretation.

Instrumentation

"Indirect" Versus "Direct" Monitoring. There are two modes of FHR monitoring. The indirect or external mode utilizes Doppler ultrasound, phonocardiograms, or abdominal wall electrocardiograms to monitor the FHR and uses a tocodynamometer to measure abdominal wall tension as an indicator of uterine contraction. The direct or internal mode utilizes a fetal electrode and intrauterine catheter to monitor FHR through fetal electrocardiograms and intrauterine cavity pressure. Both have advantages and disadvantages regarding their application and safety. Although the internal monitor has been encouraged, the external monitor remains the major mode of monitoring in the United States.

Heart Rate Averaging. When the external mode of monitoring is used, FHR signals are usually mixed with noise. Most of the FHR manufacturers have used the average FHR in order to display a better tracing. This creates a confusion where heart rate variability is concerned because the external FHR tracing is not a true representation of the beat-to-beat heart rate.

Electrode Design. During the early days of FHR monitoring, the silver-silver chloride clip electrode (Hon 1963) was used for internal monitoring. This electrode was relatively expensive to manufacture and there were some difficulties in applying and removing it. Since the stainless steel spiral electrode (Hon et al. 1972) was introduced, it has become widely accepted throughout the world. The signal obtained from the steel electrode is not as good as that from the silver-silver chlorid electrode, yet the practical aspect of this new design justifies its application in the clinical field.

Radiotelemetry. Since ambulation in labor is advantageous to the mother, there have been several attempts to utilize radiotelemetry technology to monitor labor with the patient ambulating (Neuman et al. 1979). However, due to limitations in technology and instrumentation, this mode of monitoring has not been widely accepted in the United States.

Changing Trends of Antepartum FHR Monitoring

Methodology

Oxytocin Challenge Test (OCT). There have been various antepartum fetal testing methods attempted in the past, such as maternal exercise or the hypoxia test; yet none except the contraction stress test has become an acceptable modality. Ray et al. (1972) first published a large series of data using oxytocin infusion to cause uterine contractions, and this test was called the "oxytocin challenge test." They reported that this test has great predictability regarding fetal well-being.

Nonstress Test (NST). The early experience in performing the OCT at the University of Southern California indicated that the majority of patients who showed FHR acceleration with fetal movement had a negative OCT (Freeman 1975). At the same time, several studies from Europe suggested that monitoring FHR without stress and observing FHR acceleration could provide a great predictability regarding fetal condition (Rochard et al. 1976). This test was called a "nonstress test." Due to the ease and the efficiency of this test, it became a widely acceptable device for antepartum fetal surveillance.

Contraction Stress Test (CST). The oxytocin challenge test is a form of CST. The term "CST" should be more appropriate to use because there are other methods of initiating uterine contractions for the antepartum testing. During the past 3 years, nipple stimulation has been advocated as an alternative to oxytocin infusion, and the results have been promising (Freeman 1982). This procedure does not require an intravenous line insertion, and the effect of nipple stimulation in initiating uterine contraction has been satisfactory in the majority of cases; therefore, most of the centers in the United States are using this method as a primary mode of CST. Oxytocin infusion is used only when this method fails to initiate uterine contractions.

Interpretation

CST. The original definition of CST results has remained unchanged over the years. This test requires that a minimum of three contractions/10 min be established, and consecutive late decelerations will be interpreted as a positive CST (Freeman 1975).

NST. The definition of a reactive NST has changed over the years. In the early seventies, the criteria for the reactive NST was to have five accelerations with fetal movement within a 20-min period (Martin and Schifrin 1976). A subsequent study by Evertson et al. (1979) indicated that two or more accelerations in 20 min had the same predictive values for normal babies. Therefore, the criteria for the reactive NST has been revised to two accelerations in 20 min. The majority of patients who had reactive NST had two accelerations within the first 10 min of the testing; therefore, for practical purposes, many institutions in the United States further revised this criterion to two accelerations in 10 min.

As more NSTs were carried out, there was an additional observation found during the test. Some patients had spontaneous FHR deceleration during testing. This was thought to be caused by the presence of cord occlusion or abnormal cord position (Phelan and Lewis 1981). Recent observation of this phenomenon in the postdate patient population indicated that this is associated with decreased amniotic fluid volume (Phelan et al. 1985). Therefore, intervention is recommended for postdate patients if spontaneous deceleration is noted during nonstress testing.

Timing of the Test. A preliminary study of the OCT showed that no baby died within 1 week after a negative OCT (Ray et al. 1972); therefore, the initial recommendation was to perform this test once a week for high-risk patients. However, subsequent reports from various authors indicated that some perinatal deaths occurred within 1 week of a negative test (Klapholz and Burke 1975; Evertson et al. 1978). There has been no study available; yet most institutions in the United States have made an arbitrary decision to perform antepartum FHR monitoring weekly, semi-weekly, or daily, based on indications or cost/benefit considerations.

Integration with Other Biophysical Measurements

With the development of real-time ultrasound technology, Manning et al. developed a multiobservation antepartum surveillance method called "fetal biophysical profile" (Manning et al. 1980), and they reported that this system yielded a better predictive value of the fetal condition in utero. This test includes five parameters. In addition to the conventional NST, ultrasound observations on fetal breathing, fetal body movement, fetal tone, and amniotic fluid volume were included. Each observation has a score from 0 to 2, with 2 the best and 0 the worst. The summation of the scores of five observations make a biophysical profile score. This new approach has been accepted unevenly throughout the nation. Most of the hospitals are reluctant to carry it out because of additional equipment and additional time consumed for the test. Yet most university hospitals have started to use it and are evaluating its impact in clinical practice.

Changing Trends of Social Attitude Toward FHR Monitoring

Economy

"Who should be monitored?" or "Should every patient be monitored?" has been the consistent question asked throughout the nation since the introduction of fetal monitoring. Ideally, only those patients how may develop high-risk problems during labor need monitoring. Unfortunately, there is no ideal method of predicting which patients belong to this category. Two separate studies by Hobel et al. (1973) of California and Sokol et al. (1979) of Ohio indicated that patients who had low-risk antepartum and high-risk intrapartum conditions carried a higher morbidity and mortality rate than those who had high-risk antepartum and low-risk intrapartum conditions (Table 1). Therefore, it is reasonable to assume that every pregnancy is a potential high-risk pregnancy. Although monitoring every patient is almost impossible, the majority of the hospitals in the United States are now equipped with a monitor in each labor room.

Table 1. Perinatal risk status and the perinatal outcome

Risk status		Perinatal outcome	
Antepartum	Intrapartum	Morbidity[a]	Mortality[b]
Low	Low	6.8%	3/1000
High	Low	10.0%	22/1000
Low	High	27.0%	35/1000
High	High	33.8%	145/1000

[a] Sokol et al. (1979) (morbidity: 1-min Apgar scores less than 7)
[b] Hobel et al. (1973)

Ecology

"To monitor or not to monitor?" has been one of the issues dicussed frequently in the United States during the past decade. Some are against monitoring, because they feel that the monitor is not natural, it dehumanizes the patient with multiple wires and straps, and most of the time it has to confine the patient in bed.

There have been a few publications showing that FHR monitoring did not benefit the patients. A randomized study by Haverkamp et al. (1976) concluded that there were no differences in the infant outcomes in any measured category between the electronically monitored group and the auscultated group, and the cesarean section rate was markedly increased in the monitored group. They denied the benefit of electronic fetal monitoring for improving fetal outcome. After this study was published, it was criticized heavily on the validity of the study design and outcome data. The auscultation method used, a duration of 30 s after contraction, every 15 min in the first stage, and every 5 min during the second stage, has not been the conventional obstetrical practice in the past and is not a practical and efficient way to monitor patients.

In the late seventies, the Center for Disease Control conducted an epidemiological survey regarding electronic fetal monitoring, and the result was published in 1979 (Banta and Thacker 1979). This study concluded that the benefit of electronic fetal monitoring was very limited as compared with that of auscultation. The problem with this study was that the results were derived from other publications by mathematical manipulation of the data; therefore, their conclusion was not well accepted by clinicians.

There have been numerous studies published throughout the world indicating the benefit of fetal monitoring in improving the perinatal outcome. For instance, Paul and Hon (1974) and Shamsi et al. (1979) in the United States and Renou et al. (1976) in Australia demonstrated favorable results. A recent review of the role of intrapartum fetal monitoring at the LAC/USC Medical Center during the past 10 years clearly demonstrated an important role of the monitor in reducing perinatal mortality (Yeh et al. 1982).

Medicolegal Consideration

Due to the heavy atmosphere of medicolegal problems in the United States, FHR monitoring has become one of the major issues of physicians' consideration. They often feel "damned if you do, and damned if you don't." If FHR monitoring was carried out and no proper intervention was given, the physician would be liable to a malpractice suit. On the other hand, if there was a monitor available, and the labor was not monitored, the physician could also be sued for negligence. In 1979, the National Institute of Health formed a task force to study this issue; yet no clear recommendation was made (Predictors of intrapartum fetal distress 1979). The law may regulate the use of fetal monitoring to some extent; yet it cannot dictate whether monitoring should or should not be applied.

The Impact of FHR Monitoring on Perinatal Outcome

The recent study of 10 year's experience at the LAC/USC Medical Center (Yeh et al. 1982) is one of the illustrations of the impact of FHR monitoring on the improvement of perinatal outcome. This medical center provides one of the largest obstetrical services in the United States, and it is considered the prime institution for FHR monitoring. During the 10-year period from 1970 to 1979, there were 115 000 deliveries, and 41% of them had adequate intrapartum monitoring. This monitoring rate

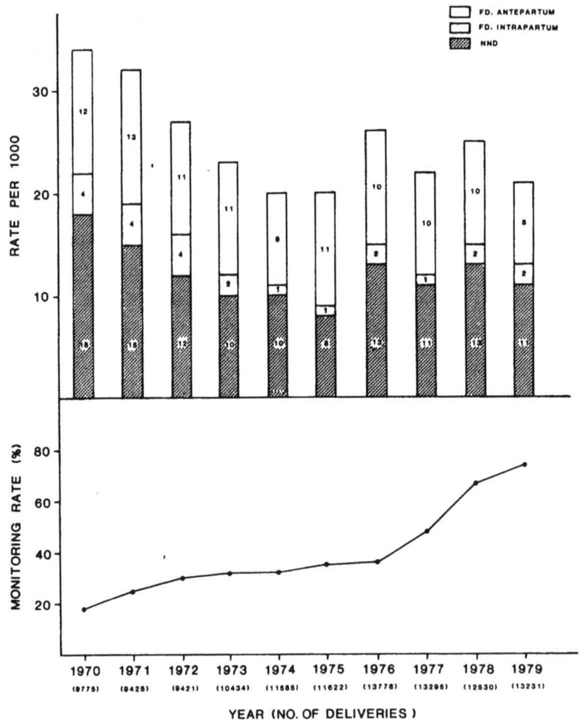

Fig. 2. Annual perinatal mortality rate and FHR monitoring rate at LAC/USC Medical Center over a 10-year period from 1970 to 1979. The monitoring rate is illustrated *at the bottom*. The *numbers in parenthesis under the year* indicate the total number of deliveries. The perinatal mortality rate (per 1000) is illustrated as the *bar graph at the top*. *FD*, fetal death; *NND*, neonatal death. (Yeh et al. 1982)

rose from 18% in 1970 to 74% in 1979 (Fig. 2). The overall perinatal mortality rate was 24.4/1000. It was 32/1000 in 1970 and decreased to 20/1000 in 1975. The rate of monitoring increased from 18% in 1970 to 36% in 1975. Due to a sudden increase in the number of deliveries in 1976, with no increase in the number of medical personnel, perinatal mortality rose to 24/1000 in 1976. During the next few years, an increase in monitoring rate and other perinatal improvements caused a gradual decrease in the mortality rate. Most of the improvement in perinatal mortality rate was in the reduction of intrapartum fetal deaths and neonatal deaths. The antepartum fetal death rate was reduced slightly over this 10-year period.

On reviewing the cesarean section rate over the same period, it showed a slight increase in primary section rate in the late seventies. The cesarean section rate in patients who were monitored declined over this period. Therefore, FHR monitoring was not considered to be the major cause of the increase in section rate.

New Developments

The application of FHR monitoring in the United States seems to have reached a plateau by the late seventies and early eighties. In order to improve the perinatal outcome, new technology and new developments are necessary. The following are some of the new developments taking place in the United States:

Fetal Scalp Stimulation

A retrospective review of previous study data from our medical center indicated that when there was FHR acceleration associated with fetal scalp puncture for blood sampling, all patients showed fetal pH values of greater than 7.28. When the fetal pH was in the range of 7.21 to 7.28, the FHR response was variable. When the fetal pH was below 7.21, there was no FHR acceleration (Clark et al. 1984). This pilot study led to a prospective study on the effect of fetal scalp stimulation. This was done with an Allis clamp pinching the fetal sclap for approximately 15 s. The initial data from approximately 200 patients showed that when FHR responded to the stimulation, all fetuses had pH values in the normal range. When there was no response, fetal pH varied (Clark et al. 1984). This result suggests that fetal scalp stimulation can be used as a screening test for those who actually need blood sampling. The responsive FHR result will possibly eliminate the need for a scalp puncture.

Other New Developments

Other fetal monitoring techniques, such as measurement of electromechanical intervals of the fetal heart (Murata and Martin 1974) and determination of fetal cardiac function with fetal echocardiograms (DeVore et al. 1982), are under intensive investigation in several institutions in the United States. Their clinical application will depend on the outcome of these studies.

In summary, the development and application of FHR monitoring in the seventies have improved the perinatal outcome by reducing intrapartum fetal deaths and neonatal deaths. The major goals of perinatologists during the eighties will be the reduction of antepartum fetal deaths.

References

Banta HD, Thacker SB (1979) Assessing in costs and benefits of electronic fetal monitoring. Obstet Gynecol Surv [Suppl] 34:627

Caldeyro-Barcia R, Poseiro JJ, Negreiros de Paiva C, et al (1963) Effect of abnormal uterine contractions on a human fetus. Mod Probl Pediatr 8:267

Clark SL, Gimovsky ML, Miller FC (1982) Fetal heart rate response to scalp blood sampling. Am J Obstet Gynecol 144:706

Clark SL, Gimovsky ML, Miller FC (1984) The scalp stimulation test. An alternative to fetal scalp blood sampling. Am J Obstet Gynecol 148:274

DeHaan J, Van Bemmel JH, Versteeg B, et al (1971) Quantitative evaluation of fetal heart rate patterns. I. Processing methods. Eur J Obstet Gynecol 1:95

DeVore GR, Donnerstein RL, Kleinman CS, et al (1982) Fetal echocardiography. I. Normal anatomy as determined by real-time-directed M-mode ultrasound. Am J Obstet Gynecol 144:249

Evertson LR, Gauthier RJ, Collea JV (1978) Fetal demise following negative contraction stress tests. Obstet Gynecol 51:671

Evertson LR, Gauthier RJ, Schifrin BS, et al (1979) Antepartum fetal heart rate testing. I. Evolution of the nonstress test. Am J Obstet Gynecol 133:29

Freeman RK (1975) The use of the oxytocin challenge test for antepartum clinical evaluation of uteroplacental respiratory function. Am J Obstet Gynecol 121:481

Freeman RK (1982) Contraction stress testing for primary fetal surveillance in patients at high risk for uteroplacental insufficiency. Clin Perinatol 9:265

Goodlin RC, Lowe EW (1974) A functional umbilical cord occlusion heart rate pattern: The significance of overshoot. Obstet Gynecol 43:22

Haverkamp AD, Thompson HE, McFee JG, et al (1976) The evaluation of continuous fetal heart rate monitoring in high-risk pregnancy. Am J Obstet Gynecol 125:310

Hobel CJ, Hyvarinen MA, Okada DM, et al (1973) Prenatal and intrapartum high-risk screening. Prediction of the high-risk neonates. Am J Obstet Gynecol 117:1

Hon EH (1963) Instrumentation of fetal heart rate and fetal electrocardiography. II. A vaginal electrode. Am J Obstet Gynecol 86:772

Hon EH, Huang HS (1962) The electronic evaluation of fetal heart rate. VII. Premature and missed beats. Obstet Gynecol 20:81

Hon EH, Quilligan EJ (1967) The classification of fetal heart rate. II. A revised working classification. Conn Med 31:779

Hon EH, Yeh SY (1969) Electronic evaluation of fetal heart rate. X. The fetal arrythmia index. Med Res Engin 8:14

Hon EH, Paul RH, Hon RW (1972) Electronic evaluation of fetal heart rate. XI. Description of a spiral electrode. Obstet Gynecol 40:362

James LS, Yeh MN, Morishima HO, et al (1976) Umbilical vein occlusion and transient acceleration of the fetal heart rate: experimental observation in subhuman primates. Am J Obstet Gynecol 126:276

Klapholz H, Burke L (1975) Intrauterine fetal demise with a negative oxytocin challenge test. J Reprod Med 15:169

Kubli FW, Hon EH, Khazin AF, et al (1969) Observation on heart rate and pH in the human fetus during labor. Am J Obstet Gynecol 104:1190

Laros RK Jr, Wong WS, Heilbron DC, et al (1977) A comparison of methods for quantitating fetal heart rate variability. Am J Obstet Gynecol 128:381

Lee CY, DiLoreto PC, O'Lane JM (1975) A study of fetal heart rate acceleration patterns. Obstet Gynecol 45:142

Lee CY, DiLoreto PC, Logrand B (1976) Fetal activity acceleration determination for the evaluation of fetal reserve. Obstet Gynecol 48:19

Manning FA, Platt LD, Sipos L (1980) Antepartum fetal evaluation: development of a fetal biophysical profile. Am J Obstet Gynecol 136:787

Manseau P, Vaquier J, Chavinie J (1972) Lerythme cardiaque foetal "sinusoidal". J Gynecol Obstet (Paris) 1:343

Martin CB Jr, Schifrin BS (1976) Prenatal fetal monitoring. In: Aladjem S, Brown AK (eds) Perinatal intensive care, chap 1. Mosby, St. Louis
Murata Y, Martin CB Jr (1974) Systolic time intervals of the fetal cardiac cycle. Obstet Gynecol 44:224
Neuman MR, Roux JF, Patrick JE, et al (1979) Evaluation of fetal monitoring by telemetry. Obstet Gynecol 54:249
Paul RH, Hon EH (1974) Clinical fetal monitoring. V. Effect on perinatal outcome. Am J Obstet Gynecol 118:529
Paul RH, Khazin-Suidan AF, Yeh SY, et al (1975) Clinical fetal monitoring. VII. The evaluation and significance of intrapartum baseline FHR variability. Am J Obstet Gynecol 123:206
Phelan JP, Lewis PE (1981) Fetal heart rate decelerations during a nonstress test. Obstet Gynecol 57:228
Phelan JP, Platt LD, Yeh SY, et al (1985) The continuing role of the nonstress test in the management of the postdates pregnancy. Am J Obstet Gynecol 151:304
Predictors of intrapartum fetal distress (1979) In: Antenatal diagnosis. U.S. Department of Health, Education, and Welfare, March 1979. National Institutes of Health, Bethesda, Maryland
Ray M, Freeman RK, Pines S, et al (1972) Clinical experience with the oxytocin challenge test. Am J Obstet Gynecol 114:1
Renou P, Chang A, Anderson I, et al (1976) Controlled trial of fetal intensive care. Am J Obstet Gynecol 126:470
Rochard F, Schifrin BS, Goupil F, et al (1976) Nonstressed fetal heart rate monitoring in the antepartum period. Am J Obstet Gynecol 126:699
Shamsi HH, Petrie RH, Steer CM (1979) Changing obstetric practices and amelioration of perinatal outcome in a university hospital. Am J Obstet Gynecol 133:855
Sokol RJ, Stojkov J, Chik L (1979) Maternal-fetal risk assessment: a clinical guide to monitoring. Clin Obstet Gynecol 22:547
Yeh SY, Betyar L, Hon EH (1972) Computer diagnosis of fetal heart rate patterns. Am J Obstet Gynecol 114:890
Yeh SY, Forsythe AF, Hon EH (1973) Quantification of fetal heart beat-to-beat interval differences. A numerical approach. Obstet Gynecol 41:355
Yeh SY, Diaz F, Paul RH (1982) Ten-year experience of intrapartum fetal monitoring in Los Angeles County/University of Southern California Medical Center. Am J Obstet Gynecol 143:496

The Dublin Randomised Controlled Trial of Intrapartum Electronic Fetal Heart Rate Monitoring

P. Boylan[1], D. MacDonald[2], A. Grant[3], M. Pereira[4], and I. Chalmers[3]

The title of my paper concerns the recently completed randomised controlled trial of electronic fetal heart rate monitoring, which was conducted at the National Maternity Hospital, Dublin, over the past 2 years. The trial was conducted because of continuing controversy about the relative merits of continuous electronic fetal monitoring (EFM) versus intermittent auscultation (IA). Although there is some evidence of a consensus that use of the more intensive methods of intrapartum monitoring is appropriate when the fetus is deemed to be at high risk, there is no such agreement concerning the application of these methods for fetuses at average or low risk of adverse outcome. The two expert committees which sat on either side of the Atlantic came to different conclusions concerning the advisability of continuous EFM for all labours:

> Periodic auscultation of the fetal heart rate is an acceptable method of assessment of fetal condition for women at low risk of intrapartum fetal distress (National Institutes of Health 1979).
> Continuous recording of the fetal heart rate should increasingly become part of the surveillance of all babies during labour (Social Services Committee 1980).

These contrasting conclusions reflect the dearth of information which has been derived from the five randomised controlled trials so far reported. The only suggestion of a beneficial effect of the more intensive methods of monitoring in these studies is the possibility that neonatal convulsions may be reduced by using continuous fetal heart rate monitoring in conjunction with fetal acid base assessment (Chalmers 1979). To set against this possible benefit, however, the evidence from these five trials suggests that continuous EFM leads to a substantial increase in the caesarean section rate, particularly if no attempt is made to assess fetal pH. We felt that the National Maternity Hospital was particularly suited to a prospective randomised controlled trial of EFM versus IA. More than 8000 babies are delivered each year at the hospital and a standard method of management of labour allows for the application of randomised procedures. The relevant figures for 1981 at the hospital are as follows:

Infants delivered	8964
Induction rate	8.2%
Forceps rate	7.0%
Caesarean section rate	5.5%

[1] University of Texas, Health Science Center at Houston, 6431 Fannin, Suite 3.270, Houston, TX 77030, USA
[2] National Maternity Hospital, Holles Street, Dublin, Ireland
[3] National Perinatal Epidemiology Unit, Radcliffe Infirmary, Oxford OX2 6HE, Great Britain
[4] Newborn Center, Children's Hospital, 1506 East 19th Avenue, Denver, CO 80218, USA

Fetal Heart Rate Monitoring
Ed. by W. Künzel

Perinatal mortality rate	12.2/1000
Deaths in labour	5
Cerebral dysfunction	32

Before the trial, selection of cases for intensive intrapartum monitoring at the hospital has been based on examination of the liquor as soon as a diagnosis of labour has been made. In 5% of cases the liquor is either absent or significantly meconium stained and a fetal scalp pH is estimated immediately. If the results are reassuring the fetal heart is monitored by EFM. In the remaining 95% of cases the fetus has been assessed at regular intervals by auscultation of the fetal heart, and by scalp pH estimation where indicated (O'Driscoll et al. 1977). The trial was to compare the latter policy of IA with EFM using a scalp electrode, with scalp pH estimation when indicated.

Full details of the prior hypotheses, methods and findings of the trial will be reported elsewhere (MacDonald et al., in preparation). This necessarily brief presentation will concentrate on the planning and execution of the trial and I will be able to give you some of the results of the initial outcome measures.

Methods

Women were eligible for inclusion in the trial if: (1) they had a live fetus of at least 28 weeks' gestation; (2) a diagnosis of labour had been made; and (3) liquor without significant meconium staining had been demonstrated at early amniotomy. Patients were excluded from the trial if: (1) they were delivered by elective caesarean section; (2) the fetus was dead; (3) there was a known fetal abnormality; (4) gestational age was less than 28 weeks; (5) there was significant meconium staining or no liquor at amniotomy; or (6) delivery occurred too rapidly to allow for randomisation. A total of 13 025 women met the entry criteria. Of these eligible women, 99.5% (12 960) were then allocated at random, by opening a sealed envelope at the time of amniotomy, to either continuous EFM or IA. All subsequent analyses are based on the unbiased comparisons between these two randomised groups (Fig. 1).

The aims of the trial were to test the following six hypotheses:

That the policy of intrapartum EFM:

1. Reduces the number of babies with Apgar scores of 2 or less at 1 min and/or 6 or less at 5 min (incidence, 10/1000)
2. Reduces the need for paediatric intervention at birth
   a) By intubation (incidence, 10/1000)
   b) By admission of normal birth weight babies to SCBU (special care baby unit; incidence, 10/1000)
3. Reduces the combined rate of
   a) Intrapartum stillbirth (incidence, 1/1000) (without severe congenital abnormality)
   b) Neonatal death (without severe congenital abnormality) (incidence, 3/1000)
   c) Cerebral dysfunction in normal birth weight babies (incidence, 2/1000)

   } Incidence, 6/1000

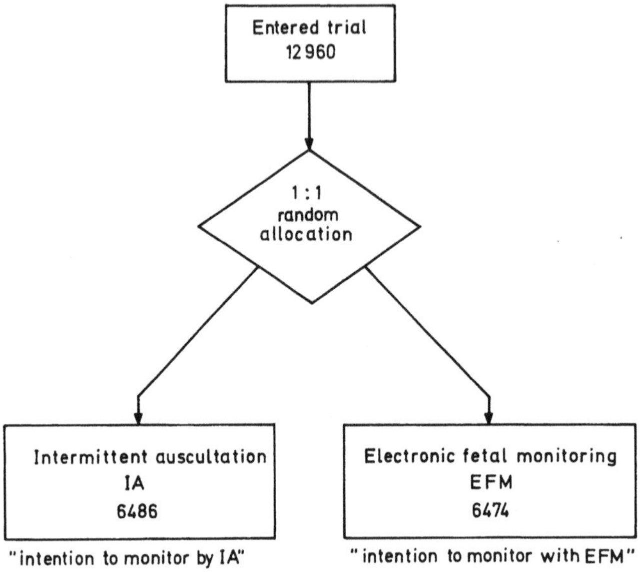

Fig. 1. The two randomized groups in the trial

4. Reduces the combined rate of 3 above + abnormal neurology which persists at day 7 (incidence, 4/1000) — Incidence, 10/1000
5. Reduces the incidence of abnormal neonatal neurology (including transient) — Incidence, 20/1000
6. Increases the caesarean section rate — Incidence, 40/1000
   and/or the forceps delivery rate — Incidence, 40/1000

The trial also aimed to assess the effect of intrapartum EFM on the following other outcome measures:

1. Condition of baby at birth:
   a) Cord pH (for 3- to 6-month period)
   b) Time to first breath and time to regular respiration
   c) Incidence of primary and terminal apnoea
2. Condition of baby in neonatal period:
   a) Incidence of respiratory distress syndrome
   b) Incidence of suspected infection
   c) Incidence of confirmed infection
   d) Incidence of injury caused by monitoring
   e) Paediatric intervention in neonatal period by:
      - Screening for infection
      - Antibiotic therapy
   f) Length of stay in hospital
   g) Subjective assessment at time of discharge from hospital
3. Labour and puerperium:
   a) Length of labour

b) Need for acceleration of labour with oxytocin
c) Need for analgesia during labour
d) Intrapartum and postpartum pyrexia
e) Length of stay in hospital

We also had the objective of assessing the long-term effects of EFM on the babies in the trial by paediatric follow-up.

During the trial there were several other side studies going on concurrently and among these was a study to assess the attitudes of mothers and hospital staff to the policy of EFM and to explore its effect on the relationship between the patient and midwife during labour, and between the mother and baby in the puerperium.

Intervention was based on abnormalities of the fetal heart. In the first stage of labour, intervention was to consist of the estimation of a scalp pH, and the decision concerning delivery or continuation of labour was based on scalp pH estimation. In the second stage of labour intervention was to consist of immediate delivery.

Results

Table 1 shows that randomisation achieved comparability between the two groups in a number of important respects.

Table 1. Descriptive variables

	IA	EFM
Maternal age—mean (years)	27.3	27.1
Married (%)	90	90
Non-Caucasian (%)	0.3	0.3
Parity (%)		
0	40	41
1–3	52	51
4+	8	8
Gestational age—mean (years)	39.9	39.9
Birth weight—mean (g)	3558	3543
Medical risk factor (%)	4.2	4.6

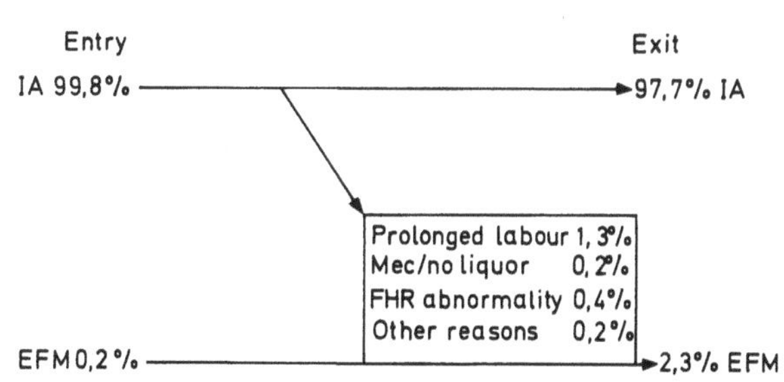

Fig. 2. IA management

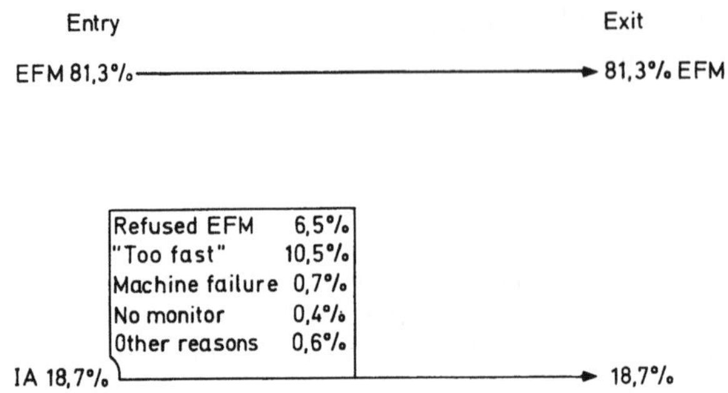

Fig. 3. EFM management

Table 2. Process variables

	IA	EFM	
Oxytocin use (%)	24	23	
Pethidine (%)	49	46	$P<0.05$
Epidural (%)	3	3	
Fetal blood sample (%) (*n*)	3.0 (194)	3.7 (240)	$P<0.05$
Randomisation to delivery interval (%)			
0– 60 min	23	27	
61–200 min	36	36	$P<0.05$
201+ min	41	37	
Duration of labour—mean (h)	4.2	3.9	$P<0.05$

The vast majority (97.7%) of women allocated to IA were monitored in this way throughout labour (Fig. 2). Of those allocated to EFM (Fig. 3), 10% delivered too rapidly for the method to be set up. A further 6% refused the technique, and a small proportion could not be monitored electronically for technical and other reasons. In all, however, more than 80% of those allocated to EFM were monitored in this way.

The rates of fetal blood sampling prompted by abnormalities of the fetal heart were 2.7% among those allocated to EFM and 1% among those allocated to IA (Table 2). Mothers allocated to EFM had significantly shorter labours and were significantly less likely to receive pethidine for analgesia (Table 1).

Discussion

The results presented in this paper indicate that it has been possible to carry out a large prospective randomised controlled trial of EFM versus IA in the busiest maternity unit in western Europe, without causing a gross disruption in the working pattern of the unit. From the initial time when the study was first mooted until the completion of the trial was a period of approximately 5 years. The trial involved considerable discussion and close cooperation between the National Perinatal Epidemiological Unit at Oxford and the National Maternity Hospital in Dublin. During the preliminary discussion stages there was active and vigorous discussion with experienced perinatologists both in the United States and in the United Kingdom. The initial results presented here enable us to say that the randomisation process worked and that EFM, backed up by fetal scalp pH estimation, did not result in a marked increase in the caesarean section rate. From the point of view of people working at the hospital, one of the most interesting findings was the reduction in requirement of analgesia and also the apparent shortening of labour associated with EFM. It is unfortunate that I am unable to present the final figures for the hard outcome variables such as fetal death in labour and neonatal convulsions, but it is hoped that the preliminary results will be presented at the British Congress of Obstetrics and Gynaecology in Birmingham in July of this year. The final results of the trial are expected to the published towards the end of this year or early in 1984.

References

Chalmers I (1979) Randomised controlled trials of fetal monitoring 1973–1977. In: Thalhammer O, Baumgarten K, Pollak A (eds) Perinatal medicine. Thieme, Stuttgart, pp 260–265

MacDonald D, Grant A, Pereira M, Boylan P, Chalmers I (to be published) The Dublin randomised controlled trial of intrapartum electronic fetal heart rate monitoring.

National Institutes of Health (1979) Report of a task force on predictors of fetal distress. In: Antenatal diagnosis. U.S. Department of Health, Education and Welfare, Washington, p 166

O'Driscoll K, Coughlin M, Fenton V, Skelly M (1977) Active management of labour: care of the fetus. Br Med J 2:1451–1453

Social Services Committee (1980) Report on perinatal and neonatal mortality. HMSO, London

The Use of Fetal Surveillance During Labor in the Federal Republic of Germany

V. M. Roemer[1], K. Bühler, and D. G. Kieback

Introduction

Medical technology has improved at a staggering pace and obstetrics is one of the fields most affected by this progress. Since its introduction in 1958 (Caldeyro-Barcia 1958) fetal heart rate (FHR) monitoring has become a widely used modality. It is estimated (Hobbins et al. 1979) that the technique is used in over half the deliveries in the United States. Recent investigations (1982) revealed that in Bavaria 88% of all fetuses during labor are monitored, 69.2% of them continously (F. K. Wulf, personal communication 1983). Similar figures (90%) have been published by Baumgarten, who reviewed 44750 deliveries in the German-speaking countries (Baumgarten 1981). Electronic fetal monitoring has been subject to criticism (Haverkamp et al. 1976; Banta and Thacker 1979a; Baumgarten 1981; Dunn 1979): the method requires application of transducers and electrodes which are connected to machines by wires or small cables. Some feel that this "confinement" of the mother detracts from the spontaneity of the experience. Others have been concerned with its contribution to the overall costs of pregnancy (Banta and Thacker 1979b). Still others have openly questioned the efficacy of this widely accepted technique (Banta and Thacker 1979b; Hobbins et al. 1979). However, during the past few years there has been increasing evidence that FHR monitoring leads to:

1. A decrease in neonatal death rate (Amato 1977; Neutra et al. 1978; Paul and Hon 1974; Paul et al. 1980; Tutera and Newman 1975; Bolte 1983; Baumgarten 1981)
2. A decrease in fetal morbidity measured by Apgar scores (Amato 1977; Ballas et al. 1980; Gabert and Stenchever 1974, 1977; Mueller-Heubach et al. 1980; Johnstone et al. 1978; Shenker et al. 1975) as well as umbilical pH values (Renou et al. 1976; Baumgarten 1981)
3. No substantial increase in cesarean section rate (Gabert and Stenchever 1977; Hughey et al. 1977; Mueller-Heubach et al. 1980; Johnstone et al. 1978; Kelso et al. 1978; Bolte 1983; Baumgarten 1981; Boehm et al. 1981; Ramzin and Weil 1981)
4. A significant reduction in the number of infants with neurological sequelae (Ingemarsson et al. 1981; Baumgarten 1981)

Thus the benefits outweigh the possible harmful effects of fetal monitoring (Hobbins et al. 1979; Banta and Thacker 1979b); therefore monitoring of each fetus during labor has been recommended (Bolte 1983; Baumgarten 1981). We do not know whether this aim has been achieved yet.

The purpose of this paper is to evaluate the situation of fetal surveillance during labor throughout the Federal Republic of Germany and—if possible—to draw clinical conclusions.

[1] Univ.-Frauenklinik, Schleichstr. 4, D-7400 Tübingen

Fetal Heart Rate Monitoring
Ed. by W. Künzel

Material and Methods

In order to collect data we sent questionnaires to every department of obstetrics in the Federal Republic of Germany. Of the 1137 questionnaires that were mailed[2], 684 were returned (60.1%) and 675 data sets were submitted to statistical analysis. Some answers (8) arrived too late to be included in the study. The data from each coding sheet were reviewed by the first author before being entered into the computer (IBM 4341/2). The majority of the questionnaires were completed correctly. Since the whole study was strictly anonymous no correction of possible erroneous data was possible. In some cases of obviously wrong answers data were omited ("lack of data"). Thus no correction of data sets took place. All quantitative variables were rounded to the next higher or lower numerical digit [exception: acidotic risk: pH<7.100 (%)]. It was possible to give special answers; all of these were encoded separately. In many questions two or more answers could be given simultaneously; in these cases the whole number of significant answers was set to 100%, not the number of departments.

From all the quantitative variables centiles were computed since nearly all variables prove not to be normally distributed (Kolmogorov-Smirnov one-sample test). Rank correlation methods were used according to Kendall to assess associations between various parameters. In order to analyze how the computed figures varied in different hospitals four categories of departments were created according to the number of deliveries per year. Figure 1 gives the distribution of the number of deliveries per year in the 675 hospitals under investigation. From this variable the 25th, 50th and 75th centiles were computed, equal to 329, 525, and 802 deliveries/year. Thus four types of hospitals were defined, differing in size. Furthermore the

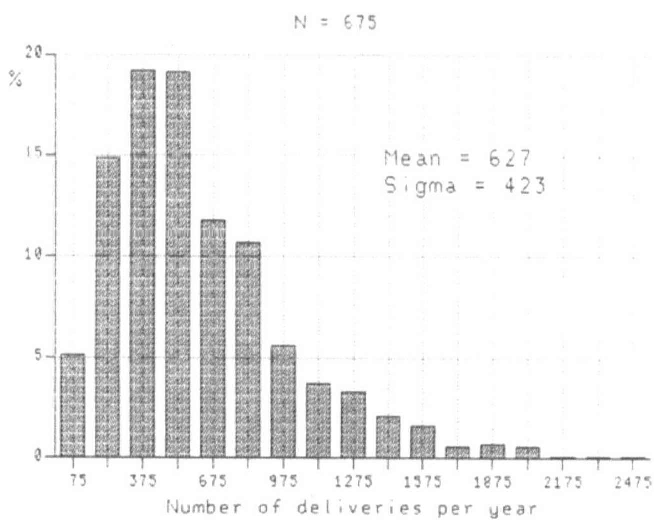

Fig. 1. Distribution of deliveries per year

---
[2] We thank Milupa for the availability and preparation of the addresses and Nestle AG for financial support in the data acquisition

ratio of the number of deliveries per year and the number of available monitors was computed; the distribution of this variable is given in Fig. 3.

Results

Table 1 gives some basic obstetrical data. Mean and median values are given since all distributions prove not to be normally distributed. From the last column *(N)* it is evident that some hospitals (29%) do not know, e.g., how many forceps deliveries are performed during a year. The uncorrected perinatal mortality figure was available from 77% and the percental rate of fetal acidemia ($pH_{UA}<7.100$) in 20.2% of hospitals, respectively. The reliability of the acidotic risk figure is not known because we have no data on the percental pH-measuring frequency in each hospital. In our own department in 88% of all deliveries acid-base measurements (pH, pCO_2, pO_2) in the umbilical blood are performed.

Table 2 gives some basic data of FHR monitoring in the Federal Republic of Germany. The median duration of its clinical use is 10 years. The majority of colleagues responding felt that nearly every fetus (99%) is monitored during labor, using external or internal methods. The distribution of this "soft" variable is given in Fig. 2.

The mean number of monitors is 3.4 and the mean number of deliveries per year and per monitor is 189; the distribution of the latter variable is given in Fig. 3.

Table 3 gives median values of some variables under investigation in the four categories of hospitals: The median number of deliveries per year is increased from 243 to 1078; the median number of deliveries per year and per monitor is significantly increased from 131 to 210. Thus the large hospitals with a higher incidence of risk

Table 1. Basic obstetrical data

	Median	Mean	SD	*N*
Number of deliveries	525	627	423	671
Cesarean section (%)	10.0	10.6	3.6	649
Forceps delivery (%)	2.0	3.6	3.6	481
Vacuum extraction (%)	7.0	8.0	5.8	620
$pH_{UA}<7.100$ (%)	1.3	1.7	1.4	137 (20%)
Perinatal mortality (‰)	4.0	5.2	4.6	520 (77%)

Table 2. Basic FHR monitoring data in the Federal Republic of Germany

	Median	Mean	SD	*N*
Duration of clinical use (years)	10	10.1	3.1	638
Monitored deliveries (%)	99.0	94.9	12.5	643
FHR monitors *(N)*	3.0	3.4	2.4	669
Deliveries/monitor	178	189	74	665

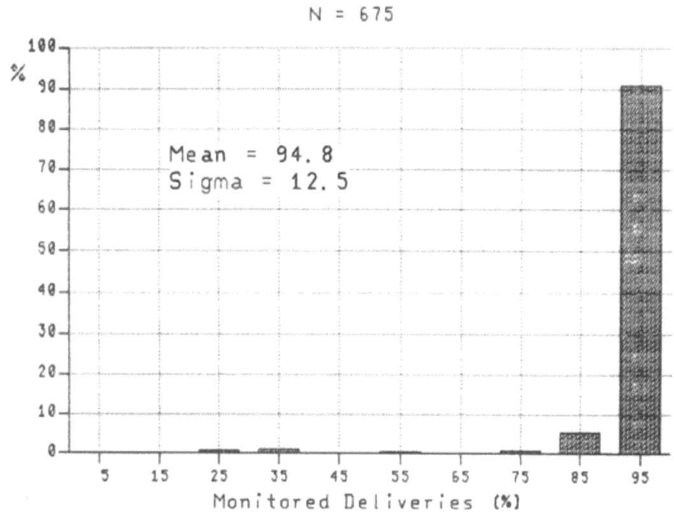

Fig. 2. Distribution of monitored deliveries

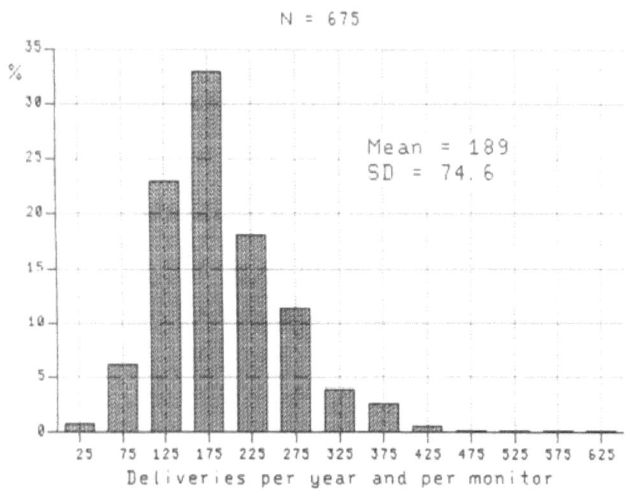

Fig. 3. Distribution of deliveries per year and per monitor

pregnancies are less well equipped when compared with the small (<25. centile) ones. The overload of obstetrical pathology is at least partly reflected in the mean perinatal mortality rates, which, at 2.4, 4.2, 6.5, and 7.2 per thousand for the four categories of hospitals, increase with hospital size. In all departments this figure amounted to 5.2 ± 4.6, *N*, 520.

Fetal monitoring is not identical with FHR monitoring: Fig. 4 shows that other methods of fetal surveillance during labor are used in 25%. However, this figure depends on the size of the department: In large hospitals (Table 4) 40.4% of all deliveries are monitored by additional methods. This means fetal blood sampling in

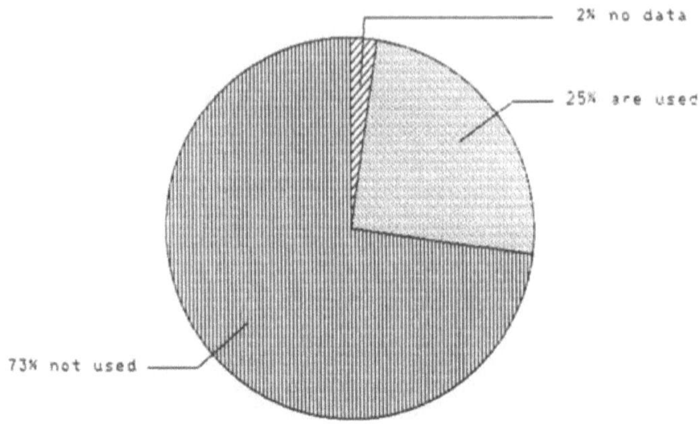

Fig. 4. Use of other methods of fetal monitoring during labor

Table 3. Basic obstetrical data

Median of	Centiles (N_{del}/year)			
	<25th	25th–49th	50th–74th	≥75th
Deliveries/year	243	420	650	1078
Cesarean section (%)	9.0	10.5	10.0	11.0
Forceps delivery (%)	2.0	2.0	1.0	3.0
Vacuum extraction (%)	8.0	7.0	7.0	6.0
Deliveries/monitor	131	158	180	210
$N_{hosp.}$	171	167	167	170

Table 4. Incidence of additional methods of fetal monitoring

	Centiles (N_{del}/year)			
	<25th	25th–49th	50th–74th	≥75th
Additional methods of fetal monitoring (%)	16.3	21.9	22.2	40.4

94%, transcutaneous pO_2 measurement in 3.9%, and transcutaneous pCO_2 and continuous pH measurements in 1%. The numerical distribution of the application of these other methods of fetal surveillance is quite constant throughout the four categories of hospitals: fetal blood sampling is the predominant additional method ranging from 90% to 94%. Consequently we may conclude that the smaller hospitals rely more upon FHR monitoring.

Figures 5 and 6 show that external methods of FHR monitoring are widely used (85%); ultrasound techniques are preferred (72%). There seems to be no important difference throughout the four categories of hospitals (Table 3).

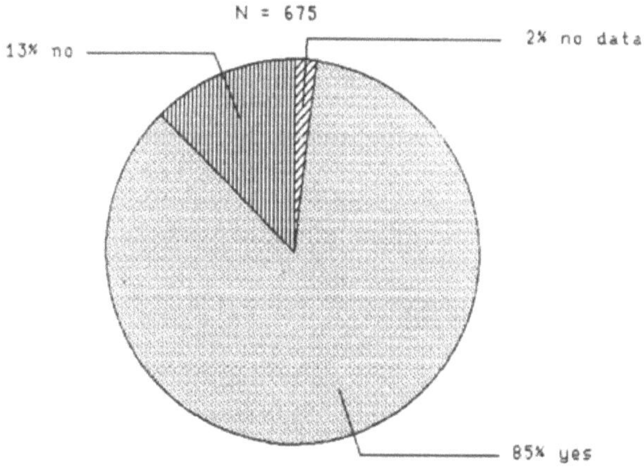

Fig. 5. Use of external methods of FHR monitoring

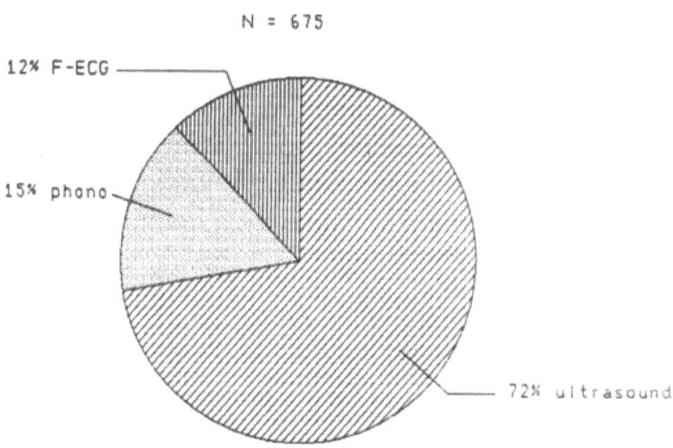

Fig. 6. Use of external methods in FHR monitoring

Table 5. Application of FHR monitoring (%)

Use of	Centiles (N_{del}/year)			
	<25th	25th–49th	50th–74th	≥75th
External methods				
Ultrasound	64.6	72.9	75.0	75.4
Phonocardiogram	21.0	14.6	12.8	14.1
Abdominal F-ECG	14.2	12.4	12.1	10.4

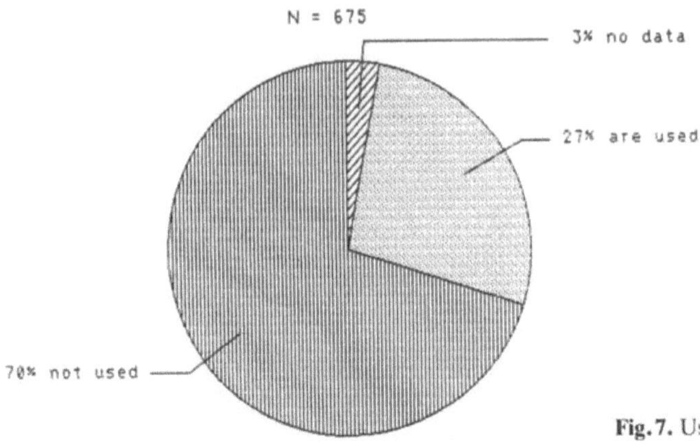

Fig. 7. Use of telemetric systems

Table 6. Application of FHR-monitoring (%)

Use of	Centiles (N_{del}/year)			
	<25th	25th–49th	50th–74th	≥75th
Telemetric system	9.8	18.0	33.5	49.1

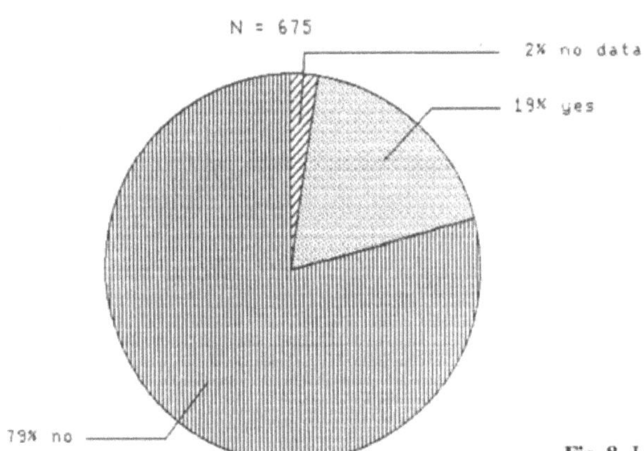

Fig. 8. Use of intrauterine catheters

Figure 7 and Table 6 indicate that telemetric systems are used in only 27% of hospitals; however, this figure is dependent on hospital size: about 50% of large hospitals are equipped with telemetric systems.

Labor monitoring is a clinically important feature of fetal surveillance: only 19% of all hospitals use intrauterine catheters to monitor labor by direct pressure measurements (Fig. 8). Again this figure is influenced by hospital size: large hospitals use

Table 7. Application of FHR-monitoring (%)

Use of	Centiles (N_{del}/year)			
	<25th	25th–49th	50th–74th	≥75th
Intrauterine catheter	7.4	20.3	18.4	29.7

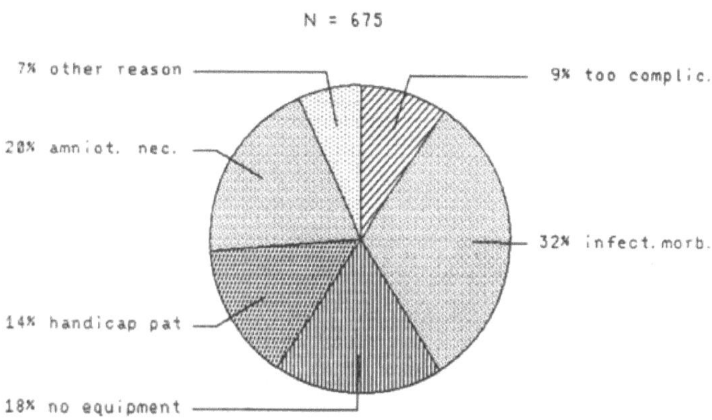

Fig. 9. Reasons for the nonuse of intrauterine catheters (more than one answer possible), see text

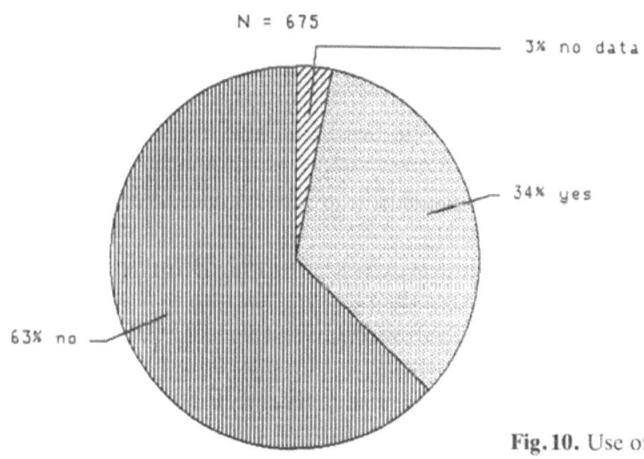

Fig. 10. Use of CTG scores

intrauterine catheters more frequently (30%, Table 7). The reasons for the nonuse of intrauterine catheters are summarized in Fig. 9: 9% of our colleagues felt that the method is too complicated, 32% mentioned possible increased infectious morbidity, 14% believed it handicaps the patient, and 20% complained about the need for early artificial amniotomy; other reasons are given by 7%.

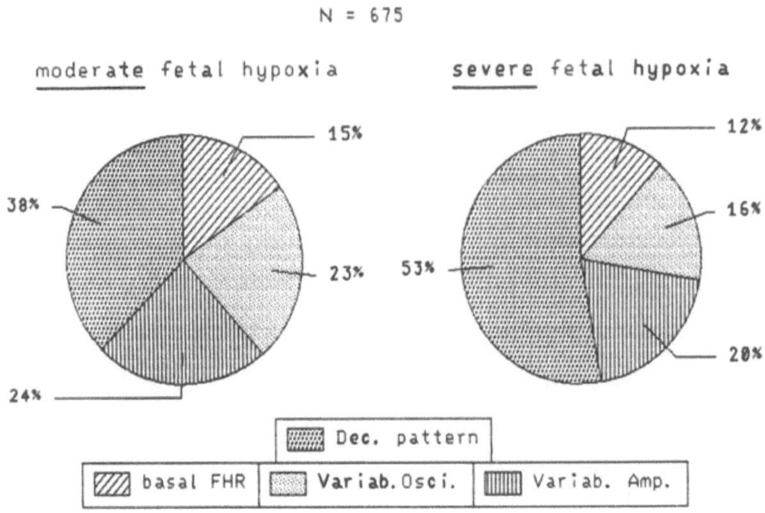

Fig. 11. Suitability of FHR monitoring for recognizing moderate or severe hypoxia

Figure 10 shows that cardiotocography (CTG) scores are used in 34% of all hospitals; this figure is fairly constant throughout the four categories of departments as defined previously.

Figure 11 gives an idea of the suitability of FHR monitoring for recognizing moderate or severe fetal hypoxia. Since no ranging was possible the percentage incidence of the answers (two were possible) may serve as an indicator: It is noteworthy that deceleration patterns seem to be most indicative in detecting both moderate and severe fetal hypoxia. FHR variability, oscillation frequency, and oscillation amplitude together are mentioned by 36% of hospitals as being suitable for detecting hypoxia. The baseline niveau is indicative in about 15%–12% of hospitals. It is difficult to decide whether these figures reflect a true picture or not. From our own studies we have concluded that deceleration pattern is a rather poor predictor of fetal well-being (Roemer et al. 1981).

It has been claimed by some authors (Haverkamp et al. 1976; Banta and Thacker 1979a, b) that FHR monitoring increases the cesarean section rate significantly. This was concluded from longitudinal studies in single hospitals. The cesarean section rate in the Federal Republic of Germany mirrored by the 675 departments which participated in the study is not extremely high: the mean value is 10.6% (Fig. 12). Instrumental vaginal deliveries (Fig. 13) total another 10%; thus about 80% of all babies are delivered vaginally and spontaneously. It must be kept in mind, however, that in a fairly large proportion of hospitals we observed "lack of data."

The question is now whether this rate of nonspontaneous deliveries is influenced by the monitoring practice.

The hospitals were asked to give the percentage incidence of electronically monitored deliveries. A large proportion of hospitals mentioned 90% or 95% (Fig. 2). This is in excellent accordance ($\bar{x} = 90.8\%$) with the data of Baumgarten (1981) analyzing 18 departments in the German-speaking countries. So there seems

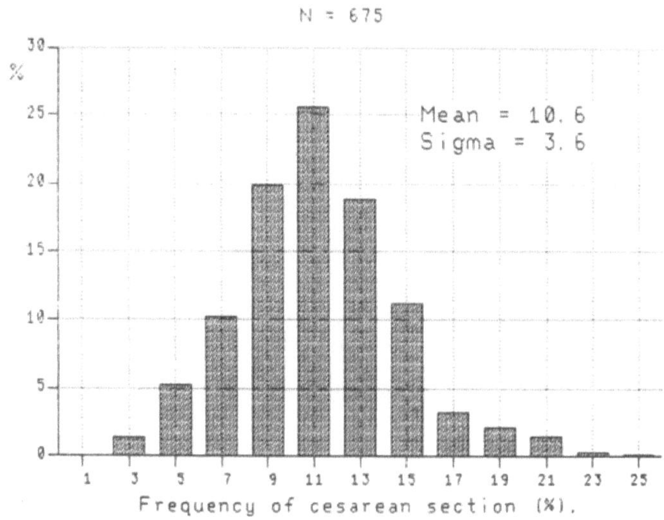

Fig. 12. Cesarean section rate

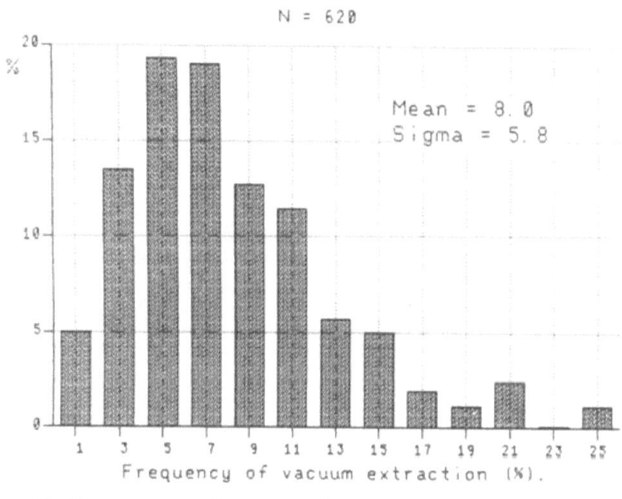

Fig. 13. Vacuum extraction rate

to exist no real distribution of this variable in the sample of the 675 participating departments. Consequently no significant associations were found in this context. Therefore we computed the number of deliveries per year and per monitor, a variable which may serve as an "index" of the monitoring frequency in each hospital. The assumption was made that the available monitors are constantly used in daily clinical routine. A low figure, around 100 deliveries/year and /monitor, would mean that every fetus could be monitored; a significantly higher value would reflect a lower incidence of electronic fetal surveillance. The mean value was 189 ± 74.6 (Fig. 3).

Table 8. All hospitals

x versus	y	τ	z
N_{del}/monitor	Cesarean section (%)	−0.020	−0.85
N_{del}/monitor	Forceps delivery (%)	−0.051	−1.67*
N_{del}/monitor	Vacuum extraction (%)	−0.045	−1.67*

τ, rank correlation coefficient
*, $P<0.05$

Table 9. Hospitals around the median number of deliveries/year (25th–75th centile)

x versus	y	τ	z
N_{del}/monitor	Cesarean section (%)	−0.087	−2.34**
N_{del}/monitor	Forceps delivery (%)	−0.159	−3.63***
N_{del}/monitor	Vacuum extraction (%)	−0.044	−1.04

**, $P<0.01$; ***, $P<0.001$

We looked first at all hospitals and found no association between the cesarean section rate and the number of deliveries per year and per monitor (Table 8). There is only a weak association between the rate of instrumental deliveries and the "index" indicating that monitoring of nearly each fetus might lead to an increased rate of instrumental deliveries.

As it is possible that in very small and very large hospitals the overall situation is somewhat different from the statistical "standard," the same analysis was carried out with the 334 departments with numbers of deliveries per year between the 25th and 75th centiles of the whole population. Thus, the quite small and large hospitals were excluded.

In this German "standard-sized department" delivering about 500 patients a year there is an association between this index and the cesarean section rate as well as the rate of forceps deliveries: Thus FHR monitoring seems to increase the rate of cesarean section and forceps delivery (Table 9).

Clinically this makes sense but one must be careful in jumping to conclusions since statistical associations, even highly significant, do not necessarily reflect causality.

Returning to clinical terms we may simply say that a higher incidence of fetal monitoring is associated with a higher rate of active obstetrical management. It is hard to believe that the beneficial effects of fetal monitoring are brought about without any alterations to these figures.

It is interesting to note that in the German "standard-sized departments" as previously defined there is a positive association ($\alpha<0.05$) between the "index" and the percentage of acidotic fetuses: lowering of the "index" leads to a smaller rate of acidotic fetuses. Thus one could argue that FHR monitoring prevents fetal acidosis.

Apgar score distributions were not available in our data sets.

There was no significant association between the index and the perinatal mortality figures in the standard-sized departments (τ, −0.04; z, −1.04; α, NS).

Conclusions

Although the reliability of each data set is questionable since only a small proportion of all departments seem to have their own data banks, the figures analyzed so far lead to the conclusion that cardiotocography is the predominant method of fetal surveillance during labor in the Federal Republic of Germany.

Fetal blood sampling is used in about 25% of all hospitals. It is the preferred additional method.

The equipment especially of the small departments seems to be excellent. Nearly every fetus (90%–95%) is monitored during labor using internal or external methods. The mean number of deliveries per year and per monitor is 189.

FHR monitoring may influence the cesarean section rate, the number of instrumental deliveries, and the incidence of fetal acidemia.

Further investigations are necessary to rule out the beneficial and possible harmful effects of FHR monitoring based on standardized data sets from each department performing obstetrics in this country.

References

Amato JC (1977) Fetal monitoring in a community hospital, a statistical analysis. Obstet Gynecol 50:269

Ballas S, Hornstein E, Jaffa AJ, Toaff R (1980) Selective versus routine intrapartum monitoring: comparison of effects on perinatal outcome. Acta Obstet Gynecol Scand 59:301

Banta HD, Thacker SB (1979a) Fetal monitoring. Letters to the editor. Obstet Gynecol 54:667

Banta HD, Thacker SB (1979b) Assessing the costs and benefits of electronic fetal monitoring. Obstet Gynecol Surv [Suppl] 34:627

Baumgarten K (1981) The benefits and hazards of feto-maternal monitoring. J Perinat Med 9:257

Boehm FH, Davidson KK, Barrett JM (1981) The effect of electronic fetal monitoring on the incidence of cesarean section. Am J Obstet Gynecol 140:295

Bolte A (1983) Der Stellenwert der intrapartualen Kardiotokographie. Ein Beitrag zur Effizienz der Methode. Verh Dtsch Ges Gynäkol Geburtshilfe, Arch Gynecol 235:641

Caldeyro-Barcia R (1958) Uterine contractility in obstetrics. 2nd Figo congress, Montreal

Dunn PM (1979) Problems associated with fetal monitoring during labour. Perinatal medicine, VI. European congress, Vienna. Thieme, Stuttgart

Gabert HA, Stenchever MA (1974) Electronic fetal monitoring as a routine practice in an obstetric service: a progress report. Am J Obstet Gynecol 118:534

Gabert HA, Stenchever MA (1977) The results of a five-year study of continous fetal monitoring on an obstetrical service. Obstet Gynecol 50:275

Haverkamp AD, Thompson HE, McFee JG, Cetrulo C (1976) The evaluation of continuous fetal heart rate monitoring in high-risk pregnancy. Am J Obstet Gynecol 125:310

Hobbins JC, Freeman R, Queenan JT (1979) The fetal monitoring dabate. Editorial. Obstet Gynecol 54:103

Hughey MJ, La Pata RE, McElin TW, Lussky R (1977) The effect of fetal monitoring on the incidence of cesarean section. Obstet Gynecol 49:513

Ingemarsson E, Ingemarsson I, Svenningsen NW (1981) Impact of routine fetal monitoring during labor on fetal outcome with long-term follow-up. J Obstet Gynecol 141:29

Johnstone FD, Cambell DM, Hughes GJ (1978) Has continuous intrapartum monitoring made any impact on fetal outcome? Lancet I: 1298

Kelso JM, Parsons J, Lawrence GF, Arora SS, Edmonds DK, Cooke ID (1978) An assessment of continous fetal heart rate monitoring in labor. Am J Obstet Gynecol 131: 526

Mueller-Heubach E, MacDonald HM, Joret D, Portman MA, Edelstone DI, Caritis SN (1980) Effects of electronic fetal heart rate monitoring on perinatal outcome and obstetric practices. Am J Obstet Gynecol 137: 758

Neutra RR, Fienberg SE, Greenland S, Friedman EA (1978) Effect of fetal monitoring on neonatal death rates. N Engl J Med 299: 324

Paul R, Hon EH (1974) Clinical fetal monitoring. V. Effect on perinatal outcome. Am J Obstet Gynecol 118: 529

Paul HR, Gauthier RJ, Quilligan EJ (1980) Clinical fetal monitoring. Acta Obstet Gynecol Scand 59: 289

Ramzin MS, Weil A (1981) Neue Aspekte der perinatalen Mortalität. In: Schmidt E, Dudenhausen JW, Saling E (Hrsg) Perinatale Medizin, Vol 8. Thieme, Stuttgart

Renou P, Chang A, Anderson I, Wood C (1976) Controlled trial of fetal intensive care. Am J Obstet Gynecol 126: 470

Roemer VM, Brühl G, Mietzner S, Heering P, Heinzl S (1981) Die Dezeleration in der direkten Kardiotokographie: Quantitative und qualitative Analyse. In: Schmidt E, Dudenhausen JW, Saling E (Hrsg) Perinatale Medizin, Vol 9. Thieme, Stuttgart

Shenker L, Post RC, Seiler JS (1975) Routine electronic monitoring of fetal heart rate and uterine activity during labor. Obstet Gynecol 46: 185

Tutera G, Newman RL (1975) Fetal monitoring: its effect on the perinatal mortality and cesarean section rates and its complications. Am J Obstet Gynecol 122: 750

Westgren M, Ingemarsson E, Ingemarsson I, Solum T (1980) Intrapartum electronic fetal monitoring in low-risk pregnancies. Obstet Gynecol 56: 301

Present and Future Technical Advances in Fetal Heart Rate Monitoring

H. D. JUNGE[1]

I would like to start with some brief statements on the technical problems and technical progress of fetal heart rate (FHR) monitoring in general, because these statements may be helpful in identifying true advances of the past, present, and future.

The introduction of electronic fetal monitoring with continuous recording of FHR and uterine activity instead of auscultation of fetal heartbeats and palpation of contractions more than a decade ago was indeed a true innovation in clinical obstetrics. In fact, it was a twofold innovation, because electronic FHR monitoring included the introduction of instantaneous, beat-to-beat heart rate recording, a method which was in contrast to the averaging effect of counting fetal heartbeats for 1 min and a method quite uncommon in cardiovascular diagnostics at that time. From the very beginning it has been and still is generally agreed that variability of FHR is a major diagnostic parameter and variability can only be documented in instantaneous FHR recordings. For that reason beat-to-beat FHR measurement to the nearest 1 ms is an absolute precondition for any form of technical functioning and clinical application of electronic FHR monitoring, and beat-to-beat measurement was and still is the major technical problem. First of all, looking at the signal properties of all source signals from the fetal heart used so far for FHR recording makes quite clear that beat-to-beat measurement without any preprocessing of signals is quite impossible. Direct fetal electrocardiography (FECG) is no exception when picked up with inappropriate electrodes. Secondly, it is of great importance that, after a brief period of discussion, FHR monitoring became generally accepted as a method of clinical routine. It is quite clear in clinical routine precise beat-to-beat measurement is much more a problem than in a laboratory setting with optimal recording conditions.

In contrast, conversion of beat-to-beat measures into instantaneous heart rate was only a minor technical problem. It was solved many years ago, and the essential technical details of ratemeters have not changed substantially since.

From these statements it is obvious that true advances in FHR monitoring could and can only be achieved by a successful search for a combination of a suitable source signal from the fetal heart and/or an optimal signal pickup method and/or a preprocessing method for beat-to-beat measuring optimally adapted to the source signal.

With these criteria in mind first let me look at the past and try to identify true advances in clinical routine FHR monitoring. To my mind, first of all the efforts of Hammacher deserve to be mentioned. He combined a microphone especially designed for fetal heart tone pickup with a preprocessing method that for the first time was especially adapted to the special signal properties of the phonocardiogram. In adding

[1] Univ.-Frauenklinik, Josef-Schneider-Str. 4, D-8700 Würzburg

Fetal Heart Rate Monitoring
Ed. by W. Künzel

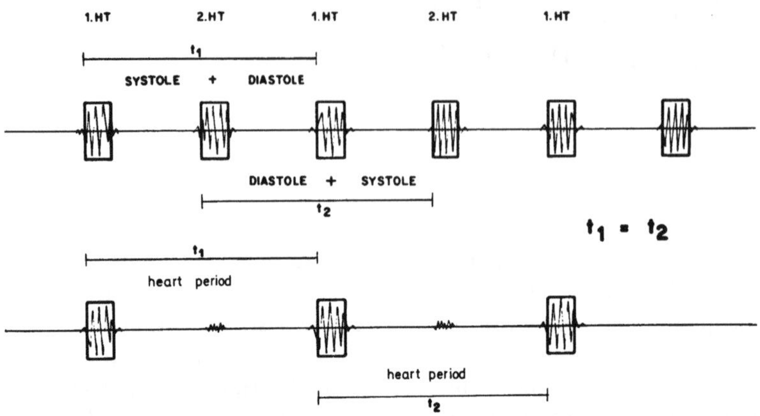

Fig. 1. Hammacher's method of comparing duration from the first to the next first heart tone and duration from the second to the next second heart tone to improve beat-to-beat FHR measurement

his "method of time comparison" from first-to-first and second-to-second heart tone (Fig. 1) to the well-established methods of amplifying, filtering, and rectifying he substantially improved beat-to-beat measurement and with it instantaneous FHR recording. Can anything prove true advance better than the fact that his success prompted the production of the first "cardiotocograph," the first commercially available machine designed especially for continuous recording of instantaneous FHR and uterine activity?

For some time it was the only machine available for clinicians, and despite the finding that it did not work as well in clinical routine as demonstrated at exhibitions it promoted the general clinical use of electronic fetal monitoring.

It cannot be denied that a substantial proportion of recordings was still insufficient for proper surveillance especially during delivery and there has been no major improvement since based on phonosignal pickup.

Obviously the latter was the reason for further efforts to improve the results of intrapartum recording. These efforts were most successful at last and there was another true advance when intrapartum FHR recording via direct FECG was established in clinical routine. To my mind the technical achievement of triggering a ratemeter with an FECG of high signal-to-noise ratio amplified with a commercially available preamplifier of EEG sensitivity could not be justifiably called an innovation. The noise-free ECG with its one sharp peak per heart cycle is an ideal source and trigger signal. The crucial point for intrapartum monitoring via FECG as the source signal was the construction of a special FECG electrode that optimally fulfilled the mechanical and electrical requirements and at the same time could be handled most easily in clinical routine. The spiral-type electrode combined with bipolar lead (Fig. 2) met these criteria and it has been in world-wide use ever since. However, to be honest it must be mentioned that intrapartum monitoring via transvaginal electrodes would not have been established as a routine method unless barriers of obstetric tradition at that time had not been torn down by those who inaugurated amnioscopy and microblood analysis of the fetus and made vaginal examination a matter of routine.

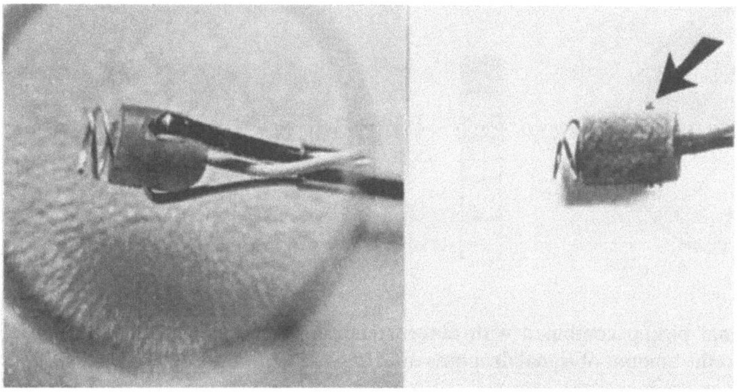

Fig. 2. Spiral-type electrode invented by Junge in 1969 *(left)* and its modification for bipolar lead (↓) by Rüttgers in 1971 *(right)*

Much ingenious work has been done on the development of methods for signal processing of the abdominal FECG. Nevertheless, I wonder whether FHR monitoring via abdominal FECG was a true advance, because for well-known reasons this method was and forever will be restricted to selected cases. It will never be available for routine application.

The introduction of the ultrasound (US) Doppler signal from the fetal heart as a source signal for FHR monitoring awaited general acceptance as a valuable innovation for many years because its advantages were balanced out by substantial disadvantages. There is the advantage of a high-source signal power because of external power input. With a narrow-beam transducer and conventional signal processing, the source signal can be shaped sufficiently for exact beat-to-beat measurement and good recording of FHR variability but the signal source often changes its position or even escapes from the US beam and the signal is lost completely. With the wide-beam transducer, escape from the beam is less frequent but poor source signal quality gives rise to much jitter, obscuring true variability.

With that I arrive at the present and future:

It was only recently that the introduction of a sophisticated preprocessing method made FHR recording via the US Doppler signal a true advance and it should be mentioned that it originates from development carried out by industry.

Fast progress in microprocessor technology in respect to storage and calculating capacity made real-time digital processing of the autocorrelation function of the Doppler signal possible, and some properties of the Doppler signal that are disadvantages for conventional preprocessing turn into advantages for autocorrelation preprocessing.

In contrast to conventional analogue methods of signal processing, which define trigger points by a peak or by a level of amplitude and/or use of a slope definition of trigger points with the autocorrelation method, are based on many points of the source signal: the influence of random noise is reduced substantially and FHR recording is improved. The improvement is documented in Fig. 3.

In nearly 400 nonstress tests from 23 to 41 weeks of gestation, 50% of recordings were excellent and 90% sufficient for interpretation. Only 4% were totally insufficient. Results are clearly dependent on gestational age (Fig. 4).

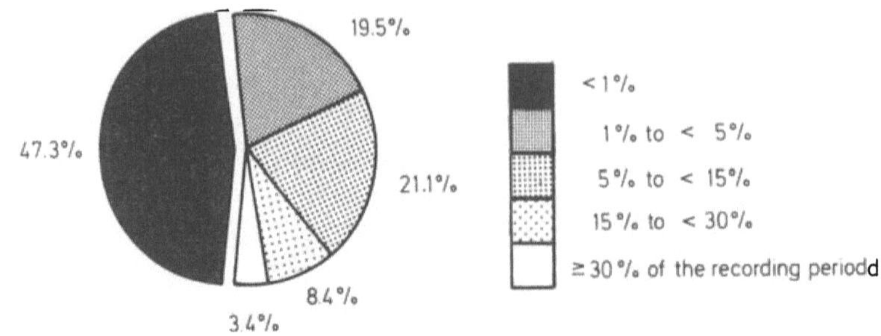

Fig. 3. Ultrasound signal pickup combined with autocorrelation preprocessing. Quality of FHR recordings according to the amount of signal dropouts of ≥ 15 s

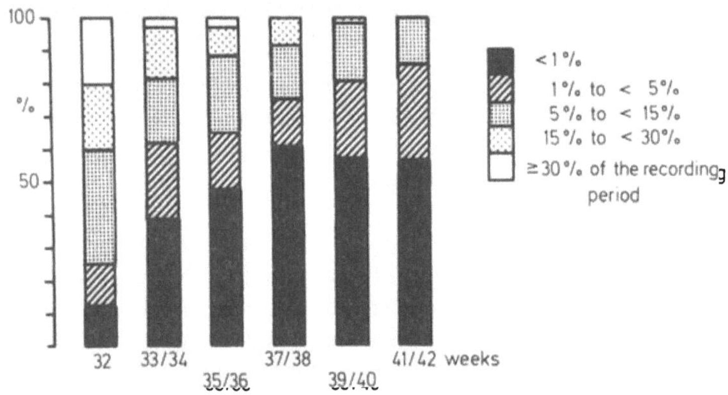

Fig. 4. Same as Fig. 3, but as a function of gestational age

In some of the insufficient recordings the source signal from the fetal heart was lost and maternal heart rate was recorded for shorter or even prolonged periods (Fig. 5). This is a potential hazard for the inexperienced nurse or doctor but not for the expert.

Signal loss in the moving fetus at present is the major shortcoming of the Doppler signal plus autocorrelation method and it needs to be overcome. In other words: a sophisticated method for constant Doppler signal pickup despite a moving signal source would be another true advance. It would complete the combination of an appropriate source signal, a specially adapted signal pickup, and a specially adapted preprocessing method for exact beat-to-beat measurement.

I have no reason to speculate that there will be an absolute and complete innovation in regard to the technique of beat-to-beat FHR recording in the near future.

In summary: FHR monitoring with the direct FECG pickup at present is the method producing the best results in respect to instantaneous FHR recording. However, direct monitoring is restricted to the phase of active labor and delivery. Moreover, due to the invasive character of direct monitoring there are potential hazards such as infection and injury and due to the invasive character this method may be rejected by patients for psychological reasons. FHR monitoring with the Doppler signal plus autocorrelation preprocessing is near perfect but awaits im-

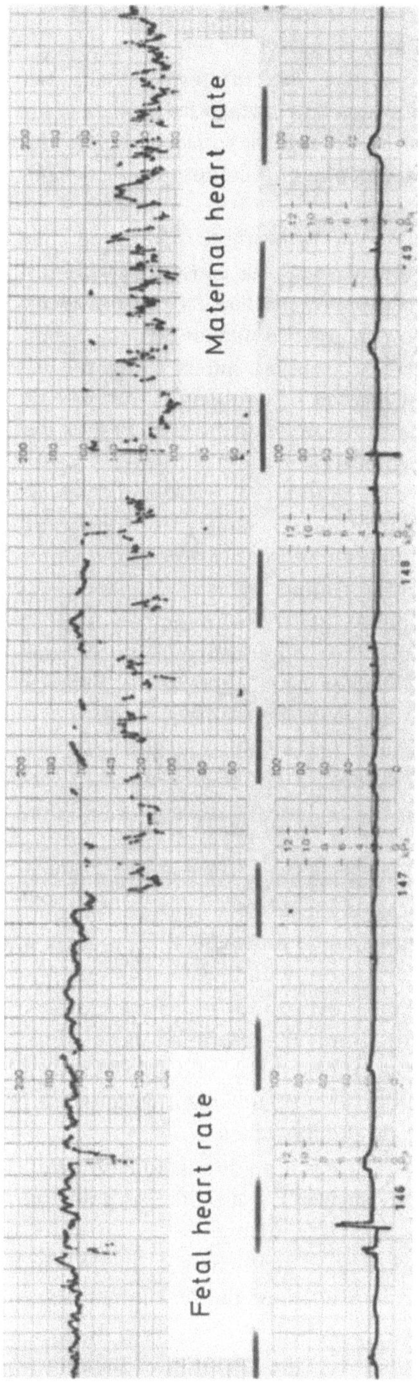

Fig. 5. Intermittent *(center)* and continuous *(right)* signal pickup from maternal vessels in a FHR recording with US signal pickup and autocorrelation preprocessing

provement of the signal pickup method. It is superior to monitoring based on phono- or abdominal FECG pickup, methods that still may be useful for selected cases.

With this summary I could end my paper but it is of some interest to discuss two additional technical features of electronic fetal monitoring, which by no means are preconditions for the success of fetal surveillance, but still they may be helpful for clinical routine. One feature is telemetry and the other is computer-aided FHR monitoring (CAFM).

A changing understanding of the role of childbirth for mother, father, and child and with that changing habits of childbirth in recent years has caused growing disapprovement of electronic fetal monitoring, its equipment, and its consequences: "confinement" of the patient and confrontation with medical machinery.

In order to adapt monitoring hardware to these changed habits telemetry was introduced and there is a trend toward miniaturization of equipment. At present, advances in this field are minimal. Radio transmission of the direct FECG and intrauterine pressure (IUP) is without major technical problems, but general limitations of direct monitoring have not been overcome. In addition, commercially available preamp + transmitter boxes are not truly miniaturized. Battery size is only part of the problem. The achievement of true miniaturization has only been documented in a few publications from biomedical centers in the United States.

There are severe problems with external signal pickup from a patient walking up and down in the labor ward because enhanced mobility will enhance electrical noise or cause signal loss. In addition, in using the Doppler signal there is the technical problem of incorporating the US generator into a patientside miniature box.

There is more than one reason to speculate that true advances in this field, real miniature radio systems for external FHR monitoring, will not be available for clinical use in the near future, and apart from the technical problems mentioned financial aspects are of growing importance.

Another field of interest in discussing technical advances of FHR monitoring is on-line computer-aided fetal monitoring (CAFM). CAFM would be the third generation of monitoring methods for fetal surveillance and with the progress in microprocessor technology monitoring can be carried out with bedside computers.

For many years and in many obstetric centers all over the world there has been much activity and much enthusiasm in this field. However, despite all these efforts CAFM today is still not established in clinical routine and there is no CAFM system commercially available. There seems to be great fear of making this large step toward the next generation of monitoring methods and machines.

All the aspects, details, and problems of CAFM cannot be discussed here. What would CAFM make a true advance? To give an answer I would like to point out some specific shortcomings of present electronic fetal monitoring.

One is data output: recording FHR continuously on strip chart is the one and only mode of display. This mode has not been changed since the first monitor was designed.

Strip chart time base is 10–30 mm/min for good visual evaluation of short-term changes. However, special features such as long-term FHR and IUP trends are more or less obscured. Computer-based adequate display of short-term changes and long-term trends and additional information in FHR will be a valuable aid for the doctor.

Table 1. Present problems of electronic fetal monitoring

Problem No. 1
Cardiotocographs record FHR and UA continuously for hours. But: who is watching and evaluating the strip charts carefully and continuously for hours for prompt detection of clinically significant CTG changes?
Solution
A CTG monitor system evaluating FHR and UA recordings continuously for detection of clinically significant CTG changes and alert output to be noticed by the doctor immediately
Problem No. 2
Detection of clinically significant CTG changes depends on the doctor's experience, physical state and environmental conditions. Will the doctor detect clinically significant CTG changes just the same when he is experienced, alert, in a relaxed situation or when he is inexperienced, tired, in a stressful situation?
Solution
A CTG monitor system evaluating FHR and UA recordings continuously for detection of clinically significant CTG changes irrespective of the doctor's experience irrespective of the doctor's physical state irrespective of environmental conditions

In any case because FHR in general is an information source of high redundancy, data reduction for easy-to-survey and adequate display of all important information and for information exchange is highly desirable. In this context it should be mentioned that, once all redundancy is removed, with progressive data reduction more and more information is lost. Therefore there are limitations for data reduction.

Other shortcomings of EFM, based on problems of clinical routine, can be overcome by CAFM (Table 1). With this, continuous evaluation of FHR records by experienced and alert personel is a precondition for EFM and shortcomings in this respect can be overcome by computer. In fact continuous operation and continuous "alertness" without failure are special properties of computers.

The meaningfulness as well as the aims and limitations in regard to an alert system in CAFM have been the matter of much controversial discussion. To my mind the quality of any alert system in CAFM has to be judged according to a good correlation between alert output and need for clinical action, and these actions may be: stand by and watch carefully, change patient's position, reposition transducer, stop or adapt oxytocin infusion rate, start tocolysis, perform a microblood analysis, or deliver the baby.

Fetal state: well-being, stress, or distress, can only be calculated from FHR according to the rules of probability. For that reason there must be some rate of false alarms. This rate of false alarms can only be influenced by the system's alert criteria, and for each rate of false alarm, i.e., for each level of intelligence of an alert system, it cannot be avoided that the rate of false-negative alerts will be raised when trying to decrease the rate of false-positive alarms.

By no means will it ever be possible in CAFM to calculate exactly actual fetal pH, predict neonatal Apgar score, or give a true long-term trend forecast for the course of gestation or delivery from FHR data.

Expecting this would be expecting miracles and not advances in FHR monitoring in the future.

Physiology of Fetal Heart Rate During Intrauterine Life

Antenatal Heart Rate Analysis at the Bedside Using a Microprocessor

G. S. Dawes[1] and C. W. G. Redman

Five years ago Dr. Chris Redman and I decided to develop a computerised technique for the numerical analysis of human fetal heart rate records. He had experienced difficulty in deriving satisfactory numerical data in high-risk pregnancies while, from observations on sheep (Dalton et al. 1977) and human fetal breathing, I suspected that these records contained more information than was extracted by visual inspection.

The results are briefly summarised. First, methods were developed to enumerate signal loss (Dawes et al. 1981b) and to fit a satisfactory baseline (Dawes et al. 1982a). The methods for recording data were improved, from using analogue tapes (accurate but slow) to data reduction onto digital tapes (faster) with analysis on a minicomputer, to on-line analysis at the bedside using microprocessors (Wickham et al. 1983). We are now beginning to use a high-resolution coloured graphical display on a fast microprocessor. The data are stored on discs and the records are plotted, with printed analyses, in a convenient form for handling on A4-size paper.

We use conventional commercial detector systems (Doppler ultrasound, maternal abdominal or scalp-clip fetal ECG, or phonocardiograph), together with their strip recorders, as the primary signal transducer. Our analyses showed that signal loss was high using conventional ultrasound equipment by manufacturers such as Sonicaid or Hewlett-Packard (8031A). It was reduced by using a range-gate to improve signal-to-noise ratio (e.g. Roche Fetasonde 5; Lawson et al. 1982) and even more by autocorrelation (e.g. Hewlett-Packard 404A; Lawson et al. 1983). Whereas conventional Doppler ultrasound instruments cause an unacceptably high (two- to threefold) spurious increase in beat-to-beat variation, autocorrelation causes an unacceptable reduction. Thus beat-to-beat variation can only be measured by detecting the fetal ECG. We also found that signal loss varies with gestational age and is increased in episodes of high heart rate variation (Dawes et al. 1981b). There are therefore good reasons for continued critical examination of methods for recording fetal heart rate and its variation.

Numerical analysis showed a prominent effect of gestational age on heart rate variation (Visser et al. 1981; Dawes et al. 1982b). This is superimposed on a diurnal variation (Visser et al. 1982). The heart rate variation is also modulated by fetal breathing and movement (Dawes et al. 1981a) and episodically by changes in fetal behaviour, as also described by Timor-Tritsch et al. (1978), Junge (1979), and Wheeler et al. (1980).

Numerical analysis allows objective measurement of the different components of fetal heart rate variation. For example, mean beat-to-beat variation of the pulse

[1] University of Oxford, Nuffield Institute for Medical Res., Headley Way, Headlington, Oxford OX3 9DS, Great Britain

Fetal Heart Rate Monitoring
Ed. by W. Künzel

interval (2.3 ms at term) is normally a small proportion of the total variation (> 30 ms over 60 min). More of the variation is associated with movements of the fetal trunk and limbs than with fetal breathing. It is possible to detect fetal breathing from analysis of a high-quality fetal ECG record, but there are better ways of doing this using ultrasound.

Analysis of fetal heart rate records can also be used to identify episodes of high heart rate variation associated with movements, as compared with episodes of low variation. It is instructive to compare the frequency distribution of accelerations (>10 or 15 bpm and 15 s) with that of episodes of high variation. Even in 64-min records from normal pregnancies there are many with less than two accelerations (16% at 28–33 weeks, 7% at 34–41 weeks) but few with no episode of high heart rate variation and movements (0.7% overall). As evidence of normality the latter is evidently a better index (Dawes et al. 1982b). But there is as yet no evidence that the compromised fetus has altered behavioural patterns.

Over the past 20 years it has been established that a substantial reduction of fetal heart rate variation may be sinister, i.e. a sign of impending death, especially when accompanied by prolonged decelerations. Two questions arise. First, is such a loss of variation a consequence of a deterioration in fetal respiration? And secondly, is fetal heart rate variation a useful prognostic index of health? We have attempted to answer these questions.

Fetal heart rate traces were compared, shortly before delivery, in 23 women delivered by Caesarean section for fetal compromise and in 49 delivered by section for other reasons (Henson et al. 1983). Fetal pulse interval variation was much reduced in the former group (mean minute range over 60 min, 22.9 ± 1.2 ms) as compared with the latter (52.3 ± 2.1 ms). The difference persisted when account was taken of gestational age yet there was no evidence of metabolic acidaemia in those fetuses delivered for suspected compromise, with low heart rate variation, as judged by the base excess of umbilical arterial blood compared with the control group. We must conclude that the low heart rate variation is due to another cause, perhaps metabolic or hormonal. It was interesting that the compromised group of fetuses, with low heart rate variation, had a high incidence of growth retardation.

To test the predictive value of fetal heart rate variation records were collected from 634 women at 32 weeks of pregnancy. In a pilot study the centile distribution of heart rate variation at 32 weeks had been estimated for heart rate records of differing durations. Analyses were subsequently made at 5-min intervals on-line to select the 5% of fetuses with the least variation, recorded over 45 min. The record duration was adjusted according to the degree of heart rate variation so that the average record length was 16 min (Lawson et al. 1984). In fact 30 records (4.7%) were collected with the lowest variation (26.1 ms mean minute range, with an observation time of 45 min; normal value 43.6 ± 1.5 ms). Nineteen of these women were delivered normally at term. Detailed analysis of the outcome showed no long-term predictive value over ordinary clinical considerations. We conclude that, as in sheep, the heart rate and its variation only gives short-term warning of fetal compromise. The reasons for the extreme variations commonly seen in fetal heart rate need further study.

There yet seems to be a place for antenatal fetal heart rate monitoring in selected high-risk patients. Indeed there is no other means of detecting impending fetal death, other than identification of fetal movements, which also modulate the heart rate. So sequential measurements on the same patient continue to have their uses. We would welcome firmer scientific proof of this generalisation and should seek a more convincing explanation of the pathophysiological changes which reduce heart rate variation than is yet available.

References

Dalton KJ, Dawes GS, Patrick JE (1977) Diurnal, respiratory and other rhythms of fetal heart rate in lambs. Am J Obstet Gynecol 127:414–424

Dawes GS, Visser GHA, Goodman JDS, Levine DH (1981a) Numerical analysis of the human fetal heart rate: modulation by breathing and movement. Am J Obstet Gynecol 140:535–544

Dawes GS, Visser GHA, Goodman JDS, Redman CWG (1981b) Numerical analysis of the human fetal heart rate: the quality of ultrasound records. Am J Obstet Gynecol 141:43–52

Dawes GS, Houghton CRS, Redman CWG (1982a) Baseline in human fetal heart-rate records. Br J Obstet Gynaecol 88:270–275

Dawes GS, Houghton CRS, Redman CWG, Visser GHA (1982b) Pattern of the normal human fetal heart rate. Br J Obstet Gynaecol 89:276–284

Henson GL, Dawes GS, Redman CWG (1983) Antenatal heart rate variability in relation to fetal acid base status at Caesarean section. Br J Obstet Gynaecol 90:516–521

Junge HD (1979) Behavioural states and state related heart rate and motor activity patterns in the newborn infant and the fetus antepartum. J Perinat Med 7:85–107

Lawson G, Dawes GS, Redman CWG (1982) A comparison of two fetal heart rate ultrasound detector systems. Am J Obstet Gynecol 143:840–842

Lawson G, Belcher R, Dawes GS, Redman CWG (1983) A comparison of ultrasound (with autocorrelation) and direct ECG fetal heart rate detector systems. Am J Obstet Gynecol 147: 721–722

Lawson GW, Dawes GS, Redman CWG (1984) Analysis of fetal heart rate on-line at 32 weeks gestation. Br J Obstet Gynaecol 91:542–550

Timor-Tritsch IE, Dierker LJ, Zador I, Hertz RH, Rosen MG (1978) Fetal movements associated with fetal heart-rate accelerations and decelerations. Am J Obstet Gynecol 131:276–280

Visser GHA, Dawes GS, Redman CWG (1981) Numerical analysis of the normal human fetal heart rate. Br J Obstet Gynaecol 88:792–802

Visser GHA, Goodman JDS, Levine DH, Dawes GS (1982) Diurnal and other cyclic variations in human fetal heart rate near term. Am J Obstet Gynecol 142:535–544

Wheeler T, Gennser G, Lindvall R, Murrills AJ (1980) Change in the fetal heart rate associated with fetal breathing and fetal movement. Br J Obstet Gynaecol 87:1068–1079

Wickham PJD, Dawes GS, Belcher R (1983) Development of methods for quantitative analysis of the fetal heart rate. J Biomed Eng 5:302–308

Fetal Hemodynamic Alterations During Advancing Gestation*

M. A. HEYMANN[1]

Introduction

Since oxygenation for the fetus occurs in the placenta the fetal circulation is arranged so that several sites of shunting are present. In addition, preferential flow and streaming take place to offset the disadvantages of intermixing of oxygenated and deoxygenated blood returning through the venous circulations. In the presence of fetal stress these patterns are changed, and the distribution of blood flow to different organs is modified. Since individual organ blood flows normally change as gestation advances an understanding and knowledge of these changes is important when considering circulatory alterations invoked by stress.

Normal Fetal Cardiac Output

Because of the various shunts normally present in the fetal circulation, and since some organs, namely those of the lower body, may be perfused by blood originating from both left and right ventricles, it has become customary to consider fetal cardiac output as the total output of the heart, i.e., the combined ventricular output. In normal fetal lambs this is approximately 400–450 ml/kg fetal body weight per minute (Rudolph and Heymann 1970). Unlike the adult circulation and also because of the various sites of shunting, the left and right ventricles do not eject in series and do not have the same stroke volume or output per minute. The right ventricle ejects about two-thirds of cardiac output (300 ml/kg fetal body weight per minute), whereas the left ventricle ejects only about one-third (150 ml/kg fetal body weight per minute) (Heymann et al. 1973). A similar relationship has been suggested in human pregnancy, based on echocardiographic measurements (Lange et al. 1980). During approximately the second half of gestation in fetal lambs cardiac output in relationship to body weight remains fairly constant (Rudolph and Heymann 1970).

Distribution of Cardiac Output and Individual Organ Blood Flows

Although cardiac output changes little with advancing gestation, the distribution of blood flow to individual organs changes significantly. In some organs there is a

* Supported in part by a grant from the U.S. Public Health Service, Program Project Grant HL 24056

[1] Cardiovascular Research Institute and Departments of Pediatrics, Physiology and Obstetrics, Gynecology and Reproductive Sciences, 1403 HSE, University of California, San Francisco, CA 94143, USA

Fetal Heart Rate Monitoring
Ed. by W. Künzel

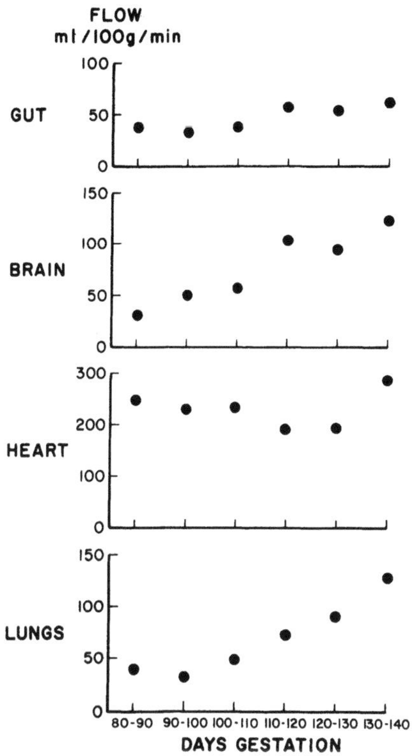

Fig. 1. Blood flow to specific organs related to gestational age (145 days is term)

relatively progressive increase in blood flow, whereas in others changes occur at specific points in gestation (Fig. 1) (Rudolph and Heymann 1970). This is true whether flow is evaluated per 100 g organ weight or, as is more usual, as a proportion of total cardiac output. Umbilical blood flow, although fairly constant over the last 20% of gestation (approximately 200 ml/kg fetal body weight per minute), does fall slightly during mid-gestation. Total fetal body flow, however, tends to increase over the last third of gestation. The percentage of cardiac output distributed to the myocardium, brain, and gastrointestinal tract all increase during the latter part of gestation, whereas that to the kidney remains fairly constant. Of great interest is the change in pulmonary blood flow, which increases from approximately 4% of total cardiac output to approximately 8% between days 120 and 130 of gestation. This is the time at which surface-active material first becomes evident in the tracheal fluid, and the increase in flow may therefore be related to increased metabolic needs. There are several other interesting gestation-related aspects of the pulmonary circulation. For example, the metabolism of prostaglandins is less in immature than in mature lungs (Clyman et al. 1981). Although the amount of pulmonary vascular smooth muscle in the resistance vessels does not change during the second half of gestation (Levin et al. 1976), the immature fetal lung does not show the same degree of pulmonary vasoconstriction to a hypoxic challenge as does the lung towards term (Lewis et al. 1976). In rhesus monkeys the number of mast cells increases during late gestation (Schwartz et al. 1974); these cells produce and release several metabolic products of arachidonic acid (e.g., prostaglandin D_2 and leukotrienes), and changing mast cell numbers might indicate developmentally related differences in the physiologic effects of these agents in the pulmonary circulation.

Factors Affecting Cardiac Output in the Fetus: The Importance of Heart Rate

Cardiac output is determined by the interrelationships of preload, mycocardial contractility, afterload, and heart rate. During situations of stress changes may occur in any or all of these to effect an improved circulation. In the fetus, the inability of the heart to respond to changes in preload and afterload and to increase myocardial contractility makes heart rate responses to stress extremely important. Compared with newborn or adult myocardium, the fetal myocardium shows immaturity of structure, function, and innervation. Friedman (1973) showed a reduction in active tension generated by fetal myocardium compared with the adult and also a higher resting tension in fetuses, suggesting reduced compliance of fetal myocardium. The ability to increase stroke work or output in response to increased preload is limited in the fetal heart (Heymann and Rudolph 1973; Kirkpatrick et al. 1976; Gilbert 1980), particularly at atrial filling pressures greater than 5 mmHg. The apparent mechanism involved in these differences between fetal and adult myocardium relates to ultrastructural differences (Sheldon et al. 1976). The diameter of fetal cells is smaller and the proportion of noncontractile mass, e.g., nuclei and mitochondria, to the number of myofibrils is significantly greater in the fetus than in the adult. In the fetus only about 30% of the total mass consists of contractile elements, whereas the corresponding proportion in the adult is approximately 60%. Individual sarcomeres, however, appear to be functionally equivalent (Friedman 1973). In newborn lambs cardiac output is decreased after increases in afterload at levels considered minimal for adults (Downing et al. 1965). In fetuses an increase in arterial pressure of only 15 mmHg depressed cardiac function to such an extent that cardiac output was 25%–30% lower than normal (Gilbert 1982). Cardiac norepinephrine concentrations in the fetus are lower than in newborns (Friedman 1973). This finding is related to the developmental differences in sympathetic innervation of the myocardium (Friedman et al. 1968; Lebowitz et al. 1972; Lipp and Rudolph 1972). Sympathetic nervous innervation starts to develop in the fetal heart by about halfway through gestation and starts at the area of the sinoatrial node, progressing towards the left ventricular apex. In most species evaluated, the left ventricular myocardium is innervated only close to term, or in some instances not until after birth. In situations of stress, therefore, increased intrinsic performance is less likely to be stimulated by reflex sympathetic routes, although sympathetically mediated increases in heart rate can occur. In contrast to the situation at term, in the immature myocardium alpha-adrenergic receptors are present in significant numbers (Cheng et al. 1980), and particularly in the immature fetus, it is possible that the myocardium is stimulated by circulating catecholamines, whereas local reflex activity is not likely to play a role in circulatory regulation.

In normal fetal lambs there is a slow progressive fall in resting heart rate during the last half of gestation (MacDonald et al. 1980). In general there is a good correlation between cardiac output and heart rate in fetal lambs. Spontaneous and induced changes in heart rate are associated with corresponding changes in either left or right ventricular output (Rudolph and Heymann 1976). An increase in heart rate from the resting level of about 180 beats per minute up to 250–300 beats per minute increased cardiac output about 20%. Likewise, a decrease in heart rate below the resting level significantly decreased ventricular output. Since many fetal stress situations are associated with bradycardia, evaluation of the heart rate may give some indication of cardiac output. Of course, the major cardiovascular changes that occur in response to stress generally are those of redistribution of blood flow rather than actual changes in total cardiac output.

References

Cheng JB, Cornett LE, Goldfien A, Roberts JM (1980) Decreased cocentration of myocardial alpha-adrenoceptors with increasing age in foetal lambs. Br J Pharmacol 70:515

Clyman RI, Mauray F, Heymann MA, Roman C (1981) Effect of gestational age on pulmonary metabolism of prostaglandin E_1 & E_2. Prostaglandins 21:505

Downing SE, Talner NS, Gardner TM (1965) Ventricular function in the newborn lamb. Am J Physiol 208:931

Friedman WF (1973) The intrinsic physiologic properties of the developing heart. In: Friedman WF, Lesch M, Sonnenblick EH (eds) Neonatal heart disease. Grune and Stratton, New York, p 21

Friedman WF, Pool PE, Jacobowitz D, Seagren SC, Braunwald E (1968) Sympathetic innervation of the developing rabbit heart. Cir Res 23:25

Gilbert RD (1980) Control of fetal cardiac output during changes in blood volume. Am J Physiol 238:H80

Gilbert RD (1982) Effects of afterload and baroreceptors on cardiac function in fetal sheep. J Dev Physiol 4:299

Heymann MA, Rudolph AM (1973) Effects of increasing preload on right ventricular output in fetal lambs in utero (Abstr). Circulation 48:IV-37

Heymann MA, Creasy RK, Rudolph AM (1973) Quantitation of blood flow patterns in the foetal lamb in utero. In: Comline KS, Cross KW, Dawes GS, Nathanielsz PW (eds) Proceedings of the Sir Joseph Barcroft centenary symposium: foetal and neonatal physiology. Cambridge University Press, Cambridge, p 129

Kirkpatrick SE, Pitlick PT, Naliboff JB, Friedman WF (1976) Frank-Starling relationship as an important determinant of fetal cardiac output. Am J Physiol 231:495

Lange LW, Sahn DJ, Allen HD, Goldberg SJ, Anderson C, Giles H (1980) Quantitative real-time cross-sectional echocardiographic imaging of the human fetus during the second half of pregnancy. Circulation 62:789

Lebowitz EA, Novick JS, Rudolph AM (1972) Development of myocardial sympathetic innervation in the fetal lamb. Pediatr Res 6:887

Levin DL, Rudolph AM, Heymann MA, Phibbs RH (1976) Morphological development of the pulmonary vascular bed in fetal lambs. Circulation 53:144

Lewis AB, Heymann MA, Rudolph AM (1976) Gestational changes in pulmonary vascular responses in fetal lambs *in utero*. Circ Res 39:536

Lipp JA, Rudolph AM (1972) Sympathetic nerve development in the rat and guinea-pig heart. Biol Neonate 21:76

MacDonald AA, Rose J, Heymann MA, Rudolph AM (1980) Heart rate response of fetal and adult sheep to hemorrhage stress. Am J Physiol 239:H789

Rudolph AM, Heymann MA (1970) Circulatory changes during growth in the fetal lamb. Circ Res 26:289

Rudolph AM, Heymann MA (1976) Cardiac output in the fetal lamb: The effects of spontaneous and induced changes of heart rate on right and left ventricular output. Am J Obstet Gynecol 124:183

Schwartz LW, Osburn BI, Frick OL (1974) An ontogenic study of histamine and mast cells in the fetal rhesus monkey. J Allergy Clin Immun 56:381

Sheldon CA, Friedman WF, Sybers HD (1976) Scanning electron microscopy of fetal and neonatal lamb cardiac cells. J Mol Cell Cardiol 8:853

Pathophysiology of Fetal Heart Rate Deceleration

Incidence and Pattern of Fetal Heart Rate Alterations During Labor

J. MELCHIOR[1] and N. BERNARD

Changes in fetal heart rate are extremely frequent during labor; methodical analysis and interpretation step-by-step through the various alterations have enabled us to draw some conclusions for better management.

We carried out a survey in a large population, investigating the incidence of changes in fetal heart rate, their grouping in different patterns, and their consequence on the condition of the neonate. In order to achieve this, we made use of computerized processing, making inquiries of our data base from the past 4 years.

The tracings were analyzed by dividing the recording into 1-h-long sections, timing backwards from the time of complete dilatation. For each 1-h section, all changes were identified and then stored in the computer. The recording was thus divided into four sections: the second stage, the final hour of dilatation (T1), the penultimate hour of dilatation (T2), and the period preceding these 2 h (T3). In the case of primiparous mothers, this time division corresponds to the first-stage progression from a dilatation of about 5 cm, and in multiparous mothers, from a dilatation of about 3 cm. The overall population included 4018 primiparas and 4168 multiparas, i.e., a total, excluding the cases of elective sections and a few women who were not recorded, of 7383 records of fetal heart rate during labor. In order to make the tables easier to understand, all results have been expressed in percentage form.

The basal rate remained normal (between 120 and 160 bpm) in 90% of cases until the final hour and at that time in only 82%. The mean normal rate was the same throughout dilatation (136 bpm). There was little change in the incidence of tachycardia (above 160 bpm for more than 10 min) as labor progressed, but, in contrast, the level of bradycardia (below 120 bpm) doubled from 6% at the beginning of labor to reach 13.8% by the end of labor. At that time, 1.4% were severe, below 100 bpm.

The oscillations were analyzed on the basis of their amplitude and frequency. Their incidence remained unchanged throughout labor. Different types of oscillation could be detected simultaneously in a single recording: 71.2% of recordings presented "small oscillations" (5–10 bpm) and 62.9% "moderate oscillations" (10–25 bpm). "Large" ones, exceeding 25 bpm, were observed in only 2% of cases. They reflect an overreactivity, but should not be considered pathological. For severely reduced variability, we suggest a subdivision into two cases, since we believe they are of differing significance: "minimal oscillations" (3–5 bpm), which occurred in 4.9%, and true "flat pattern" ($\leq$ 2 bpm) in 0.2%, which is always extremely pathological.

The frequency of the oscillations was normal (2–6 cycles) in 82.5% of recordings, and in 23.1% it exceeded 6/min. In 0.2% of cases it was less than 2, typifing the true flat pattern.

[1] Service de Gynecologie et Obstetrique, Centre Medico-Chirurgical FOCH, 40 Rue Worth, F-92151 Suresnes Cedex, France

Fetal Heart Rate Monitoring
Ed. by W. Künzel

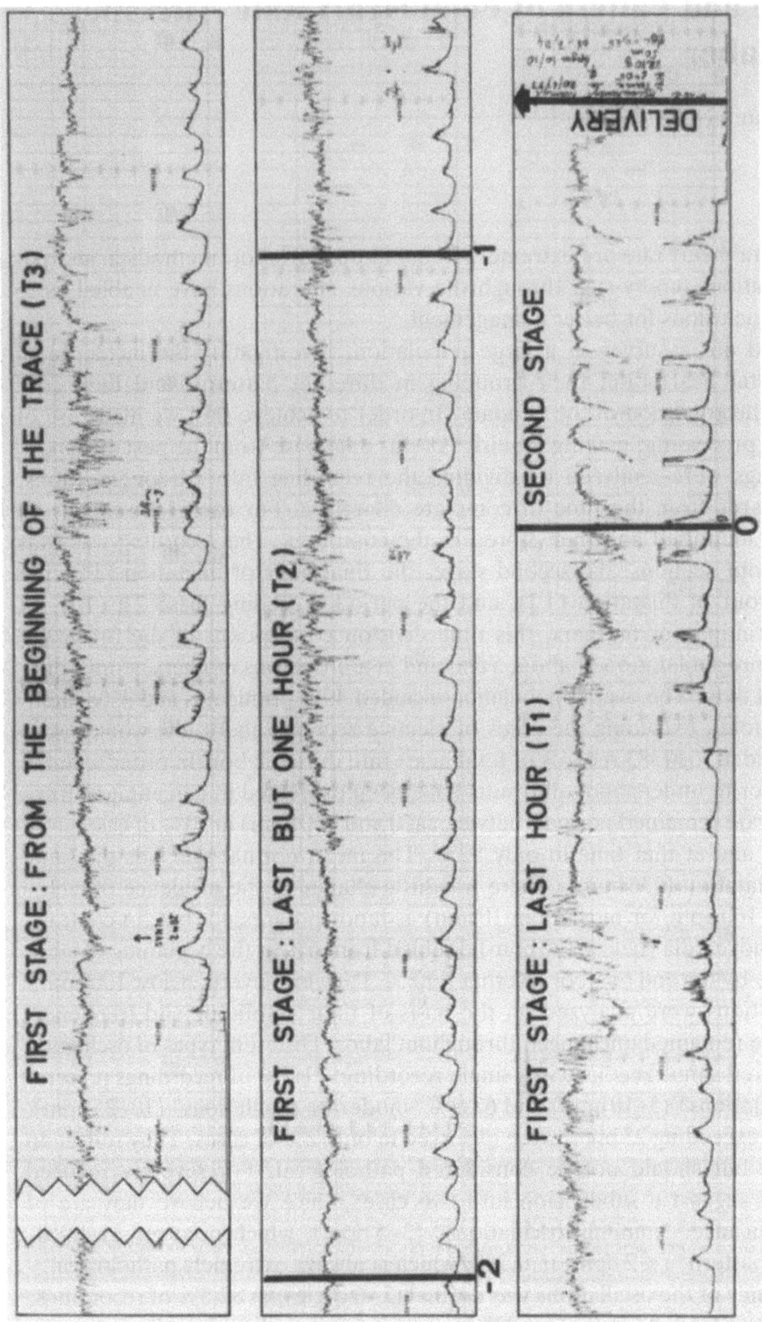

Fig. 1. Division of recording into 1-h-long sections

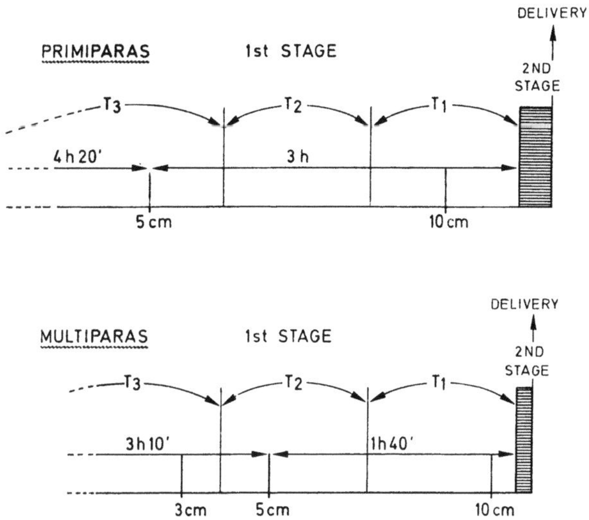

Fig. 2. Time division and first-stage progression

Table 1. Baseline during labor

bpm	T3	T2	T1
Tachycardia	4.7%	3.4%	4.2%
160			
Normocardia	89.3	89.2	82
120			
Bradycardia	6	7.4	13.8 (1.4% < 100 bpm)

Table 2. Oscillations. Different types of oscillations may be observed on the same trace

Amplitude		Frequency	
• small	71.2%	2–6/min	82.5%
• medium	62.9	> 6/min	23.1
• large	2.1		
• reduced (3–5 bpm)	4.7	< 2/min	0.2
• flat pattern (≤ 2 bpm)	0.2		

Table 3. Accelerations during labor. Different types of accelerations may be observed on the same trace

	T3	T2	T1
• Sporadic	65.3%	31%	14.1%
• Associated with uterine contractions	46.7	36.4	26.6
• Before deceleration	18.8	36.8	54.7
• After deceleration	2.8	5	14.8

Table 4. Decelerations

	T3	T2	T1
• None	51%	37.4%	11.7%
• Early	0.4	0.5	0.9
• Late	0.3	0.5	0.5
• Variable			
• non resid.	38.2	53.4	79
• resid.	2	2.8	5.5
• Sporadic	10.4	6.2	2.6

Though accelerations are associated with fetal well-being, it is of interest to note the evolution of their occurrence during labor. The incidence of sporadic accelerations fell from 65% to 14%, depending on the active movements of the fetus during labor. When they were isolated during contractions their incidence fell from 46% to 26%. This decrease is linked to the appearance of decelerations. Two other types of accelerations accompanied the decelerations: the first one preceding a deceleration rose from 18% to 54%, and less frequently the second one followed a deceleration, prior to the return to the basal rate. It increased from 2.8% at the beginning of the first stage to 14.8% at the end of it.

The predominant type of fetal heart rate alteration is that of deceleration. No such change can be considered normal since it always means stress on the fetus.

The possible diagnostic or prognostic value of their interpretation, their type, their amplitude, the time at which they occur, and the number of times they are repeated must be taken into account.

The classification we use, among the different ones that have been described, is derived from Hon (1971). Considering the start of deceleration in relation to the beginning of the uterine contraction, the decelerations were distinguished as early, late, and variable. We made a subdivision for the latter into two classes, depending on the presence of a residual phase after the end of the contraction. Finally we characterized "prolonged decelerations," from 3- to 10-min duration, related to some particular clinical circumstance.

During the labor, there was no deceleration in more than half of the recordings, but in only one trace out of ten during the final hour. The percentage of early deceleration seems perhaps to be very low in our analysis. As a matter of fact, they were often mistaken for nonresidual deceleration and that tendency corresponds to the important number of cord complications (40%) detected at birth. Variable decelerations were noted in 40% at the time of a dilatation to 5 cm, in 83% at the end of the first stage, but the most dangerous, i.e., the residual ones which reflect hypoxia, were present in only 2%–5% of cases. The incidence of late deceleration was very low (0.5%) since in these cases they had already occurred during pregnancy and led to an elective cesarean section, before the onset of labor.

The various alterations were combined and thus we could evaluate the fetal heart rate significance. Each period was classed as normal, suspicious, or pathological. The earlier the onset of changes in fetal heart rate, the more serious they were considered to be. Thus, a change which would be suspicious, hence acceptable, if it occurred during the 2 final hours would be pathological if it occurred before. This was not an arbitrary interpretation, but one based on our findings with respect to the condition of the neonate.

At the beginning of the trace, there were 76.6% normal fetal heart rates, 21.5% suspicious, and 1.9% pathological. In the penultimate hour, their frequencies were respectively 65%, 30.9%, and 3.9% and at the end of labor 43%, 51.7%, and 5.3%. Throughout labor, 67% of recordings showed no change. Very few improved but 27.8% deteriorated. If a pathological pattern is considered to correspond to fetal distress, as we have just seen above, 5.3% of such recordings were detected during the final hour and they resulted in 22% acute cesareans, 37% vaginal operative deliveries, and only 41% spontaneous deliveries.

The condition of the neonate may be considered on the basis of this classification of the fetal heart rate during the final hour. We found that the Apgar score at 1 min was ≥8 in 93% of normal patterns, in 86% of suspicious ones, and in less than 50%

Table 5. Suspicious, fetal heart rate pattern. (Last hour of the first stage)

	• B.L.: Bradycardia		100–120 bpm > 10 min or < 100 bpm 3–10 min
or	• Decelerations	• early : repeated • nonresidual variable : repeated	
or	• Reduced oscillations > 30 min (3–5 bpm)		

Table 6. Pathological fetal heart rate pattern. (Last hour of the first stage)

	• B.L.	_Bradycardia	< 100 bpm > 10 min
		_Tachycardia	• 160–180 bpm > 10 min associated with other alterations • > 180 bpm > 10 min isolated
or	• Decelerations		• late • residual variable (moderate or marked)
or	• Flat Pattern > 10 min		

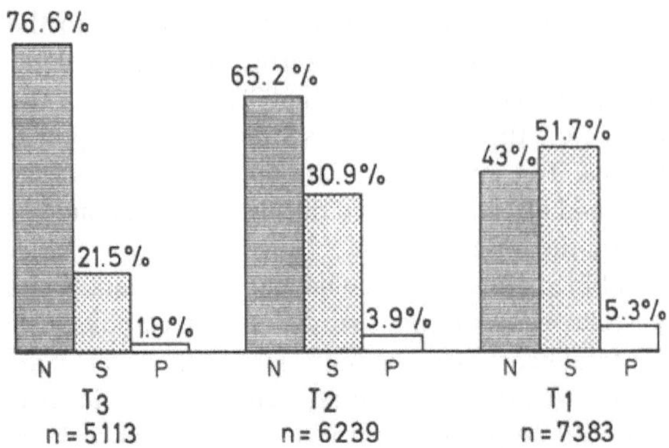

Fig. 3. Evolution of fetal heart rate pattern during the first stage. *N*, normal; *S*, suspicious; *P*, pathological

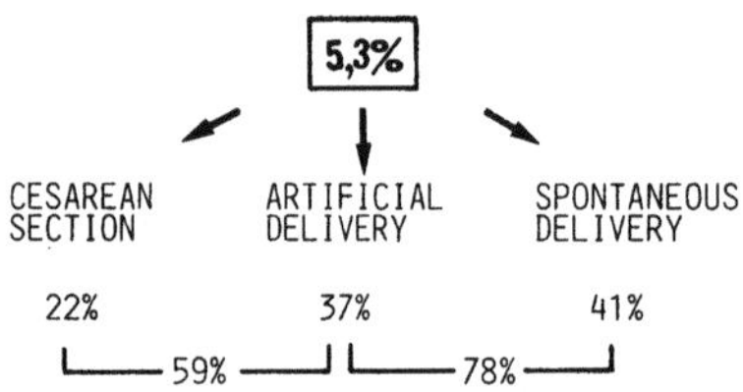

Fig. 4. Fetal distress during the last hour of the first stage

Table 7. Condition of the neonates according to fetal heart rate pattern (last hour)

	Apgar 1′ ⩾8	Apgar 5′ ⩾9	Ph > 7.20
• Normal	92.6%	95.5%	71.6%
• Suspicious	85.9	93.9	60.4
• Pathological	47.7	71.2	37.9

of pathological ones. The same was true of the 5-min Apgar score and even more decisively of the pH, measured in the umbilical artery at birth.

However, these findings do not take into account the second stage, which, despite its short duration, constitutes the period of greatest aggression on the fetus, as shown by the traces. The rapid succession of events and the need to make urgent clinical decisions demand different methods of analyzing the recording than during dilatation. To this end, we identified five different patterns (Melchior 1974). They were unevenly distributed:

Type 0 is characterized by stability of the heart rate. The baseline level is normal and it is usually found following a trace generally unchanged during dilatation. But this pattern occurred in only 1.4% of deliveries, and this indicates the very small number, and hence the unpredictability, of deliveries devoid of any risk to the fetus.

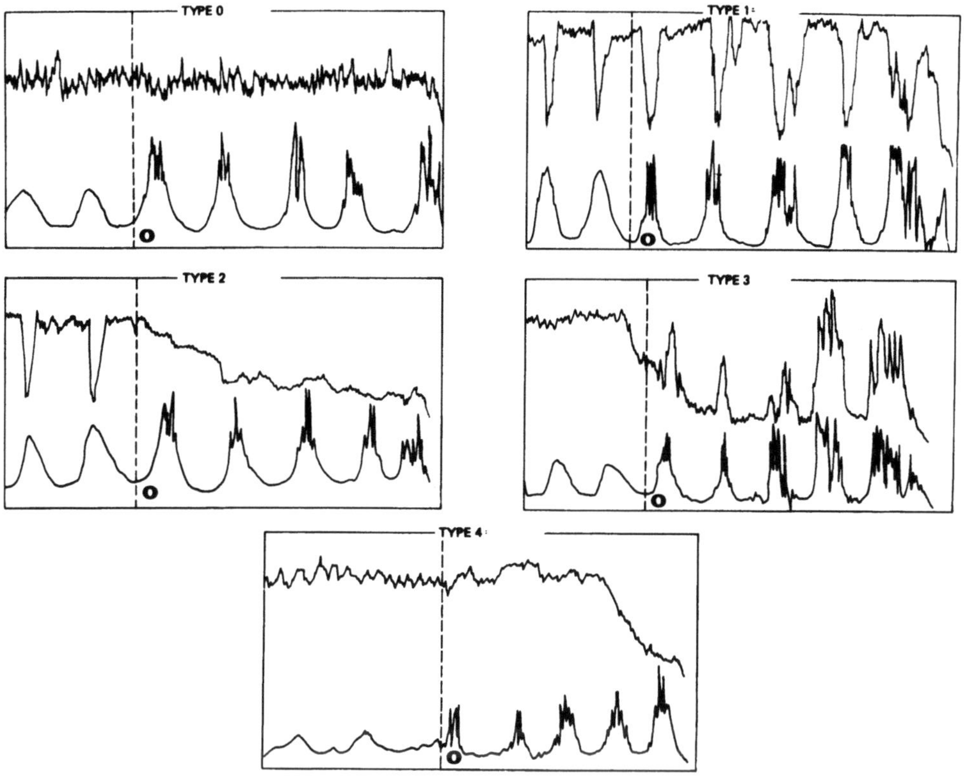

Fig. 5. Fetal heart rate patterns during the second stage

This establishes the need for close monitoring of fetal condition, in all cases and not only in high-risk pregnancies.

Type 1 is characterized by successive decelerations often becoming progressively more severe with each successive bearing-down effort. An important feature is the return to the preexisting baseline during the short intermission between contractions; this shows the recovery of the fetus. These were usually variable decelerations related to cord complication often obvious at birth. This was the most usual type of second stage, since it accounted for 65% of the deliveries.

Type 2 is defined by a fairly rapid fall in the basal rate, resulting in permanent bradycardia in addition to which there may also be episodes of deceleration during pushing efforts. The recordings also present a flattening of the oscillations, which may culminate in a flat trace. This pattern was observed in 23.7% of recordings.

Type 3 is a less common variant of the previous one. It is characterized by the onset of marked accelerations during each contraction over a background picture of bradycardia, itself often severe.

The last, *type 4,* is another variant. This has the appearance of being diphasic. Initially the heart rate remains normal, with or without decelerations, then it slows and develops into a bradycardia, like that of type 2.

The distribution of these patterns according to the number of previous births showed that a pattern with no change in fetal heart rate (type 0), or with deceleration (type 1), was more common in primiparous mothers. Those presenting with bradycardia (type 2), on the other hand, were more frequent in multiparous women.

We established some rules by reducing the duration of the second stage according to each pattern: 15–20 min for the pattern with decelerations (1) after which if spontaneous delivery has not occurred forceps outlet must be performed. For the patterns with bradycardia (2; 3) the second stage must be shorter, about 10 min, without going beyond 5 min in case of a fall below 100 beats/min. The management is the same in type 4 after onset of bradycardia. No limit is set for type 0 as long as the heart rate remains normal.

Dellenbach et al. (1983) also confirmed that the duration of the second stage is correlated to the rise in lactate level detected in the fetal scalp during full dilatation and in the umbilical artery at birth. If the acceptable limit for this rise is considered to be 3 mmol/liter, then they found the same limits for the duration as we did.

If these morphological limits are respected, the condition of the neonate varies little in relation to pattern of second stage.

The value of this classification is in providing a rapid estimation of the risks facing the fetus and to limit this period to an acceptable duration.

However, a pattern which does not remain stable does not imply so-called fetal distress. This would amount to stating that there is 98% incidence of fetal distress. If retrospectively one wishes to detect only from the trace fetuses exposed to greater distress during the second stage, then the criteria selected must be more limited. We consider that there has been fetal distress in cases presenting type 1 recording accompanied by late deceleration or residual variable ones lasting over 20 min; in cases presenting type 2 traces with bradycardia of less than 80 beats/min for over 5 min, or of 80–100 beats/min for over 10 min; and in cases presenting a type 3 trace

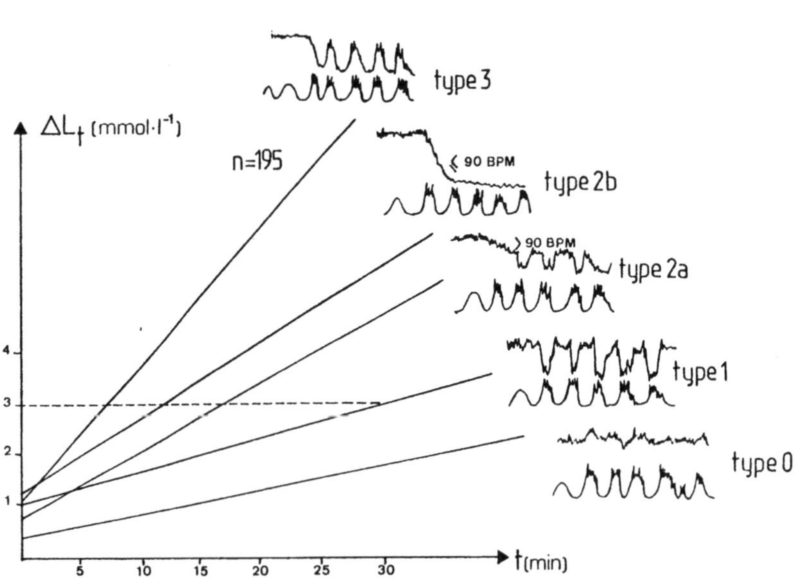

Fig. 6. Increase in lactate level according to the duration and the fetal heart rate pattern during the second stage. (Dellenbach et al. 1983)

Table 8. Fetal distress during the second stage

Type 1	• with late deceleration • or resid. var. dec. >20 min (moderate, marked)	13.7%
or		
Type 2	• with B.L. <80 bpm >5 min • or B.L. 80–100 bpm >10 min	68.1%
or		
Type 3	• with B.L. <100 bpm >5 min	18.2%

Table 9. Fetal distress in vaginal deliveries

First stage	→	Second stage		
• without F.D. ($n = 6045$)	96%	↗ without F.D.	85.9%	
		↘ with F.D.	10.1%	11.3%
• with F.D. ($n = 254$)	4%	↗ with F.D.	1.2%	
		↘ without F.D.	2.8%	

with bradycardia of below 100 beats/min for over 5 min. This fetal distress would be present in 11.3% of cases.

In the 96% of fetuses in good condition during the final hour of dilatation, 10% presented fetal distress during the second stage. Of the 4% of the cases which had already suffered distress during the preceding hour, 1.2% underwent additional distress during the second stage. The condition of these neonates at birth was markedly different from the condition of the general population of neonates.

The fetal heart rate is a powerful indication of the condition of the fetus during the first and second stages. The onset of suspicious or pathological changes, the frequency of which rises as labor progresses, argues in favor of careful monitoring during all deliveries, whether of high-risk cases or not, as we already have discussed at Berlin in 1981 (Melchior and Bernard 1982).

Monitoring of the fetal heart rate provides information about actual fetal well-being and makes it possible to give the risk facing the neonate at birth and, hence, to detect indications for fetal extraction in time and also to avoid hasty interventions.

References

Dellenbach P, Hsiung R, Piquard F, Schaefer A, Haberey P (1983) Apport du dosage du lactate à la surveillance du foetus. Arnette, Paris, pp 131–145

Hon EH (1971) An introduction to fetal heart rate monitoring. Harty, New Haven

Melchior J (1974) Die fetale Herzfrequenz in der Austreibungsperiode. 6. Deutscher Kongreß für Perinatale Medizin, Berlin, 1973. Thieme, Stuttgart, S 235

Melchior J, Bernard N (1982) Occurrence of fetal complications during labor in a so-called "non risk" group. 2nd Int Berlin Meeting of Perinatal Medicine. J Perinat Med [Suppl 2] 10:52–54

Fetal Hemodynamic Responses to Reduced Uterine Blood Flow in the Sheep Fetus*

J. T. Parer[1]

Introduction

This paper will cover two separate aspects of fetal heart rate monitoring:

1. Fetal responses to short periods of reduced uterine blood flow (UBF), of 10–60 min, particularly with respect to alterations in the distribution of blood flow within the fetus
2. Fetal responses to brief, e.g., 20 s, reductions in UBF, in an attempt to mimic changes such as one might see with uterine contractions

I will at times refer to studies involving hypoxia, induced by decreasing maternal inspired oxygen, as opposed to asphyxia, induced by controlled reductions of UBF. The latter includes an increase in carbon dioxide, as well as decrease in oxygen. The responses in general are qualitatively similar, with one important difference (described below), although there may be quantitative differences.

This review will use illustrations of work in our own laboratory, though numerous other workers have similar findings.

Reduction of Uterine Blood Flow or Fetal O_2 Supply for 10–60 min

Fetal compensatory responses to acute moderate asphyxia are:

1. Redistribution of blood flow favoring vital organs
   a) Brain
   b) Heart
   c) Adrenal gland
   d) Umbilical circulation
2. Bradycardia
3. Decreased fetal oxygen consumption
4. Anaerobic metabolism

Each of these responses may be considered to be protective to the fetus, tending to limit the detrimental effects of O_2 insufficiency on certain "priority" or vital organs. The degree of hypoxia achieved is variable in different studies, but in general the PO_2 of distal aortic blood is reduced to approximately 12 mmHg. This corresponds to a reduction in uterine blood flow of approximately 50%.

* Supported by NIH Grants HD 13764 and HD 18016

[1] Department of Obstetrics, Gynecology and Reproductive Sciences, University of California, San Francisco, CA 94143, USA

Fetal Heart Rate Monitoring
Ed. by W. Künzel

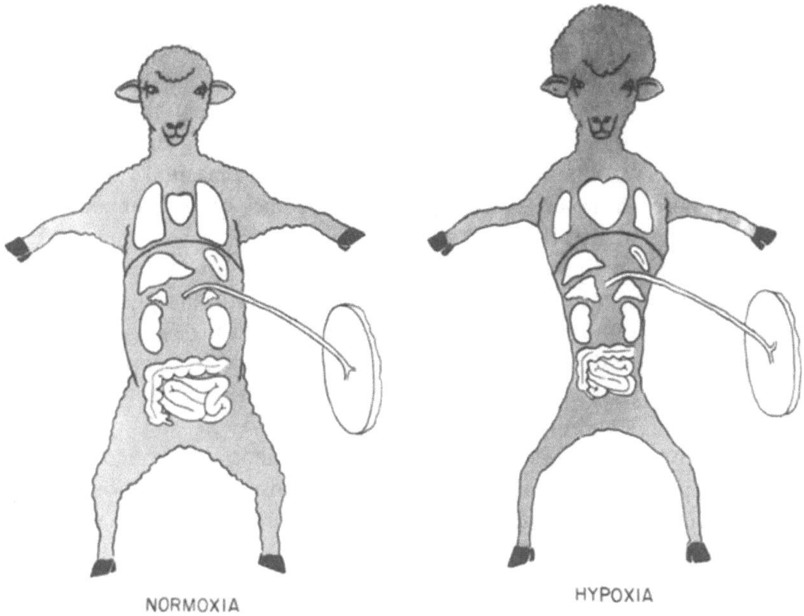

Fig. 1. Schematic illustration of the redistribution of blood flow during fetal hypoxia. The size of the organs and regions of the body are in proportion to the quantity of blood flow. The head, heart, and adrenal glands are larger, the placental size remains unchanged, and the other organs and body are smaller. (Courtesy of Dr. M. Lynne Reuss)

Redistribution of Fetal Blood Flow

A number of investigators have now shown that during hypoxia or asphyxia there is a redistribution of fetal cardiac output such that blood flow (a) increases to the brain, heart, and adrenal gland, (b) is maintained to the placenta, and (c) decreases to the carcase, gut, liver, spleen, and kidney (Cohn et al. 1974; Peeters et al. 1979).

This is illustrated in Fig. 1, where the fetal organs and regions of the body are drawn in proportion to their flow during normoxia and then hypoxia.

Mechanisms Producing Shifts in Blood Flow

The reduction of blood flow to the "nonpriority" organs, with the exception of the carcase, is caused by alpha-adrenergic activity. This has been demonstrated with the use of the alpha-adrenergic blocker phenoxybenzamine in chronically catheterized fetal sheep during induced hypoxia. The hypoxia-induced increase in vascular resistance to the gut, liver, lungs, spleen, and kidney was either fully or partially reversed following such blockade (Reuss et al. 1982).

The vasoconstriction of the carcase is likely to be due to vasopressin. The evidence for this is twofold: (a) vasopressin levels increase in the fetus during hypoxia (Rurak 1978) and (b) vasopressin infusion into the normoxic fetus causes vasocostriction of the carcase (Iwamoto et al. 1979). There is a counteracting effect of endogenous opioids during hypoxia, which tends to vasodilate the carcase. This was shown by an increase in carcase vascular resistance in the hypoxic fetus following administration of the opioid blocker naloxone (Llanos et al. 1983). This may be explained by endogenous opioids inhibiting vasopressin release, and appears to be a push-pull, balancing mechanism.

The vasodilatation of "vital" organs has received relatively little attention. Recent studies in fetal sheep utilizing propranolol blockade suggest that there is active beta-adrenergic vasodilatation in the myocardial and placental vascular beds during hypoxia. There was no consistent change in resistance of the brain or adrenal vascular beds (Court et al. 1984).

It has been shown that an increase in carbon dioxide pressure causes an increase in cerebral blood flow in the fetus, as it does in the adult (Rosenberg et al. 1982). However, it is clear that other mechanisms are also at work during asphyxia, because substantial rises in cerebral blood flow occur with relatively brief periods (several minutes) of isocapnic hypoxia. This also holds true even before the development of a metabolic acidemia (Cohn et al. 1974).

In summary, alpha-adrenergic activity and vasopressin cause vasoconstriction, and endogenous opioids and beta-adrenergic activity cause vasodilatation of some vascular beds during fetal asphyxia or hypoxia, but there are other as yet undescribed mechanisms.

Blood Flow Distribution During Severe Asphyxia

The compensatory changes described in the preceding section must require an intact series of sensors and effectors, which depend on a certain minimum supply of substrates (including oxygen) for integrity. It seems obvious that at profound degrees of uterine blood flow reduction the compensatory mechanisms break down. Such a breakdown is seen in Fig. 2, where the percentage of change in blood flow to four fetal regions is related to different degrees of reduced uterine blood flow (25%–75% reduction) for approximately 10 min (Yaffe et al. 1982). At each degree of reduction of UBF fetal arterial blood pressure increases, until at 25% of normal UBF it

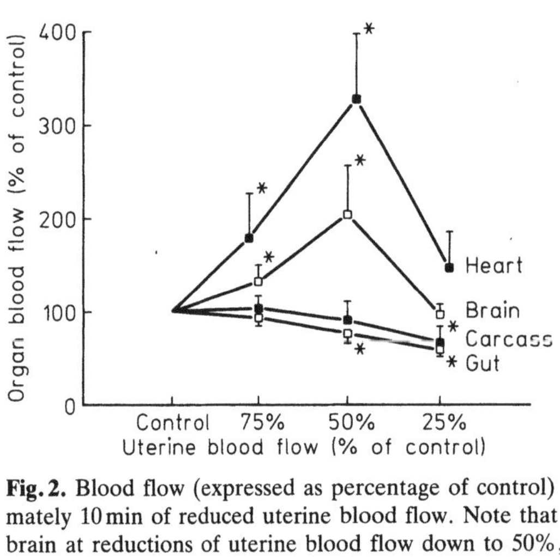

Fig. 2. Blood flow (expressed as percentage of control) to four regions of the fetus after approximately 10 min of reduced uterine blood flow. Note that the blood flow increases to the heart and brain at reductions of uterine blood flow down to 50%, but this cannot be maintained at 25% of normal uterine blood flow. *Points* are means; *bars* are SDs; *, $P<0.01$. (Yaffe et al. 1982)

averages 69 mm Hg (the control value was 50 mm Hg). At this stage there is an intense vasoconstriction, with reduction of cardiac output, and reduced blood flow to the "vital" organs: heart, brain, adrenal gland, and placenta. This reduction is presumed to be due to incipient or actual hypoxic myocardial failure.

Oxygen Consumption During Fetal O_2 Insufficiency

Total Fetal O_2 Uptake. Reduction of oxygen supply to the fetus by a moderate amount (e.g., fetal distal aortic O_2 tension 10–12 mm Hg) results in a stepwise, sustained reduction in fetal O_2 consumption which is at least approximately related to the degree of O_2 reduction (Parer 1980). Mean values of one such study are depicted in Fig. 3, when umbilical venous and arterial O_2 pressure, O_2 content, and pH values are shown during the control period and during hypoxia, superimposed on an oxygen dissociation curve. The umbilical blood flow did not alter with hypoxia (209 ml/min per kg), and the decrease to 56% of control O_2 consumption was entirely explained by a decline in the umbilical venous-umbilical arterial O_2 difference (Fig. 3, numbers in brackets). At severe reduction of uterine blood flow (see previous section), when fetal cardiac output and umbilical blood flow is reduced, the reduction of fetal O_2 consumption would be even greater, but this latter must be regarded as a stage of decompensation.

O_2 Uptake by Specific Organs. It has already been stated that during hypoxia blood flow to the brain and heart increases. In both organs it has been shown that the increase in blood flow matches the decrease in arteriovenous O_2 concentration differences across the organ so as to maintain the O_2 uptake by the organ, at least during moderate degrees of hypoxia (Jones et al. 1977; Fisher et al. 1982). Thus even during hypoxemia of moderate degree, e.g., fetal distal aortic O_2 pressure values of 12 mm Hg (normal is about 20–24 mm Hg in fetal sheep), these vital organs can be quite adequately oxygenated. This has important implications in the clinical interpretation of values obtained during fetal blood sampling.

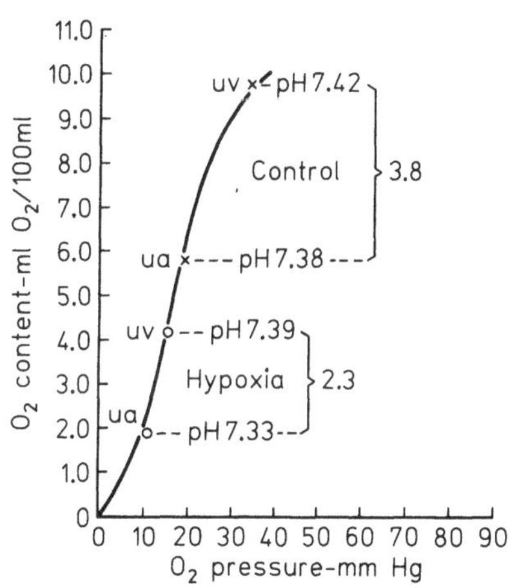

Fig. 3. Oxygen dissociation curve of fetal blood relating oxygen content to oxygen partial pressure, adjusted to pH 7.4. Superimposed are points for umbilical venous (*uv*) and umbilical arterial (*ua*) blood and actual pH values. The *numbers to the right of the brackets* are venous-arterial oxygen content differences (ml O_2/100 ml). The "hypoxia" values were obtained at a mean maternal arterial blood PO_2 of ca. 35 mm Hg

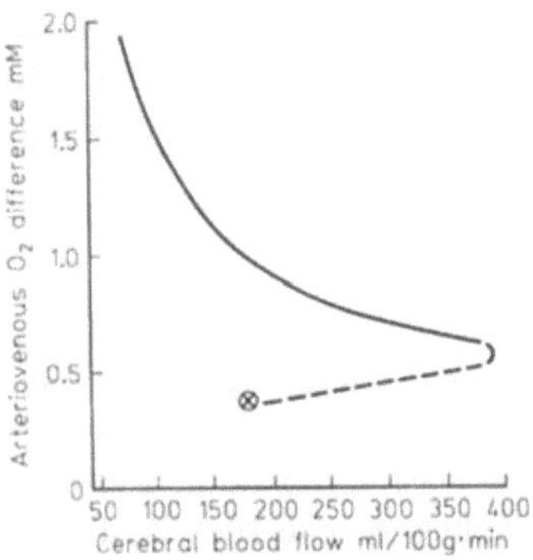

Fig. 4. The relationship between ascending aortic-sagittal sinus oxygen content difference and cerebral blood flow under conditions of progressive hypoxia. The *solid line* is from Jones et al. (1977) and describes constancy of cerebral oxygen consumption. The point *X* is from Yaffe et al. (1982) and is reconstructed from measured cerebral blood flow and an arteriovenous oxygen content difference calculated from arterial oxygen content, using data from Jones et al. (1977) and Jones et al. (1978)

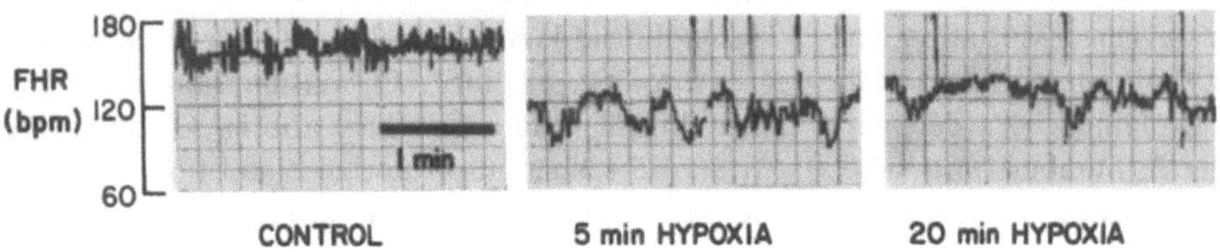

Fig. 5. Heart rate of fetal sheep before (distal aortic O_2 pressure 21 mm Hg) and during acute hypoxia (distal aortic O_2 pressure 11 mm Hg). Note the sustained bradycardia

Because the blood flow to the nonpriority organs declines during asphyxia or hypoxia and the oxygen extraction is known to decline across organs where it has been measured (Jones et al. 1977; Fisher et al. 1982), it is clear that O_2 consumption to such organs (e.g., gut, carcase) will decline. The fetus can apparently tolerate such periods of decreased O_2 uptake if they are limited, e.g., less than 1 h. These organs are probably the source of the progressive increase in lactate during hypoxia, due to anaerobic metabolism (Mann 1970).

Oxygen uptake by the priority organs during severe asphyxia has not been extensively studied. However, as mentioned above, it is known that eventually their blood flow does not continue to increase, and if fact declines (Yaffe et al. 1982). The arteriovenous O_2 concentration difference must continue to decline so O_2 consumption must decrease. This is illustrated for the cerebral circulation in Fig. 4. We speculate that this stage of decompensation is where progressive fetal cerebral damage occurs. We have also speculated that the presence of normal fetal heart rate variability depends on the integrity (and therefore normal O_2 consumption) of the central nervous system, so this point of decompensation may be where fetal heart rate variability decreases or is lost (Parer 1983).

Effect on Fetal Heart Rate

The initial response to acute asphyxia or hypoxia in the chronically prepared, unanesthetized fetus is invariably bradycardia (Fig. 5). This is in contrast to some earlier experimental animal work on acutely operated and anesthetized animals, where the response was sometimes a tachycardia, but was unpredictable. Apparently the normal control mechanisms can be disrupted by anesthesia and surgery.

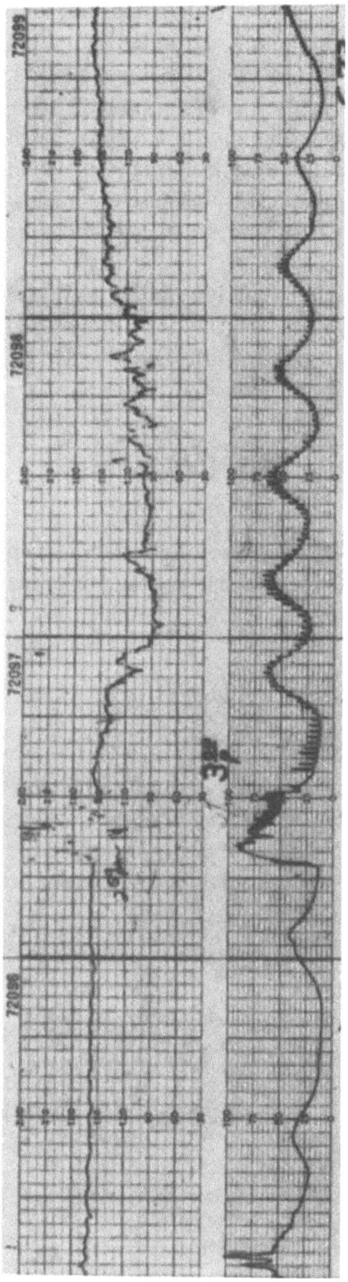

Fig. 6. Fetal heart rate and uterine contraction tracing during an eclamptic seizure (at 2:59 p.m.) of about 50 s duration. The mother is apneic during the convulsion and has about 8 min of excessive uterine activity afterwards. As a result, oxygenation is decreased in the fetus, which responds with a bradycardia. (Paul et al. 1978)

The bradycardia may be prolonged during milder degrees of hypoxia, but with increased severity of hypoxia, when substantial catecholamine secretion occurs, the ultimate result after 15 or 30 min may be a tachycardia (Jones and Robinson 1975). We have also noted that during controlled reduction of uterine blood flow to 30%–50% of normal in fetal sheep there is an initial bradycardia and then a recovery of heart rate to control levels by 10 min with a subsequent mild tachycardia (Gu Wei et al. 1982). This is not entirely explained by catecholamine levels, because the highest heart rates are found after release of the uterine artery occlusion, when catecholamine levels are returning toward normal.

The human fetus undoubtedly responds similarly to acutely imposed asphyxia with a bradycardia, as seen from the fetal bradycardia in association with material apnea and excessive uterine activity following an eclamptic seizure (Fig. 6).

Brief Uterine Blood Flow Reduction (20 s), Simulating Uterine Contractions

Uterine contractions in the sheep and primate are accompanied by a decrease in UBF (Greiss 1973). We surgically prepared pregnant sheep so that we could examine fetal cardiorespiratory responses and control mechanisms during 20 s reductions of UBF virtually to zero by inflating a balloon-tipped catheter in the distal maternal aorta (Parer et al. 1980).

The Normoxic Fetus

Maternal aortic occlusion for 20 s in the normal fetus consistently produced a transient reduction in fetal heart rate averaging 40 bpm (Fig. 7). The nadir of the deceleration occurred 30 s after commencement of the occlusion, and the duration of the deceleration averaged 60 s. This "late deceleration" in normoxic fetuses could be

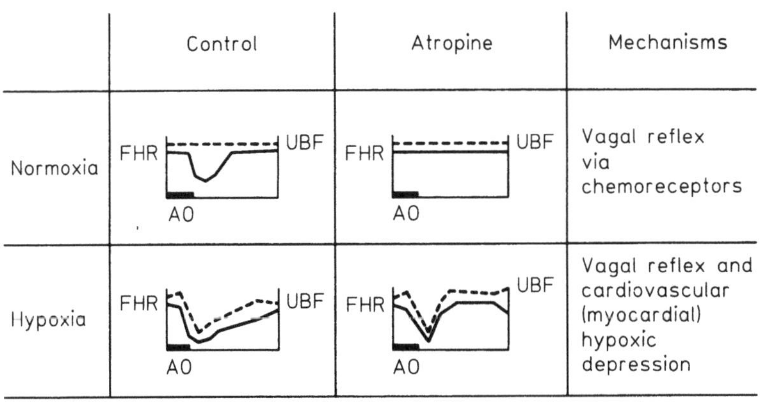

Fig. 7. Mechanisms of the two types of late decelerations of the fetal heart rate *(FHR, solid line)*. The reflex late deceleration occurs in the centrally (nervous system and myocardium) normoxic fetus during brief 20-s reduction of uterine blood flow (*AO*, maternal aortic occlusion). The second type of late deceleration is seen in the fetus which is already hypoxic and is due to both reflex mechanisms and transient hypoxic myocardial failure. (Harris et al. 1982)

completely abolished by pretreatment with atropine, so we concluded that it was of vagal origin. (After atropine treatment aortic occlusion in fact resulted in a small late acceleration, which could in turn be abolished by beta-adrenergic blockade with propranolol.)

These late decelerations were not accompanied by any consistent change in fetal arterial blood pressure or umbilical blood flow, but concomitantly with the occlusion there was a transient decrease in fetal O_2 consumption to less than 50% of control because of narrowing of the umbilical venous-umbilical arterial O_2 content difference. The most dramatic decline was seen in umbilical venous O_2 pressure and content.

We concluded that these reflex late decelerations in the normoxic fetus were due to sensing of the brief period of hypoxemia by either peripheral or central chemoreceptors, and not by baroreceptors.

The Hypoxic Fetus

When maternal aortic occlusion was performed in the fetus whose mother was already made hypoxemic by lowering her F_{IO_2} to approximately 0.1 (fetal distal aortic O_2 pressure of 12 mm Hg), there was a more profound and prolonged late deceleration (Harris et al. 1982). There were significant decreases in both fetal arterial blood pressure and umbilical blood flow. Fetal cardiac output was not measured.

Pretreatment with atropine caused a fetal tachycardia (mean fetal heart rate 255 bpm), and modified the deceleration such that it was briefer and not so profound. The product of peak systolic pressure and heart rate declined to 76%, and this, being an index of myocardial metabolism, suggested that myocardial oxygen consumption was similarly depressed (Harris et al. 1982). We therefore theorized that during hypoxia the mechanism of the late deceleration was both vagal (because atropine modified it) and also due to a second mechanism—transient hypoxic myocardial failure (Fig. 7).

Early studies by Caldeyro-Barcia and his colleagues (1966) are in support of this view, that there are two separate mechanisms for late decelerations. When atropine was given subcutaneously to a fetus with type I dips there was a tachycardia and abolition of the dips. There appeared to be fetal heart rate variability in this case, although it was difficult to discern at the slow paper speed used by these investigators. When atropine was given to another fetus with type II dips (and apparent decreased variability) the late decelerations were modified, but not abolished.

It is our tentative hypothesis, which has utility in clinical management, that in the presence of fetal heart rate (FHR) variability late decelerations are of the reflex type, signifying adequate cerebral and myocardial oxygenation (Parer 1983). With absent FHR variability, the late decelerations are also due to transient hypoxic myocardial failure, and subsequent inadequacy of cerebral oxygen supply and uptake because of compromised fetal cardiac output. Although this has not been rigidly demonstrated experimentally, it is consistent with widespread clinical observations. Thus babies which at the moment of birth have normal FHR variability, despite their "ominous" late decelerations, are almost invariably vigorous in terms of the 5-min Apgar score (Fig. 8). Those babies with late deceleration and absent FHR variability are usually depressed (Fig. 9).

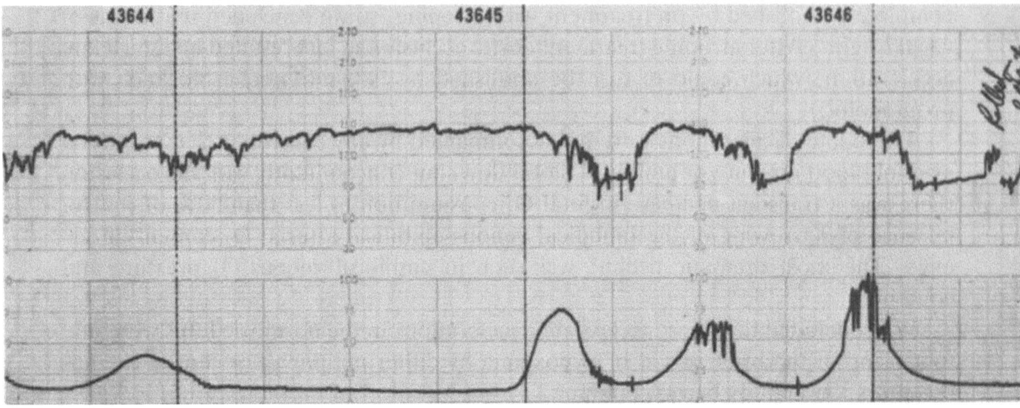

Fig. 8. Reflex late decelerations. The FHR pattern previously had been normal, but late decelerations appeared following severe maternal hypotension, 70/30 mm Hg, which was preceded by sympathetic blockade caused by a caudal anesthetic. Note that the FHR variability is maintained, signifying adequate cardiorespiratory compensation and maintenance of cerebral oxygen uptake. This stressed, but not decompensated, fetus was delivered vaginally by forceps shortly after this tracing, with Apgar scores of 2 (1 min) and 7 (5 min)

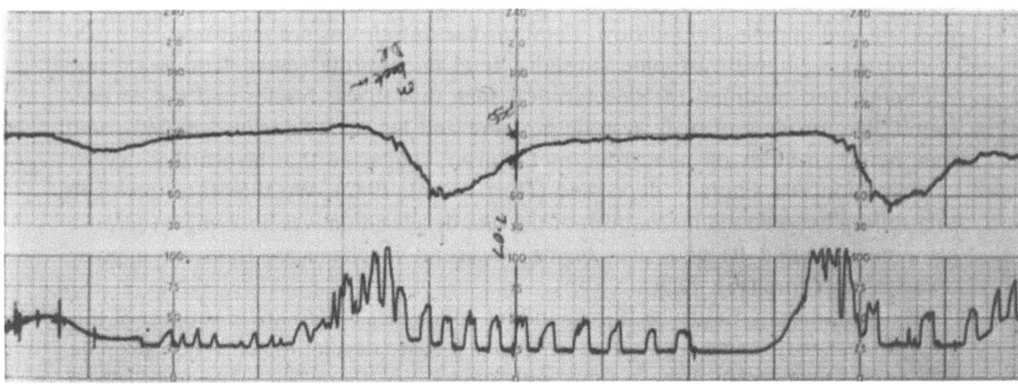

Fig. 9. Late decelerations with virtually absent FHR variability. These findings represent transient asphyxial myocardial failure as well as intermittent vagal decreases in heart rate. The lack of FHR variability also signifies a decreased cerebral oxygenation. Note the acidosis in fetal scalp blood (pH, 7.07). A 3340-g girl with Apgar scores of 3 (1 min) and 4 (5 min) was delivered soon after this tracing was made. Cesarean section was considered to be contraindicated because of a severe pre-eclamptic coagulopathy

"Early decelerations," commonly discussed in North American FHR monitoring, are probably a variant of reflex late decelerations, signifying a transient reflex response to peripheral, but not central, hypoxemia.

Mechanisms of Variable Decelerations

Variable decelerations are commonly ascribed to umbilical cord compression; indeed they are sometimes even called (we believe erroneously) "cord compression"

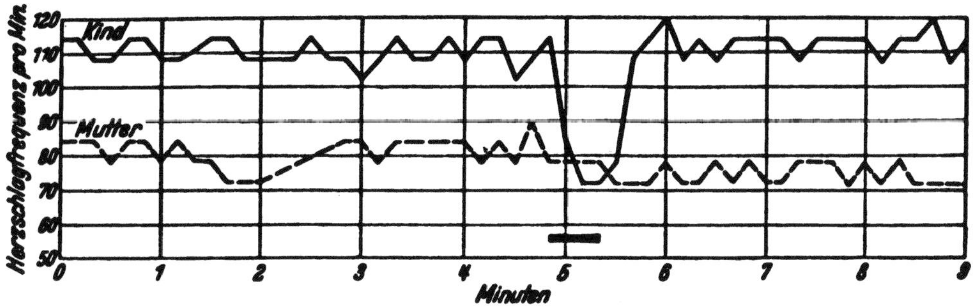

Fig. 10. The fetal response to 30 s of pressing the fetal head against the sacral promontary is a rapid drop in heart rate. It has a similar appearance to the variable decelerations often seen in the second stage of labor. (Rech 1933)

patterns. This arose from the observation that one can produce abrupt and profound decreases in FHR by squeezing the umbilical cord (Hon 1968). However, it does not necessarily follow that all variable decelerations are due to cord compression. Wulf in his paper "History of Fetal Heart Rate Monitoring" in this volume shows a tracing of Rech's (1933) work demonstrating an abrupt drop in FHR with head compression, so this is likely to be another mechanism (Fig. 10). The prevalence of variable decelerations in the second stage of labor, or on application of forceps or traction on a vacuum extractor, all support the view that head compression, and therefore dural stimulation, stimulates abrupt vagal discharge. Goodlin and Haesslein (1977) have shown that a fetal valsalva maneuver will also produce a variable deceleration.

Clinically the mechanism is not too important; maternal position change will often abolish the pattern. What is important is that if the deceleration is prolonged (e.g., greater than 60 s) or profound (e.g., 60 bpm or lower) it is almost certain to be associated with a decrease in umbilical blood flow either due to direct cord compression or due to a decrease in fetal cardiac output because of inability of the fetus to increase stroke volume adequately. Thus we believe that it is appropriate to consider the clinical correlate of variable decelerations to be insufficiency of umbilical blood flow.

Clinical Implications

The term "fetal distress" is used rather loosely, and is defined sometimes as simply "late decelerations," or "severe variable deceleration," or "absence of FHR variability" (Haverkamp et al. 1979). We believe this is inappropriate, as it does not take into account the dynamic nature of fetal oxygenation during labor, or the physiologic significance of various FHR patterns. A better definition is:

> "Progressive fetal asphyxia, which, if not reversed or averted, will ultimately result in neurologic damage or death."

Thus the indication for emergency delivery of a fetus when FHR patterns signify this condition should be termed "fetal intolerance of labor."

In summary, it is now apparent that the continuous FHR tracing has encoded upon it a large amount of data, including the three common mechanisms of fetal asphyxial stress during labor, and information about adequacy of organ (heart and brain) blood flow and oxygenation. Clinical correlates are:

1. Acute maternal hypoxemia, or sustained stepwise reduction of uterine or umbilical blood flow, is recognized by prolonged fetal bradycardia.
2. Inadequate UBF is recognized by late decelerations, initially vagal, but, if asphyxia is prolonged, they may be due to hypoxic myocardial failure. The two types are distinguished by the presence or absence of FHR variability (see below).
3. Inadequate umbilical blood flow is recognized as variable decelerations. This is possibly due to umbilical cord compression with contractions, or, especially during the second stage and expulsion of the head, to dural compression.
4. Inadequate cerebral oxygen consumption is recognized as decreasing or absent FHR variability. This is almost certainly due to a decrease in fetal cardiac ouput, due to inadequate myocardial blood flow and oxygenation, because of one or other of the above asphyxial mechanisms.

References

Caldeyro-Barcia R, Mendez-Bauer C, Poseiro JJ, Escarcena LA, Pose SV, Bieniarz J, Arnt I, Gulin L, Althabe O (1966) Control of human fetal heart rate during labour. In: Cassels DE (ed) The heart and circulation in the new born and infant. Grune and Stratton, New York

Cohn HE, Sacks EJ, Heymann MA, Rudolph AM (1974) Cardiovascular responses to hypoxemia and acidemia in fetal lambs. Am J Obstet Gynecol 120: 817–824

Court DJ, Parer JT, Block BSB, Llanos AJ (1984) Effects of beta-adrenergic blockade on blood flow distribution during hypoxemia in fetal sheep. J Dev Physiol 6: 349–358

Fisher DJ, Heymann MA, Rudolph AM (1982) Fetal myocardial oxygen and carbohydrate consumption during acutely induced hypoxemia. Am J Physiol 242: H657–H661

Goodlin RC, Haesslein HC (1977) Fetal reacting bradycardia. Am J Obstet Gynecol 129: 845–856

Greiss FC (1973) Concepts of uterine blood flow. In: Wynn RM (ed) Obstetrics and gynecology annual. Appleton-Century-Crofts, New York

Gu Wei, Parer JT, Jones CT (1982) Fetal tachycardia: the role of catechoalmines during experimental asphyxia. Abstracts of scientific papers, Xth World congress of gynecology and obstetrics, San Francisco

Harris JL, Krueger TR, Parer JT (1982) Mechanisms of the late decelerations of the fetal heart rate during hypoxia. Am J Obstet Gynecol 142: 410–415

Haverkamp AD, Orleans M, Langendoerfer S, McFee J, Murphy J, Thompson HE (1979) A controlled trial of the differential effects of intrapartum fetal monitoring. Am J Obstet Gynecol 142: 399–408

Hon EH (1968) An atlas of fetal heart rate patterns. Harty, New Haven

Iwamoto HI, Rudolph AM, Keil LC, Heymann MA (1979) Hemodynamic responses of the sheep fetus to vasopressin infusions. Circ Res 44: 430–436

Jones CT, Robinson RO (1975) Plasma catecholamines in foetal and adult sheep. J Physiol (Lond) 248: 15–33

Jones MD Jr, Sheldon RE, Peeters LL, Meschia G, Battaglia FC, Makowski EL (1977) Fetal cerebral oxygen consumption at different levels of oxygenation. J Appl Physiol 43: 1080–1084

Jones MD, Sheldon RE, Peeters LL, Makowski EL, Meschia G (1978) Regulation of cerebral blood flow in the ovine fetus. Am J Physiol 235: H162–H166

Llanos AJ, Court D, Holbrook RH, Block RS, Vega R, Parer JT (1983) Cardiovascular effects of naloxone during asphyxia in fetal sheep. Abstracts of scientific papers, 30th Annual meeting of society for gynecologic investigation, Washington, DC, p 300

Mann L (1970) Effects of hypoxia on umbilical circulation and fetal metabolism. Am J Physiol 218: 1453–1458

Parer JT (1980) The effect of acute maternal hypoxia on fetal oxygenation and the umbilical circulation in the sheep. Eur J Obstet Gynecol Reprod Biol 10:125–136
Parer JT (1983) Handbook of fetal heart rate monitoring. Saunders, Philadelphia
Parer JT, Krueger TR, Harris JL (1980) Fetal oxygen consumption and mechanisms of heart rate response during artificially produced late decelerations of fetal heart rate in sheep. Am J Obstet Gynecol 136:478–482
Paul RH, Koh KS, Bernstein SS (1978) Changes in fetal heart rate—uterine contraction patterns associated with eclampsia. Am J Obstet Gynecol 130:165–169
Peeters LLH, Sheldon RE, Jones MD, Makowski E, Meschia G (1979) Blood flow to fetal organs as a function of arterial oxygen content. Am J Obstet Gynecol 135:637
Rech W (1933) Untersuchungen über die Herztätigkeit des Fetus, Teil 3. Die Wirkung des Kopfdruckes auf die Frequenz des fetalen Herzschlages. Arch Gynäkol 154:47–57
Reuss ML, Parer JT, Harris JL, Krueger JR (1982) Hemodynamic effects of alpha-adrenergic blockade during hypoxia in fetal sheep. Am J Obstet Gynecol 142:410–415
Rosenberg AA, Jones MD, Traystman RJ, Simmons MA, Molteni RA (1982) Response of cerebral blood flow to changes in pCO_2 in fetal, newborn, and adult sheep. Am J Physiol 242:H862–H866
Rurak DW (1978) Plasma vasopressin levels during hypoxaemia and the cardiovascular effects of exogenous vasopressin in foetal and adult sheep. J Physiol 277:341–357
Yaffe H, Parer JT, Llanos A, Block B (1982) Fetal hemodynamic responses to graded reductions of uterine blood flow in sheep. Abstracts of scientific papers, 29th Annual meeting of society for gynecologic investigation, Dallas, p 113

Variability of Fetal Heart Rate Deceleration, Blood Pressure, and Acid Base Alterations During Defined Repetitive Hypoxic Stress

E. KASTENDIECK[1], W. KÜNZEL[2], and A. JENSEN[3]

Complete reduction of uterine blood flow (UBF) results in a decline of oxygen saturation (SO_2) in the fetal arterial blood. Fetal heart rate (FHR) starts to decelerate when oxygen saturation falls about 10%–15% (Künzel et al. 1983) independent of the status of fetal oxygenation prior to the reduction of uterine blood flow. There was no critical limit of oxygen saturation for the induction of deceleration. The decrease in FHR is accompanied by a rise in blood pressure and respiratory and metabolic acidosis with considerable variability in quantity and in time (Künzel et al. 1983).

The aim of this study was to investigate the cardiovascular and metabolic alterations *in repetitive intermittent* hypoxic episodes to simulate repeated decelerations as they can often be observed during labor. For the obstetrician the question arises of precisely how decelerations indicate fetal hypoxia and acidosis and in which way FHR and blood pressure response change in defined intermittent hypoxic periods.

Methods

In an acute preparation of eight near term pregnant sheep (ten experiments) the UBF was completely reduced 11 times for 60 s during a period of 30 min. The maternal aorta was occluded with an inflatable balloon catheter as described previously (Künzel et al. 1981, 1983). Total reduction of UBF could be secured by measuring the blood pressure distal to the site of occlusion.

Catheters were inserted into the fetal aorta for blood sampling and for continuous recording of systolic and diastolic blood pressure and FHR. FHR was triggered by the blood pressure waves. In addition, a fiberglass optic system was inserted into the fetal aorta to measure the oxygen saturation continuously (in vivo hemoreflectometer IVH 3, Schwarzer).

Lactate, pH, PCO_2, PO_2, and SO_2 were measured as previously described (Künzel et al. 1983).

[1] Universitäts-Frauenklinik, Josef-Schneider-Str. 4, D-8700 Würzburg
[2] Frauenklinik und Hebammenlehranstalt der Justus-Liebig-Universität Gießen, Klinikstr. 28, D-6300 Gießen
[3] University of California, San Francisco, School of Medicine, Cardiovascular Research Institute, San Francisco, CA 94143, USA

Fetal Heart Rate Monitoring
Ed. by W. Künzel

Results

Repetitive Fetal Heart Rate Decelerations and Fetal Oxygenation

In Fig. 1 an original recording of FHR, SO_2, and transcutaneous (tc) PO_2 is demonstrated. Reduction of UBF for 60 s repeated at intervals of 3 min generates decelera-

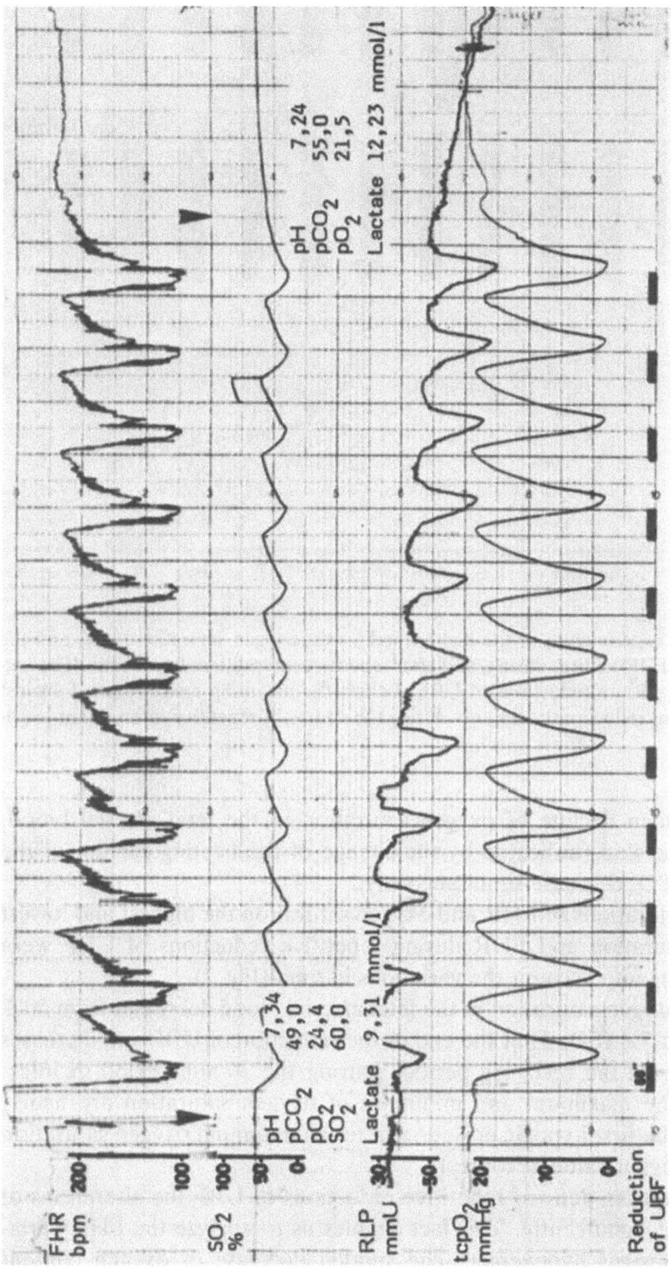

Fig. 1. Original recording of FHR, oxygen saturation of fetal arterial blood (*SO_2*), relative local skin perfusion (*RLP*), and transcutaneous PO_2

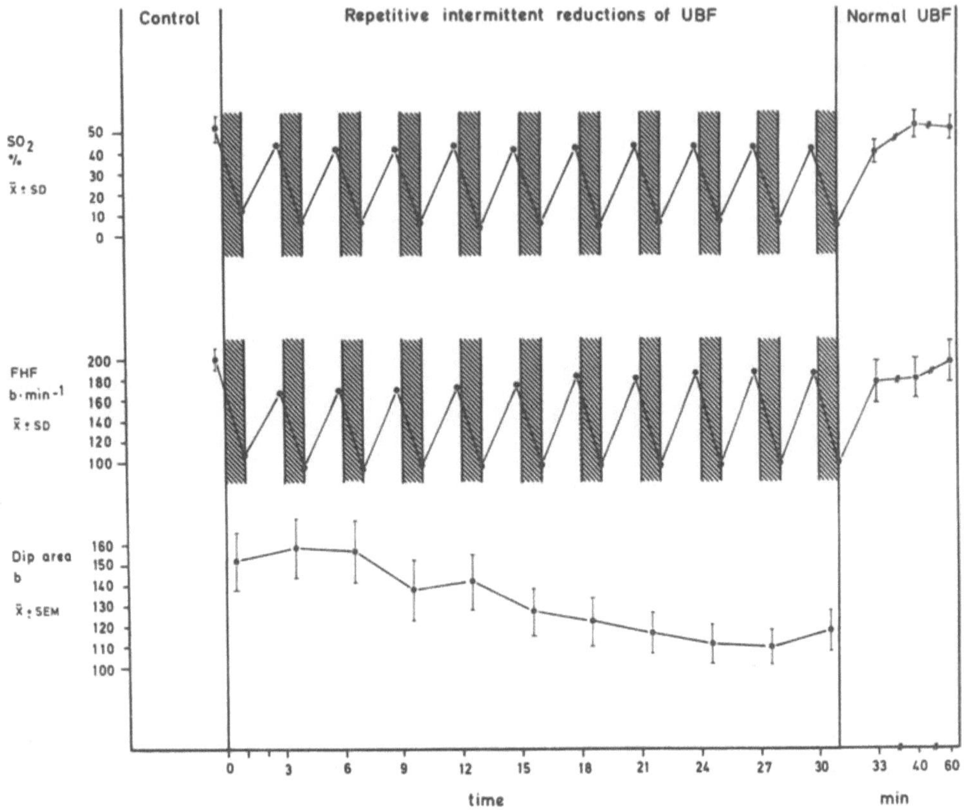

Fig. 2. Mean values (ten experiments) of the highest and lowest oxygen saturation (SO_2) and the maximum and minimum FHR before, during, and after repetitive intermittent hypoxemia. The *hatched columns* indicate the 1-min reductions of UBF. Below, the mean dip area is plotted against time. There is a significant reduction in dip area during the course of repetitive intermittent hypoxemia ($2P<0.01$)

tions due to the sudden decline of oxygen saturation in the fetal arterial blood. The blood flow of the skin (indicated by the change of the heating current of the electrode) and the $tcPO_2$ decrease simultaneously.

To quantify the alterations of FHR and oxygen saturation the highest and lowest values of oxygen saturation and FHR during repetitive reductions of UBF were determined, not taking into account the variations in time (Fig. 2).

On average, the oxygen saturation in the fetal arterial blood decreases from 50% (SD, 11) at control to 5% (SD, 5) at the end of the reduction of UBF and increases to 40% (SD, 12) during the recovery period. During the 30-min period of intermittent hypoxemia the maximum and minimum of oxygen saturation are nearly constant, except for the first hypoxic episode where the minimum oxygen saturation is higher due to the higher value at control.

It is evident that during defined repetitive reductions of UBF the alterations of oxygen do not change significantly. This fact enables us to analyze the FHR variability in constant transient hypoxemia. The sudden decrease of oxygen content results in deceleration of FHR. The mean amplitude and the mean depth of the decelerations do not change during the 30 min of repetitive hypoxemia (Fig. 2).

There is, however, a change of FHR response during the recovery period. In the course of 30-min repetitive hypoxemia the rise of FHR during the "normoxic" intervals accelerates, i.e., the duration of deceleration during a period of repetitive hypoxemia is reduced. This means that the FHR maximum during the recovery intervals increases after defined repetitive hypoxic episodes. Consequently, the dip area, i.e., the area between FHR baseline and deceleration (dimension, b/min · min), measured by planimetry, significantly diminishes (Fig. 2).

Similar results were found in previous experiments in acute and chronic pregnant sheep preparations (Künzel et al. 1981).

How much does the FHR response vary in the different experiments? Do the FHR alterations reflect the fetal oxygenation? Does the quantitative analysis of deceleration enable the diagnosis of the degree of hypoxia in the different experiments to be made?

As a result of the variability of FHR response to hypoxic stress no significant correlations can be found between:

1. Decrease of SO_2 (range, 25%–60%) and amplitude of deceleration (range, 60–140 b/min) (*r*, 0.12; *n*, 10) (mean values of 11 decelerations)
2. Minimum values of SO_2 (range, 0%–20%) and depth of deceleration (range, 90–130 b/min) (*r*, 0.2; *n*, 10) (mean values of 11 decelerations)

   In a wider range of observations, however (besides the 60-s also taking into account the 30-s (*n*, 2) and 90-s (*n*, 3) reductions of UBF) a relationship between the minimum of SO_2 (min SO_2; range, 0%–30%) and the depth of deceleration (min FHR; range, 80–150 b/min) can be demonstrated (min SO_2, 1.5; min FHR, +95; *n*, 15; *r*, 0.73; *P*, <0.01).
3. No correlation between dip area (range, 500–2500 b) and oxygen saturation preceding the hypoxic period (range, 20%–65%) (*r*, 0.1; *n*, 10)

In summary: Decelerations indicate intermittent acute reduction of oxygen in the fetal arterial blood. It is, however, impossible to appreciate the degree of hypoxemia accurately by the amplitude, the depth, and the area of decelerations. Besides the sudden decrease of oxygen other factors may be involved in regulating the FHR response. There is some evidence that FHR decelerations are also influenced by the blood pressure increase via baroreceptor stimulation.

Repetitive Decelerations and Blood Pressure Alterations

The repetitive intermittent hypoxemia generates an increase and a fall in the fetal arterial blood pressure which are variable in time as well as in magnitude.

In order to quantify blood pressure response the mean values of systolic and diastolic blood pressure have been calculated at defined conditions (see Fig. 3). The mean values of FHR and the corresponding systolic and diastolic blood pressure before, during, and at the end of 11 hypoxic episodes and during the recovery intervals are shown in Fig. 4. During the 30-min period of intermittent hypoxia the blood pressure is elevated due to a stimulation of the adrenosympathetic system followed by peripheral vasoconstriction. This vascular response correlates with a 10- to 50-fold increase of catecholamine concentrations and decrease of transcutaneous PO_2 and relative local skin perfusion (Jensen et al. 1982).

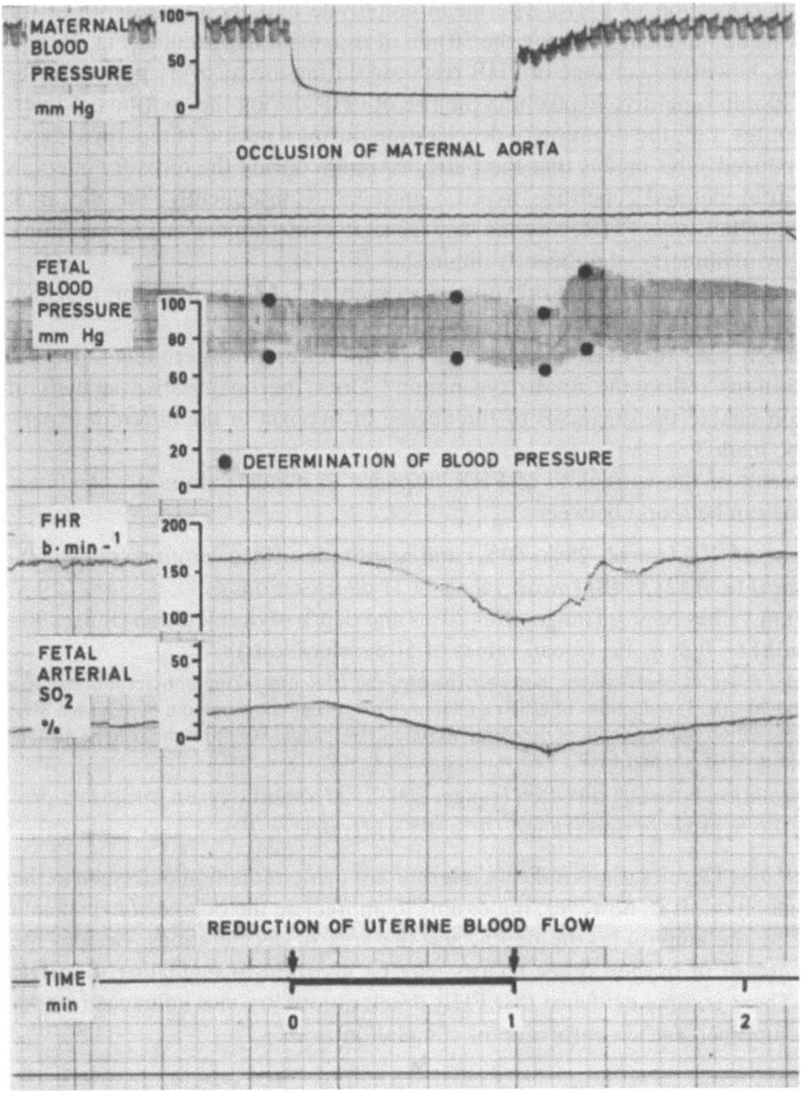

Fig. 3. Original recording of maternal and fetal arterial blood pressure, FHR, and fetal arterial SO_2 during a 1-min reduction of UBF. The *filled circles* indicate the defined conditions for determination of blood pressure: (1) before reduction of UBF, (2) the maximum value during the fall of FHR, (3) the minimum blood pressure at the lowest SO_2, and (4) the maximum blood pressure after restoration of UBF and fetal oxygenation

The maximum response of the blood pressure rise occurs at the second and third deceleration. The systolic blood pressure increases from 70 mmHg (SD, 11) at control to 100 mmHg (SD, 18) and the diastolic blood pressure from 48 mmHg (SD, 10) to 60 mmHg (SD, 11).

During the following hypoxic episodes the systolic blood pressure gradually declines probably due to the reduction of cardiac output since there is no evidence

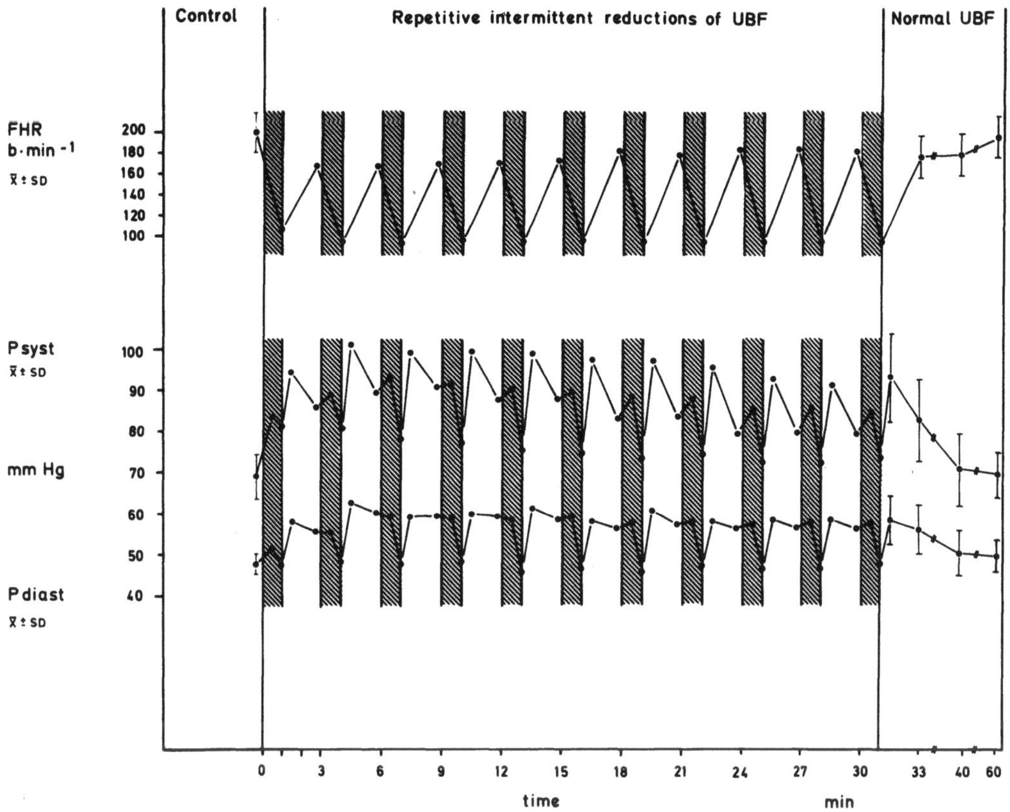

Fig. 4. Maximum and minimum FHR and systolic and diastolic blood pressure before, during, and after the 30-min period of repetitive intermittent hypoxemia (*n*, 10). The *hatched columns* indicate the 1-min reductions of UBF. The blood pressure is elevated, showing a decreasing tendency of systolic blood pressure during the 30 min of hypoxia while the diastolic pressure remains nearly constant. Repetitive intermittent hypoxemia causes fluctuations of blood pressure: a slight increase during slowing of FHR, a distinct decrease at the end of reduction of UBF, and a marked increase again when fetal oxygenation and FHR are improving after restoration of UBF

for diminution of peripheral vasoconstriction as can be shown by $tcPO_2$ and skin perfusion monitoring. Furthermore, the pulse pressure gradually declines from 35 mm Hg (SD, 10) (first deceleration) to 26 mm Hg (SD, 10) (eleventh deceleration) indicating that during repetitive hypoxic episodes the stroke volume becomes smaller.

The extensive blood pressure elevation at the beginning of about 30 mm Hg coincides with a great dip area. The delayed recovery of FHR during the first decelerations seems to be caused by an increased blood pressure response at the beginning of the 30-min intermittent hypoxic period via a stronger stimulation of baroreceptors. With this assumption, the baroreceptor-induced vagal stimulation leads to the prolongation of deceleration. The decrease in the dip area during the course of repetitive hypoxemia may be caused by the decline of blood pressure response resulting in a reduced stimulation of the baroreceptors. It may, however, also be possible that the sensitivity of baroreceptors during the repetitive hypoxic stress changes.

In the following the fluctuation of blood pressure is analyzed in detail. During the decline in FHR only in the first deceleration a remarkable increase in the systolic blood pressure (13 mm Hg; SD, 5; range, 7–26) is evident. In the following decelerations there is only a slight increase of 4 mm Hg (SD, 5.4; range, 10–15; *n*, 100). The increase in blood pressure is related neither to the amplitude nor to the depth of deceleration.

These results suggest that the blood pressure increase of a few mm Hg (in 30% of the cases even a slight blood pressure decrease can be observed) is too small to induce deceleration by baroreceptor stimulation. In addition, the onset of deceleration precedes the blood pressure alteration in 40% of the decelerations.

The adequate stimulus for FHR deceleration seems to be the acute reduction of oxygen with chemoreceptor response. Similar results and conclusions were obtained by Künzel et al. (1983) and Parer et al. (1980).

At the end of deceleration and at the lowest oxygen saturation the blood pressure decreases about 14 mm Hg (SD, 13; range, 35–15; *n*, 100; $2P$, <0.001). This is obviously due to a reduction in cardiac output generated by myocardial hypoxia (Itskovitz et al. 1982).

After the release of the aortal occlusion a marked rise in blood pressure of about 22 mm Hg (SD, 12; range, 1–50) is evident as a result of increasing cardiac output during the recovery interval. Thus, FHR and stroke volume (indicated by a pulse pressure rise of about 10 mm Hg) increase in parallel to the improvement in fetal oxygenation.

During the further course of the 2-min recovery periods the fetal arterial blood pressure declines again (13 mm Hg; SD, 9; range, 0–33).

In conclusion, during repetitive hypoxic episodes:

There is a considerable increase in systolic and diastolic blood pressure. The blood pressure decreases during the 30-min period of repetitive hypoxia probably due to myocardial depression and consecutive reduction of cardiac output. Nevertheless, at the end of the hypoxic period the blood pressure still exceeds the value of the control.

During the intermittent hypoxic intervals there is a fluctuation of blood pressure with great variability. On average, there is a minor increase in blood pressure at the beginning of deceleration. During severe oxygen deprivation at the depth of FHR deceleration the blood pressure declines. It starts to increase again to a maximum value after fetal oxygenation has been recovered.

The decrease in dip area of the consecutive decelerations might be explained by the reduction in blood pressure and reduced stimulation of baroreceptors.

Repetitive Decelerations and Acid Base Alterations

The acid base and blood gas measurements before and after the period of repetitive hypoxemia are shown in Table 1. The fetal arterial pH falls 0.004 (SD, 0.002) and lactate concentration rises by 0.1 (SD, 0.08) mmol/liter per minute, i.e., a tenfold smaller change per unit time than in acute persistent anoxia measured in other experiments (Künzel et al. 1983; Moll and Kastendieck 1978).

Table 1. Acid base balance and blood gas values ($\bar{x} \pm SD$) before and after the 30-min period of repetitive intermittent hypoxemia

	At control	Posthypoxic period		
		33 min	40 min	60 min
pH	7.34 (0.05)	7.24 (0.10)	7.25 (0.09)	7.30 (0.08)
PCO_2 (mm Hg)	49.4 (5.5)	56.7 (11.3)	54.2 (10.1)	50.0 (6.2)
PO_2 (mm Hg)	21.3 (3.1)	20.4 (3.1)	22.6 (2.8)	22.4 (2.7)
Base deficit (mmol/liter)	1.4 (2.9)	6.7 (5.5)	5.1 (5.5)	3.9 (4.9)
Lactate (mmol/liter)	5.0 (2.5)	9.7 (3.6)	9.7 (3.9)	8.9 (3.4)

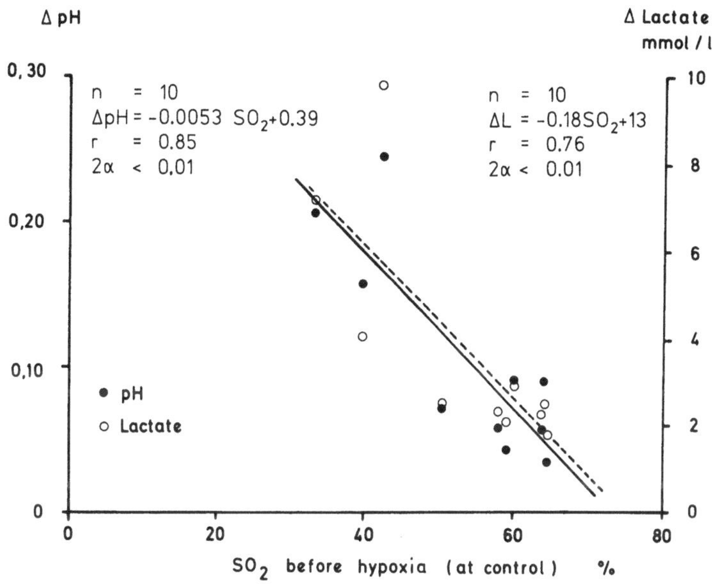

Fig. 5. The decrease of pH (ΔpH) and the increase of lactate (Δlactate) during the 30-min period of hypoxia correlated to the fetal oxygen saturation prior to reduction of UBF (SO_2 at control). The oxygen-deprived fetus accumulates lactic acid more than the well-oxygenized fetus

The increase in lactic acid per minute varies from 0.06 to 0.3 mmol/liter and is not related to FHR alterations as far as the dip area, baseline, amplitude, and depth of decelerations are concerned.

The increase in lactate is inversely related to fetal oxygenation before hypoxia is induced (Fig. 5). These results suggest a greater accumulation of lactic acid in the oxygen-deprived fetus than in the well-oxygenated fetus. Different rates of utilization and/or production of lactic acid may provide an explanation.

In the guinea pig fetus (Moll and Kastendieck 1978) and in the sheep fetus (Kastendieck et al. 1982), lactate utilization depends on oxygen saturation in the fetal arterial blood. The half-life ($t_{1/2}$) of lactate is 30 min when SO_2 is 60% and extends to 60 min when SO_2 is 30%. In the experiments reported here it is evident that the maximum oxygen saturation during repetitive hypoxic episodes is about

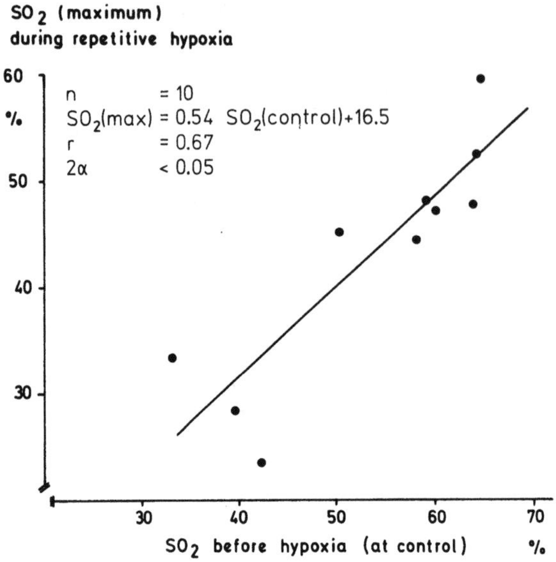

Fig. 6. The fetal SO_2 during the recovery intervals (SO_2 maximum) correlated to SO_2 prior to the reduction of UBF (SO_2 at control). The well-oxygenized fetus obtains nearly normal SO_2; the oxygen-deprived fetus obtains only a SO_2 (maximum) of 30% during the recovery intervals

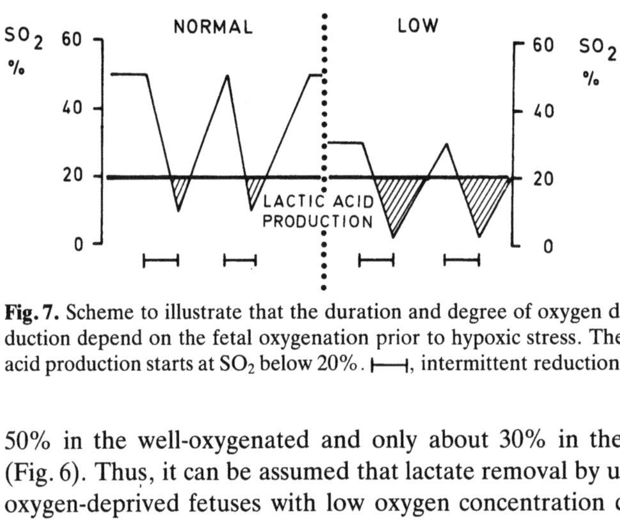

Fig. 7. Scheme to illustrate that the duration and degree of oxygen deprivation with lactic acid production depend on the fetal oxygenation prior to hypoxic stress. There is some evidence that lactic acid production starts at SO_2 below 20%. ├─┤, intermittent reductions of UBF

50% in the well-oxygenated and only about 30% in the oxygen-deprived fetuses (Fig. 6). Thus, it can be assumed that lactate removal by utilization is reduced in the oxygen-deprived fetuses with low oxygen concentration during the recovery intervals.

In addition, the production of lactic acid is probably enhanced in the oxygen-deprived fetus because the duration and the degree of oxygen deprivation during repetitive reductions of uterine blood flow is more excessive than in the fetus with normal oxygenation at control (Fig. 7). There is some evidence that in the fetus anaerobic glycolysis starts at a critical limit of SO_2, i.e., about 20%–25% (Moll and Kastendieck 1978; Kastendieck et al., unpublished observation in chronic sheep experiments). Thus, the rate of lactic acid production depends on the duration and degree of oxygen deprivation below 20%–25%.

Summary and Conclusions

1. Decelerations are induced by a sudden decrease in oxygen content in fetal arterial blood, indicating acute alterations in fetal oxygenation.
2. The amplitude and the depth or area of deceleration are not an accurate measure of the severity of hypoxia.
3. Repetitive intermittent hypoxia during a period of 30 min causes fluctuations in systolic and diastolic blood pressure on an elevated blood pressure level due to strong adrenosympathetic stimulation. The alterations during a single deceleration show a slight increase in blood pressure at the onset of deceleration followed by a decrease at the depth of oxygen deprivation. Parallel to the improvement of oxygenation the blood pressure rises again reaching a maximum value. During the course of 30-min repetitive intermittent hypoxemia the systolic blood pressure and the pulse pressure gradually decrease probably due to a reduction in cardiac output while the diastolic blood pressure as an indicator of total peripheral resistance remains constant.
4. The reduction in systolic blood pressure at the end of the 30-min period occurs simultaneously with the reduction in dip area, suggesting that the duration of deceleration is influenced by baroreceptor stimulation. Extensive blood pressure elevation seems to delay the recovery of FHR, and inversely the decline in blood pressure accelerates the FHR increase.
5. During 30 min of repetitive intermittent hypoxemia the pH falls (0.004) and lactate rises 0.01 mmol/liter per minute. The metabolic acidosis is not closely related to the dip area but depends on the fetal oxygenation prior to hypoxia.

References

Itskovitz J, Goetzmann BW, Rudolph AM (1982) The mechanism of late deceleration of the heart rate and its relationship to oxygenation in normoxemic and chronically hypoxemic fetal lambs. Am J Obstet Gynecol 142:66

Jensen A, Künzel W, Kastendieck E (1982) Epinephrine and norepinephrine release in the fetus after repeated hypoxia. J Perinat Med [Suppl 2] 10:109

Kastendieck E, Künzel W, Kurz CS (1980) Utilization of lactic acid and cardiovascular response in the sheep fetus receiving an infusion of lactic acid. Arch Gynäkol 230:21

Kastendieck E, Paulick R, Martius J, Jensen A (1982) Einfluß der metabolischen Azidose auf Herzfrequenz, Blutdruck, Oxygenation, Säure-Basen-Status, Glucose- und Elektrolytkonzentrationen des Feten und Geschwindigkeit der fetalen Milchsäureelemination im chronischen Schaftexperiment. In: Dudenhausen JW, Saling E (Hrsg) Perinatale Medizin, Vol 9. Thieme, Stuttgart

Künzel W, Kurz CS, Kastendieck E (1981) Die Variabilität der fetalen Herzfrequenzreaktion auf die Reduktion der uterinen Durchblutung. Z Geburtshilfe Perinat 185:343

Künzel W, Kastendieck E, Hohmann E (1983) Heart rate and blood pressure response and metabolic changes in the sheep fetus following reduction of uterine blood flow. Gynecol Obstet Invest 15:300

Moll W, Kastendieck E (1978) Accumulation and disappearance of lactate in a fetus with a hemochorial placenta. The role of placental transfer and fetal metabolism. J Perinat Med 6:246

Parer JT, Krueger TR, Harris JL (1980) Fetal oxygen consumption and mechanisms of heart rate response during artificially produced late decelerations of fetal heart rate in sheep. Am J Obstet Gynecol 136:478

Fetal Heart Rate Response to Hypoxia in the Subhuman Primate

E. Mueller-Heubach[1]

Study of fetal heart rate response to hypoxia in the subhuman primate has particular applicability to the clinical situation in the human. Most studies have been carried out in the fetal rhesus monkey, which has a hemochorial placenta, a uterus similar in configuration to the human uterus, and a growth rate almost identical to that of the human fetus. The fetal brain, our major concern during hypoxia, constitutes about 12% of birth weight in the rhesus monkey and in man compared with 1.3% in the lamb (Dawes 1968). Accordingly, about 16% of cardiac output in the near term fetal monkey supplies the brain under normoxemic conditions (Behrman et al. 1970) compared with 3% in the fetal lamb (Cohn et al. 1974).

Experimental Preparation

Surgical preparation of fetal monkeys for study of cardiovascular physiology is usually done under ketamine or sodium pentobarbital anesthesia. Laparoscopy and hysterotomy are performed. Catheters are implanted into fetal vessels and into the uterine cavity. Electrodes are placed subcutaneously on both shoulders. For umbilical cord compression an inflatable occluding device is placed around the umbilical cord. For interruption of uterine blood flow, an inflatable balloon catheter is inserted into a maternal femoral artery with the tip just below the level of the renal arteries. The experimental procedure is difficult due to the small size of the rhesus monkey fetus, which weighs about 450 g at term. The fetus is placed back into the uterus and uterine and abdominal incisions are closed. Studies are carried out after a 1-h recovery period. The surgical procedure usually results in uterine activity. Establishing a chronic preparation of fetal monkeys has been very difficult with limited success (Martin et al. 1973).

Baseline Fetal Heart Rate

The baseline fetal heart rate in the rhesus monkey fetus is higher than in the human. A decrease in baseline fetal heart rate is seen in the rhesus monkey with decreasing oxygen tension in fetal arterial blood. In the PO_2 range between 23 and 31 mm Hg, the decline in fetal heart rate is small. When fetal arterial PO_2 falls below 23 mm Hg, baseline fetal heart rate decreases significantly; however, even with extreme degrees of hypoxemia, the maximal decline in fetal heart rate amounts only to 20% of the

[1] University of Pittsburgh, School of Medicine, Department of Obstetrics and Gynecology, Magee-Womens Hospital, Forbes and Halket Streets, Pittsburgh, PA 15213, USA

Fetal Heart Rate Monitoring
Ed. by W. Künzel

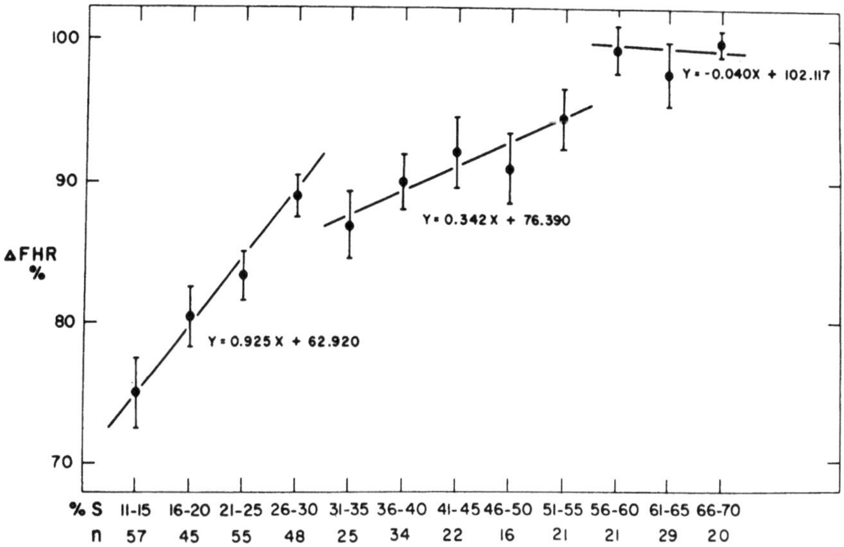

Fig. 1. Mean ± SE of hemoglobin saturation with oxygen *(S)* of carotid arterial blood and heart rate *(FHR)* in the fetal monkey. Changes in FHR are expressed in percent (100% = 220.5 bpm). *n*, number of observations in each group of *S* values. (Mueller-Heubach et al. 1980)

baseline during normoxemia (Mueller-Heubach et al. 1980). When hemoglobin saturation with oxygen of fetal arterial blood and baseline fetal heart rate are compared, no significant heart rate change is present when hemoglobin saturation is 56% or above. At saturations of 31%–56% there is some decline in baseline fetal heart rate which becomes more pronounced in the saturation range of 11%–30%. Maximal decline in fetal heart rate with extreme desaturation of fetal hemoglobin is 25% (Fig. 1).

Beat-to-Beat Variability

The effect of hypoxemia and respiratory acidosis on variability of fetal heart rate in monkeys has been studied by Ikenoue and his co-workers in a chronic preparation (Ikenoue et al. 1981). These investigators have demonstrated the effect of fetal hypoxemia produced by allowing the mother to breathe a 10% oxygen mixture on long-term and short-term variability of fetal heart rate. There was an increase in both short-term and long-term variability with fetal hypoxemia. The increase in short-term variability was more pronounced. When fetal hypoxemia was produced after pretreatment of the monkey fetus with atropine, changes in short-term and long-term variability were markedly attenuated. Carbon dioxide tension was unchanged during these episodes of experimental fetal hypoxemia. When respiratory acidosis was produced by maternal breathing of a 12% carbon dioxide gas mixture, long-term and short-term variability of fetal heart rate increased in a similar fashion. Atropine blocked this increase in long- and short-term variability with a greater effect on long-term variability. These observations suggest a reflex mechanism for control of fetal heart rate variability which is mediated via the vagus nerve. Stimulation of peripheral and/or central chemoreceptors by falling PO_2 or increasing PCO_2 appears to be the cause for this increased vagal activity.

Variable Deceleration

In obstetrical practice the most frequently observed decelerative pattern of fetal heart rate is the variable deceleration which is the result of compression of the umbilical cord. Depending on the degree of cord compression, the changes in the fetal circulation as well as blood flow between placenta and fetus vary. With partial compression of the umbilical cord, the low pressure circulation in the umbilical vein is more likely to be affected, resulting in a decrease in venous return from the placenta. When pressure on the umbilical cord exceeds the higher pressure in the umbilical arteries, there is a sudden marked increase in peripheral vascular resistance in the fetal circulation and flow between fetus and placenta is interrupted. The effect of partial occlusion of the umbilical cord as well as the isolated umbilical vein has been examined by James and co-workers in the pregnant baboon (James et al. 1976). Partial cord occlusion produced a small fall in fetal blood pressure which was accompanied by a significant increase in fetal heart rate. There was a concomitant limited decrease in fetal arterial PO_2 but no significant change in arterial pH or PCO_2. This response was similar whether the intact umbilical cord or the isolated intra-abdominal portion of the umbilical vein were occluded. This fetal heart rate response to partial umbilical cord compression is the likely mechanism of the transient increase in fetal heart rate frequently seen before and after variable deceleration in the human fetus.

We have investigated cardiovascular changes and alterations in transcutaneous oxygen tension in the fetal monkey with complete experimental umbilical cord occlusion (Mueller-Heubach and Battelli 1982). Figure 2 illustrates a 30-s umbilical cord occlusion resulting in a variable deceleration in fetal heart rate. Fetal blood pressure is increased and transcutaneous PO_2 decreases during umbilical cord occlusion. Return of transcutaneous (tc) PO_2 to baseline occurs slowly after the end of the cord occlusion. When the changes which occur with umbilical cord occlusion are examined at a higher paper speed of the recording polygraph providing higher resolution, it is apparent that fetal blood pressure increases about 1 s after the start of umbilical cord occlusion followed within 1–2 s by a decrease in fetal heart rate. The initial increase in fetal blood pressure above baseline lasts about 19 s until fetal blood pressure falls below the preocclusion level. Transcutaneous oxygen tension begins to decline 12 s after the start of umbilical cord occlusion and does not return to its baseline value until 75 s after the end of the cord occlusion. The relative heat output of the transcutaneous PO_2 electrode, which is thought to reflect skin perfusion indirectly, is unchanged. Even at very high amplification of the relative heat output signal there are no consistent changes in relative heat output of the $tcPO_2$ electrode, thus permitting no conclusions about skin perfusion during hypoxemia. To identify the relationship between fetal $tcPO_2$ and fetal heart rate more precisely, we have summarized data from 24 umbilical cord occlusions of 15- or 30-s duration in Table 1. During a 15-s cord occlusion fetal heart rate decreases by 55 beats/min;

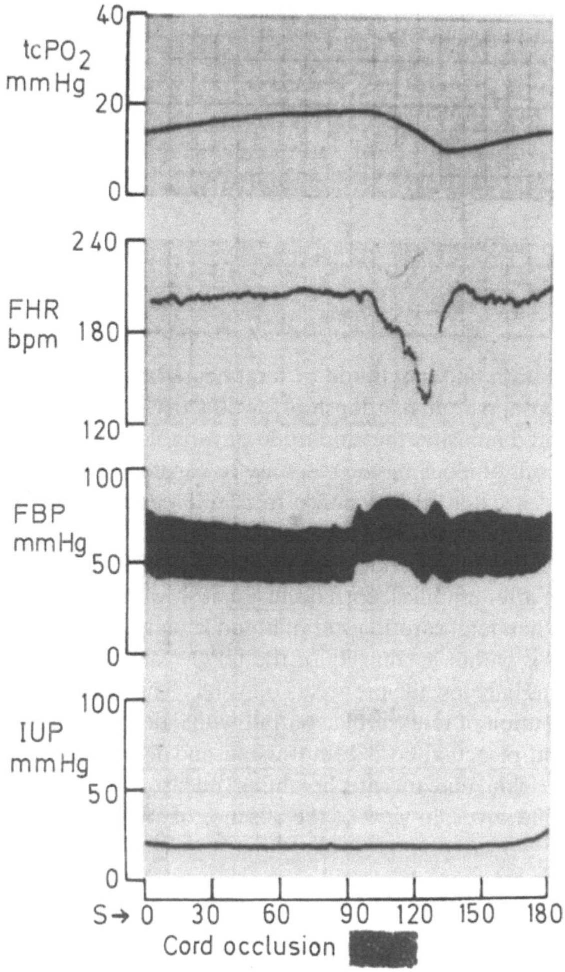

Fig. 2. $tcPO_2$, fetal heart rate *(FHR)*, fetal blood pressure *(FBP)*, and intrauterine pressure *(IUP)* during a 30-s umbilical cord occlusion at a paper speed of 30 mm/min. (Mueller-Heubach and Battelli 1982)

doubling of the period of cord occlusion produces a 78-beat/min decline in fetal heart rate. At the same time, $tcPO_2$ falls by 6 and 11 mm Hg respectively. Accordingly, the decline in fetal heart rate compared with the fall in $tcPO_2$ is less for a 30-s than for a 15-s cord occlusion.

Based on these observations, the probable physiological mechanism of variable deceleration of fetal heart rate is an initial baroreceptor stimulation producing a rather immediate and rapid decline in fetal heart rate. This baroreceptor stimulation ceases when fetal blood pressure returns to baseline about 19 s after the start of the cord occlusion and the further fetal heart rate decline of lesser magnitude is likely caused by chemoreceptor stimulation in view of a continued fall in $tcPO_2$. This contention is supported by the fact that there is no relationship between $tcPO_2$ at the

Table 1. Relationship between fetal heart rate and $tcPO_2$ during umbilical cord compression. (Mueller-Heubach and Battelli 1982)

Cord compression (s)	ΔFHR$\downarrow$ (bpm)	$\Delta tcPO_2\downarrow$ (torr)	ΔFHR$\downarrow$/ $\Delta tcPO_2\downarrow$ (bpm/torr)	$t/\Delta tcPO_2\downarrow$ (s/torr)
15	55 ± 19	6.0 ± 1.6	9 ± 3.6	10 ± 2.3
30	78 ± 20	11.5 ± 3.3	7 ± 2.4	8 ± 2.8

All values are means ± SD

beginning of umbilical cord occlusion and amplitude of fetal heart rate decline for 15-s occlusions, while there is an apparent relationship for 30-s occlusions. Vagal blockade with atropine delays and diminishes the amplitude of variable deceleration of fetal heart rate, mainly as a result of blocking the response to baroreceptor stimulation but probably also to a lesser extent the response to chemoreceptor stimulation. Other investigators have described myocardial conduction defects with umbilical cord occlusions for durations longer than in our study (Yeh et al. 1975). Recovery of transcutaneous oxygen tension after umbilical cord occlusion is slow, taking 8–10 s for each millimeter Hg $tcPO_2$. When fetal carotid arterial blood is sampled 30 s after the end of cord occlusion, PaO_2 is within ±1 mm Hg of the $tcPO_2$ value before occlusion while $tcPO_2$ is still 3–7 mm Hg below the preocclusion value. This discrepancy indicates alterations in the distribution of fetal cardiac output with a decrease in skin perfusion well beyond the period of actual cord compression and fetal heart rate change. Vasoconstriction of the skin due to catecholamine release is a possible mechanism for this observation; however, in view of the absence of systemic hypertension once the cord occlusion is over, it is more likely that local factors may be responsible for this phenomenon.

Late Decelerations

During labor intervillous space perfusion and, as a result, placental gas exchange between maternal and fetal circulation are interrupted with each uterine contraction. When an interruption of intervillous space blood flow is produced by occlusion of the maternal aorta below the level of the renal arteries, the fetal heart rate will remain unchanged or exhibit the pattern of late deceleration depending on the oxygenation of the fetus before maternal aortic occlusion. With continuing partial constriction of the maternal aorta, late decelerations of fetal heart rate following uterine contractions will develop as illustrated in Fig. 3. Changes in fetal arterial pH, PO_2, PCO_2, base deficit, and hemoglobin saturation with oxygen and carbon dioxide over the course of the tracing are indicated. There is no change in fetal heart rate following the first uterine contraction. Thereafter each contraction is followed by a late deceleration of increasing amplitude. Progressively greater decreases of fetal blood pressure can be seen concomitant with each deceleration. At the same time the degree of hypercapnia decreases, leading to an increase in arterial pH.

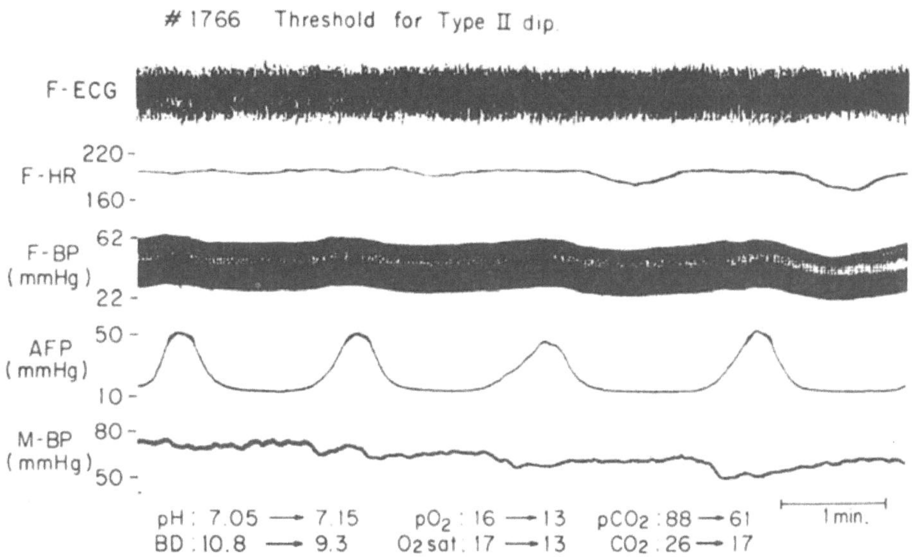

Fig. 3. Late deceleration (type II dip) onset. Fetal partial asphyxia was produced by: (1) earlier infusion of oxytocin into the maternal bloodstream and (2) lowering the maternal blood pressure by aortic constriction. (Myers 1972)

Several years ago we examined the relationship between fetal arterial pH, PO_2, hemoglobin saturation with oxygen, and the appearance of late decelerations of fetal heart rate (Myers et al. 1973). Fetal arterial blood was sampled before uterine contractions. The lowest values of pH, PO_2, and saturation were determined which were not associated with a late deceleration after the uterine contraction which followed fetal arterial blood sampling. In addition, pH, PO_2, and saturation values were measured before uterine contractions which were followed by late decelerations amounting in amplitude to 5% and 10% of baseline fetal heart rate. There was no relationship between fetal arterial blood pH and the appearance and magnitude of late decelerations. In contrast, oxygen tension of fetal arterial blood was progressively lower when uterine contractions provoked late decelerations of increasing amplitude. The relationship between late decelerations and fetal oxygenation became even clearer when hemoglobin saturation with oxygen of fetal arterial blood was considered (Table 2). A normal uterine contraction in the rhesus monkey was not followed by a late deceleration of fetal heart rate unless saturation of fetal arterial blood before a uterine contraction was about 25% or less. We also assessed the relationship between the interval of onset of contraction and onset of late deceleration. Figure 4 illustrates that late deceleration of fetal heart rate occurred earlier in the contraction cycle when oxygen tension of fetal arterial blood was low before a uterine contraction which elicited a late deceleration. A most important relationship is illustrated in Fig. 5. The amplitude of late deceleration of fetal heart rate was related to the hemoglobin saturation with oxygen of fetal arterial blood before a uterine contraction. When saturation was 50% or more, a normal uterine contraction was not followed by a late deceleration. Figure 6 illustrates that the degree of fetal hypotension was related to the amplitude of late deceleration. From a teleological

Table 2. Lowest values of arterial blood hemoglobin saturation with oxygen (abdominal aorta) of mature fetal monkeys at which uterine contractions failed to elicit decelerations and the highest values at which the magnitudes of late decelerations were 5% and 10% of baseline heart rate. Control values at the onset of the experiment ranged from 68% to 74%. (Myers et al. 1973)

	Late deceleration (%)		
	0	5	10
No	9	12	14
Mean	34.1	25.6[a]	18.9[b]
SD	6.8	5.6	5.3
Range	25–45	20–40	10–29

[a] Statistically different from the mean of the zero deceleration group at the level of $P<0.001$

[b] Statistically different from the means of zero and 5% deceleration groups at the level of $P<0.001$

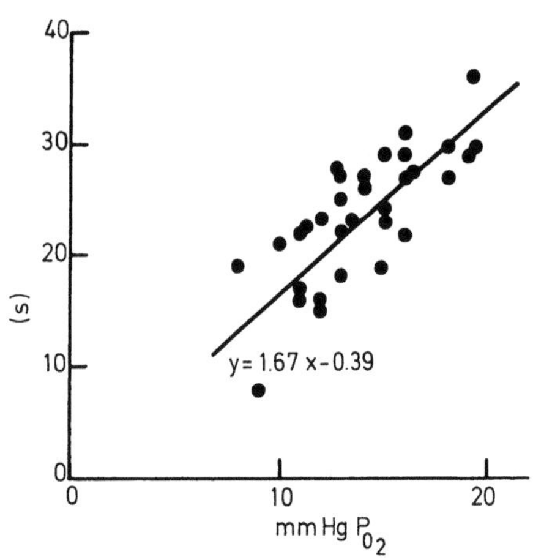

Fig. 4. Interval *(s)* between the onset of uterine contractions and the onset of late decelerations as a function of the fetal arterial blood oxygen tension (mmHg). (Myers et al. 1973)

point of view, this is a sensible arrangement because myocardial oxygen consumption is related to the product of heart rate and blood pressure.

In order to elucidate further the mechanism by which fetal oxygenation and the appearance of late deceleration of fetal heart rate are related, we have recently used a model of well-quantitated interruptions of uterine perfusion using an inflatable balloon catheter of the Swan-Ganz type inserted via a maternal femoral artery into the maternal aorta (Mueller-Heubach et al. 1982). Late decelerations of fetal heart rate produced by inflation of the balloon catheter in the maternal aorta are comparable to those seen after spontaneous uterine contractions. It is of note that the configura-

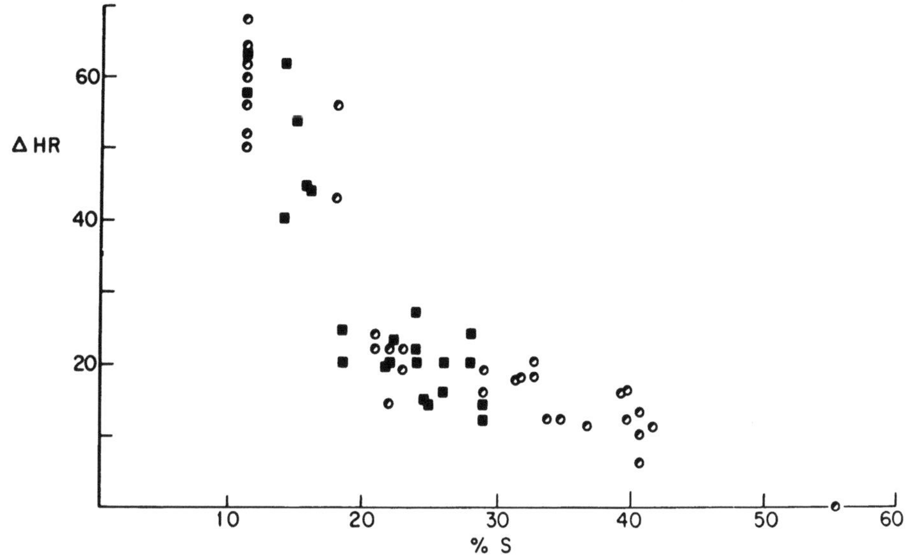

Fig. 5. Decreases in the heart rate (beats/min) of two fetal monkeys during late decelerations as a function of the fetal arterial blood hemoglobin saturation with oxygen (percent) before the onset of the uterine contractions. (Myers et al. 1973)

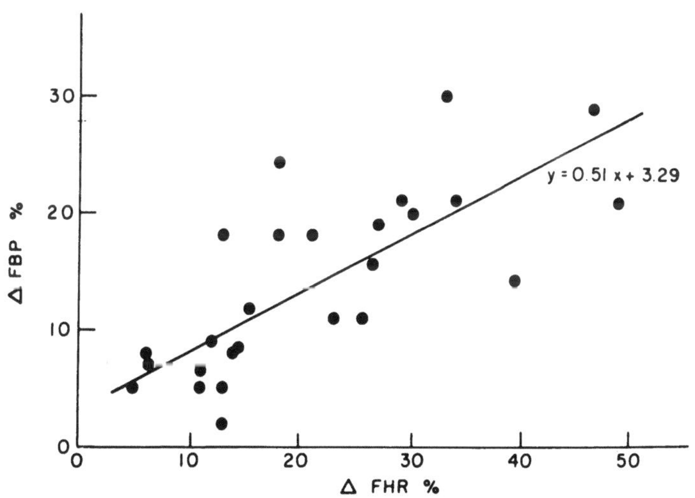

Fig. 6. Relative decrease in the fetal blood pressure as a function of the heart rate decrease of the fetal rhesus monkey during late decelerations. (Myers et al. 1973)

tion of these late decelerations is similar to that seen in the human fetus and very different from the configuration of heart rate decelerations produced in the fetal lamb by different investigator groups, namely those headed by Künzel (Künzel et al. 1980), Martin (Martin et al. 1979), Parer (Parer et al. 1980), as well as ourselves (Mueller-Heubach et al. 1981). Transcutaneous PO_2 decreased with late deceleration followed by a prolonged return to baseline after the late deceleration. As mentioned in the description of our studies on variable decelerations, there was also a discrepancy between PaO_2 and $tcPO_2$ during this recovery period with an earlier return of PaO_2 to baseline. These recent studies were done under ketamine anesthesia, whereas our earlier work on late decelerations (Myers et al. 1973) was done under pentobarbital anesthesia, which is thought to have a more depressant cardiovascular effect. However, late deceleration of fetal heart rate under ketamine anesthesia was also accompanied by hypotension. This is in contrast to our observations (Mueller-Heubach et al. 1981) and those of others (Künzel et al. 1980; Martin et al. 1979; Parer et al. 1980) in the fetal lamb in which experimental late deceleration is accompanied by an increase in blood pressure. In order to investigate the role of reflex mechanisms versus direct myocardial depression during late deceleration, we produced vagal blockade using atropine. At a fetal arterial pH of 7.22 and a PO_2 of 15 mm Hg before inflation of the balloon in the maternal aorta for 45 s, late deceleration was markedly decreased in amplitude and duration after atropine administration (0.2 mg). However, when late deceleration was produced in an extremely asphyxiated fetal monkey with a fetal arterial pH of 6.93 and a PO_2 of 11 mm Hg, late deceleration decreased in magnitude to a much lesser extent even at twice the dose of atropine (0.4 mg). These observations suggest that late deceleration of fetal heart rate is largely mediated by the vagus nerve in response to chemoreceptor stimulation. The nature and location of these chemoreceptors is unknown. However, with extreme degrees of fetal asphyxia, an element of direct myocardial depression appears to be added to this reflex mechanism.

The work done by investigators using the subhuman primate as a model has greatly expanded our understanding of fetal heart rate changes during fetal hypoxia and thus has aided the clinician in the management of the human fetus at risk.

References

Behrman RE, Lees MH, Peterson EN, DeLannoy CW, Seeds AE (1970) Distribution of the circulation in the normal and asphyxiated fetal primate. Am J Obstet Gynecol 108:956

Cohn HE, Sacks EJ, Heymann MA, Rudolph AM (1974) Cardiovascular responses to hypoxemia and acidemia in fetal lambs. Am J Obstet Gynecol 120:817

Dawes GS (1968) Foetal and neonatal physiology. Year Book Medical, Chicago, p 16

Ikenoue T, Martin CB Jr, Murata Y, Ettinger BB, Lu PS (1981) Effect of acute hypoxemia and respiratory acidosis on the fetal heart rate in monkeys. Am J Obstet Gynecol 141:797

James LS, Yeh MN, Morishima HO, Daniel SS, Caritis SN, Niemann WH, Indyk L (1976) Umbilical vein occlusion and transient acceleration of the fetal heart rate. Am J Obstet Gynecol 126:276

Künzel W, Kastendieck E, Kurz CS, Paulik R (1980) Transcutaneous PO_2 and cardiovascular observations in the sheep fetus following the reduction of uterine blood flow. J Perinat Med 8:85

Martin CB Jr, Murata Y, Parer JT (1973) A method for obtaining biochemical and biophysical measurements from rhesus monkey fetuses for prolonged periods. Am J Obstet Gynecol 117:126

Martin CB Jr, DeHaan J, Van der Wildt B, Jongsma HW, Dieleman A, Arts THM (1979) Mechanisms of late decelerations in the fetal heart rate. A study with autonomic blocking agents in fetal lambs. Eur J Obstet Gynecol Reprod Biol 9:361

Mueller-Heubach E, Battelli AF (1982) Variable heart rate decelerations and transcutaneous PO_2 ($tcPO_2$) during umbilical cord occlusion in the fetal monkey. Am J Obstet Gynecol 144:796–802

Mueller-Heubach E, Myers RE, Adamsons K (1980) Fetal heart rate and blood pressure during prolonged partial asphyxia in the rhesus monkey. Am J Obstet Gynecol 137:48

Mueller-Heubach E, Caritis SN, Edelstone DI, Huch R, Huch A (1981) Comparison of continuous transcutaneous PO_2 measurements with intermittent arterial PO_2 determinations in fetal lambs. Obstet Gynecol 57:248

Mueller-Heubach E, Caritis SN, Edelstone DI (1982) Mechanisms of late deceleration in fetal monkeys: transcutaneous PO_2 ($tcPO_2$), fetal blood pressure and vagal blockade. Society for Gynecologic Investigation, Program and Abstract No. 176

Myers RE (1972) Two patterns of perinatal brain damage and their conditions of occurrence. Am J Obstet Gynecol 112:246

Myers RE, Mueller-Heubach E, Adamsons K (1973) Predictability of the state of fetal oxygenation from quantitative analysis of components of late decelerations. Am J Obstet Gynecol 115:1083

Parer JT, Krueger TR, Harris JL (1980) Fetal oxygen consumption and mechanisms of heart rate response during artificially produced late decelerations of fetal heart rate in sheep. Am J Obstet Gynecol 136:478

Yeh MN, Morishima HO, Niemann WH, James LS (1975) Myocardial conduction defects in association with compression of the umbilical cord. Experimental observations in fetal baboons. Am J Obstet Gynecol 121:951

Fetal Heart Rate Alterations in Partial and Total Cord Occlusion

W. Künzel[1]

Fetal life in utero is protected against environmental influences by a number of mechanisms. The fetus is sheltered from mechanical disturbances by the amniotic fluid. This protective mechanism becomes understandable if the uterus is considered as a sphere (Fig. 1). The placenta is attached on the inner wall of the sphere. The fetus is connected to the placenta by a compressible tube freely floating in the amniotic fluid, the umbilical cord. An increase in pressure inside this sphere during uterine contractions increases the pressure in all compartments: the fetus, including the fetal vessels, the placenta, and the intervillous space. The blood pressure in the umbilical artery increases during uterine contractions by the same amount that the amniotic fluid pressure rises. The increase is paralleled by the elevation of the blood pressure in the umbilical vein and in the intervillous space. The driving pressure for the umbilical circulation therefore remains unchanged during uterine contractions.

Uterine blood flow, however, decreases if the uterus contracts due to uterine vein occlusion and the rise of the vascular resistance exerted by the compression of the radial and spiral arteries passing through the myometrium (Borell et al. 1965; Greiss 1965).

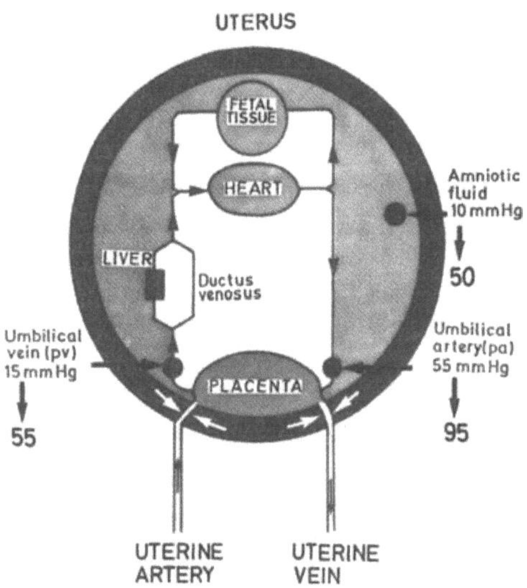

Fig. 1. The uterus and its contents considered as a sphere. The amniotic fluid protects the umbilical blood flow during uterine contractions. Uterine blood flow, however, decreases due to compression of the arteries and veins passing the myometrium

[1] Frauenklinik und Hebammenlehranstalt der Justus-Liebig-Universität Gießen, Klinikstr. 28, D-6300 Gießen

Fetal Heart Rate Monitoring
Ed. by W. Künzel

The loss of amniotic fluid in cases of early rupture of membranes or in cases of oligohydramny leads to the presumption that disorders of umbilical circulation occur. Cord prolapse, cord around the fetal neck, and cord around the body are similar situations which lead to cord occlusion. Partial and total cord occlusion are always accompanied by fetal compromise, depending on the severity and duration of occlusion.

The concern of this paper is to analyze the cardiovascular response of the fetus to varying degrees of umbilical vein and total cord occlusion.

To investigate the response of umbilical vein occlusion on fetal heart rate and umbilical blood flow an experimental model in the sheep was used. The experiments were performed on 11 sheep with a dated gestational age of 126–137 days (Künzel et al. 1977).

A catheter was advanced into the fetal aorta from the femoral artery and into the umbilical vein. The blood pressure was measured in these vessels and the arterial blood pressure waves were used to trigger the continuous fetal heart rate monitoring.

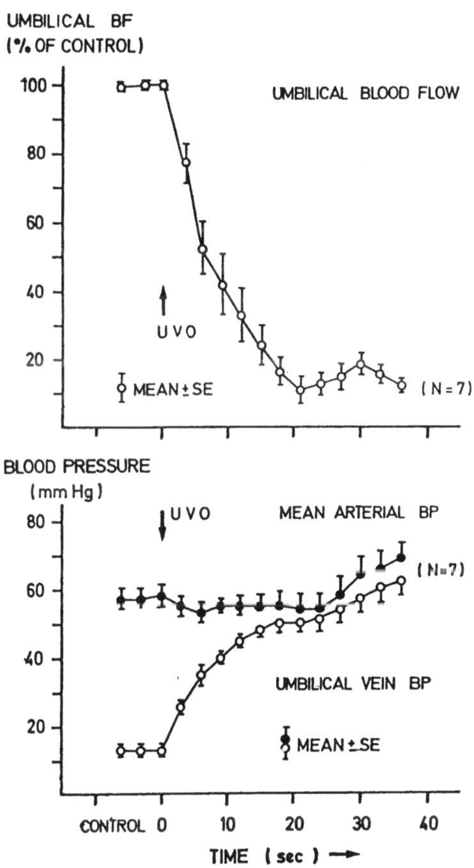

Fig. 2. Umbilical blood flow (% of control), mean arterial blood pressure, and umbilical vein blood pressure, following umbilical vein occlusion *(UVO)*. Umbilical blood flow falls as a response to the fall in perfusion pressure (= mean arterial BP − umbilical vein BP) across the placenta. (Künzel et al. 1977)

Umbilical blood flow was measured with an electromagnetic flow probe which was placed around the common umbilical vein. Total and partial cord occlusions were performed with an inflatable cuff placed around the umbilical cord. Fetal heart rate, blood pressure, and umbilical blood flow were continuously recorded throughout the experiments. Both before and during occlusion of the umbilical cord blood samples were obtained from the fetal aorta for pH, PCO_2, and oxygen saturation measurements. In additional experiments the mechanism of umbilical cord occlusion on umbilical blood flow was investigated.

The Mechanism of Umbilical Blood Flow Reduction During Labor

Umbilical blood flow can be simply reduced by compressing the umbilical vein, by constricting the umbilical artery, or both. In both cases a high extrinsic pressure increasses the resistance to flow that is located around the vessels of the umbilical cord. If the resistance is located in the umbilical vein, flow is reduced by a fall of the perfusion pressure (Fig. 2).

Figure 2 shows the response of the mean arterial blood pressure and the blood pressure in the umbilical vein in seven experiments if the umbilical vein is completely occluded. Within several seconds the umbilical vein blood pressure distal to the occlusion rises followed by a small drop in the arterial blood pressure. Umbilical blood flow falls as a result of the reduced perfusion pressure. The rise in blood pressure after 25 s might be a response to the fall in fetal oxygen saturation, because the umbilical blood flow was near to zero at this time.

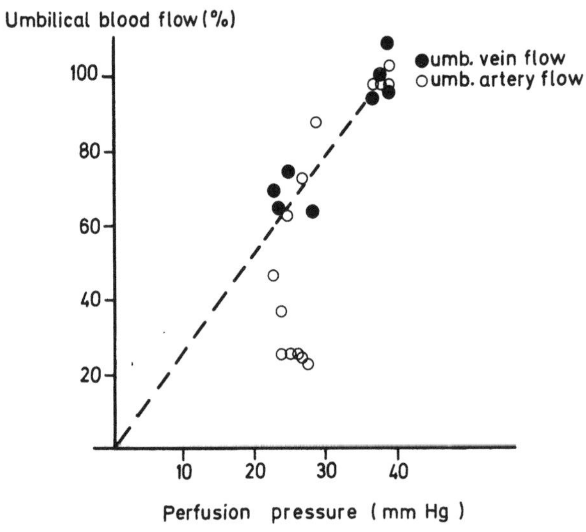

Fig. 3. Umbilical blood flow in the umbilical vein and umbilical artery. An inflatable cuff was placed around the umbilical cord. Slow inflation of the cuff shows decrease in both flows as a response to the fall in perfusion pressure. Decreasing pulsations in the umbilical artery indicate an increased resistance to flow in this vessel. This is demonstrated by the deviation of the flow measurements from the line of identity

By extreme external force exerted on the umbilical cord it might be possible that both vessels become occluded. An example of such a situation is shown in Fig. 3. The blood flow and blood pressure from both umbilical vessels were recorded. By inflation of a cuff placed around the cord, the flow in both vessels decreased in proportion to the reduction of the perfusion pressure from 40 to 25 mm Hg. From this time on a steep fall of blood flow occurred in parallel with an increase in resistance to flow in the umbilical artery evident by the ceasing pulsations in this vessel and an increase of resistance in the umbilical circulation.

The responses of the blood pressure in the fetal aorta, the umbilical artery, and the umbilical vein under these particular circumstances are shown in Fig. 4. Following cord compression, the blood pressure distal to the location of the occlusion rose in the umbilical vein and fell in the umbilical artery. This led to a perfusion pressure of zero. Heart rate fell in response. After the release of the occlusion umbilical artery blood pressure rose accompanied for a short time by a further increase of umbilical vein blood pressure. The complete release of occlusion was then followed by the restoration of all parameters.

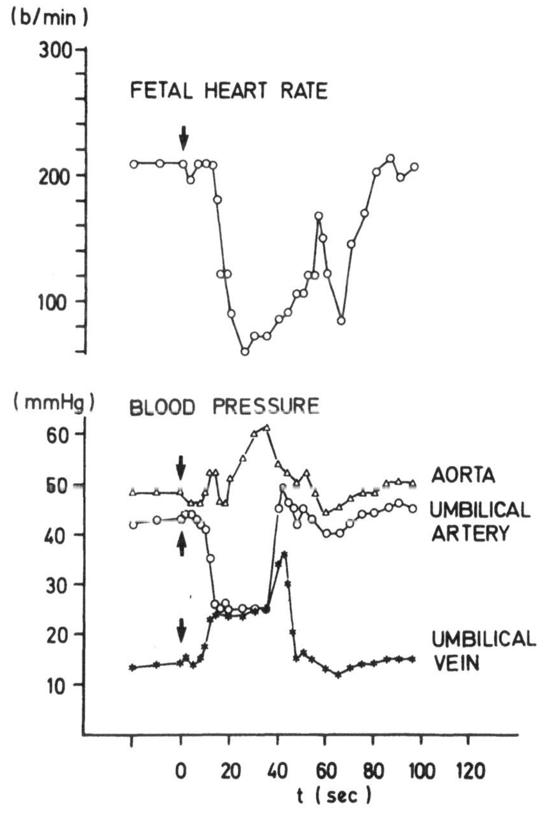

Fig. 4. Total umbilical cord occlusion (introduced slowly at the *arrow*) is accompanied by a fall in blood pressure in the umbilical artery and a rise in BP in the aorta and the umbilical vein. Fetal heart rate fell as a response to total cord occlusion

The Response of Fetal Heart Rate and Blood Pressure to Umbilical Vein Occlusion

The fall in fetal heart rate is closely related to the reduction in umbilical blood flow and fetal oxygen deprivation (Künzel et al. 1977). Following umbilical vein occlusion, the blood pressure in the umbilical vein increased, followed by reduction in pulse pressure and delayed onset of heart rate deceleration (Fig. 5). The late onset of heart rate deceleration was generated by a fall in oxygen saturation (SO_2) in the fetal blood.

As already pointed out by Acheson et al. (1957), fetal oxygen consumption is compromised if the SO_2 in the fetal arterial blood falls below 40%. We have therefore grouped the experiments to the fetal SO_2 that was reached after 2 min umbilical vein occlusion. In the first group of experiments oxygen saturation following uterine vein occlusion was above 40% and in the second group oxygen saturation was below 40%. Umbilical blood flow was reduced in the first group by 48% and in the second group by 73%. Fetal heart rate responded in relation to the fall in blood flow. In cases of moderate hypoxia fetal heart rate showed no or just a slight change. In cases of severe reduction of umbilical blood flow the fetal heart rate dropped from 185 to 140 beats/min.

The alteration of the systolic, the diastolic, and the umbilical vein blood pressure was also dependent on the reduction of umbilical blood flow. The blood pressure increase was more pronounced in cases where the umbilical blood flow was reduced by 73%.

The fall in fetal heart rate as a percentage of the control showed a direct relationship to the fall in umbilical blood flow as a percentage of the control. A small change in umbilical blood flow was not followed by alterations in the fetal heart rate. If the flow, however, dropped below 60% of control, heart rate decreased significantly. During the recovery period fetal heart rate was in the normal range 2 min after

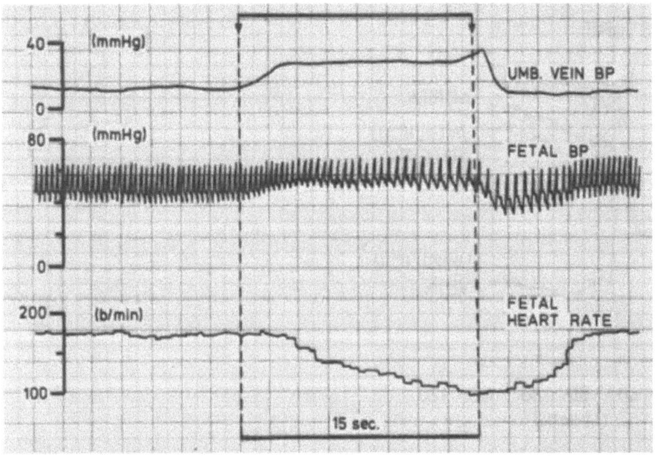

Fig. 5. Blood pressure in the umbilical vein and fetal aorta and fetal heart rate following umbilical vein occlusion over 15 s

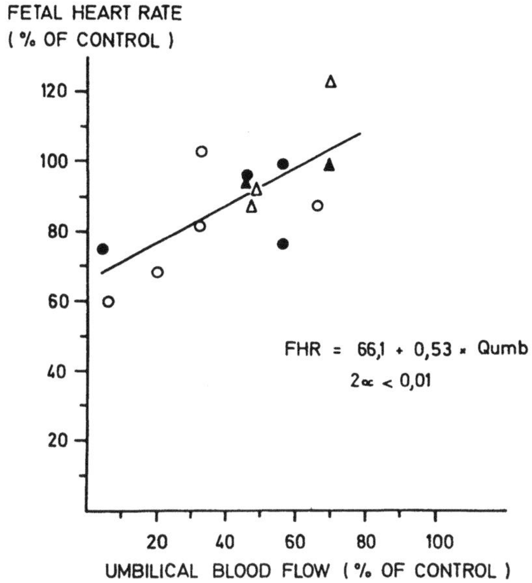

Fig. 6. Relationship between fall in umbilical blood flow and decrease in fetal heart rate

umbilical vein occlusion had been released and fetal blood pressure decreased within 3 min to values prior to occlusion.

The Response of Fetal Heart Rate and Blood Pressure to Total Cord Occlusion

Total cord occlusion where the umbilical artery and vein are occluded within seconds are very rare occasions during parturition. It has been tempting, however, to look at the differences of the cardiovascular response to total cord occlusion and umbilical vein occlusion in a sheep model (Künzel et al. 1980).

Eleven sheep with a dated gestational age of 126–137 days were used for the experiments. The studies were conducted on an acute preparation, where each sheep was anesthetized with 0.5%–1.0% halothane in nitrous oxide and 30% oxygen. After relaxation the sheep was mechanically ventilated. The preparation of the animal was the same as in umbilical vein occlusion. Total cord occlusion was performed within 1 s by inflating the cuff which was placed around the umbilical cord. An original recording of a total cord occlusion over 6 s is shown in Fig. 7. Umbilical blood flow decreased to zero and fetal heart rate fell within 0.2 s paralleled by a rise in blood pressure. The magnitude of the fall in fetal heart rate was dependent on the duration of flow reduction. If the flow was reduced for less than 10 s fetal heart rate fell from 190 to 150 beats/min. It decreased, however, to 90 beats/min, if the flow was reduced for 60–120 s. The increase in blood pressure was also related to the time of flow reduction.

After release of the complete reduction of umbilical blood flow there was a steep fall in systolic and diastolic blood pressure within 20 s (Fig. 8). This was more

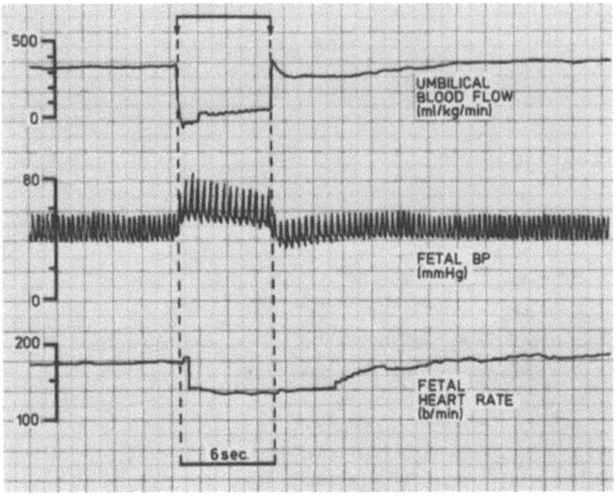

Fig. 7. Original recording of umbilical blood flow, fetal arterial blood pressure, and fetal heart rate following total cord occlusion over 6 s

pronounced in the group where umbilical blood flow had been reduced for 120 s. Blood pressure and fetal heart rate were in the range of the control 5–10 min after the occlusion had ceased.

Heart Rate and Blood Pressure Immediately After Cord Occlusion

In total cord occlusion the immediate increase in blood pressure and fall in heart rate are caused by the abrupt rise in vascular resistance in the umbilical circulation, followed by alterations which are caused by the subsequent developing hypoxia. We have carried out a preliminary analysis of the heart rate and the blood pressure response immediately after the cord had been occluded.

In 12 observations (Table 1) the acid base values of the control were in the normal range. The pH was 7.37 (group A). The respective umbilical blood flow was 148 ml/kg per min. In seven experiments (group B) the pH was 7.21–7.30 and the umbilical blood flow 88 ml/kg per min; seven fetuses were in poor condition with a pH of 7.20 and less and a blood flow of 50 ml/kg per min (group C).

Fetuses with severe acidosis had the lowest blood pressure at control and the lowest blood pressure response following total cord occlusion. The systolic blood pressure was 40 mm Hg in the control and increased by 5 mm Hg. In contrast the normal oxygenated fetus had a systolic blood pressure of 55 mm Hg. It rose to 70 mm Hg, reaching its maximum after 2–3 s. After a short decline it exhibited a further rise after 8–10 s as a response to the fetal hypoxemia.

The fetal circulation time from the umbilical vein to the carotid artery is 1.9 s (SD, 0.2) (Power and Longo 1975). That observation permits one to conclude that after total cord occlusion the baroreceptors generate the initial response of fetal heart rate deceleration, followed by the stimulation of the chemoreceptors as a response to hypoxemia.

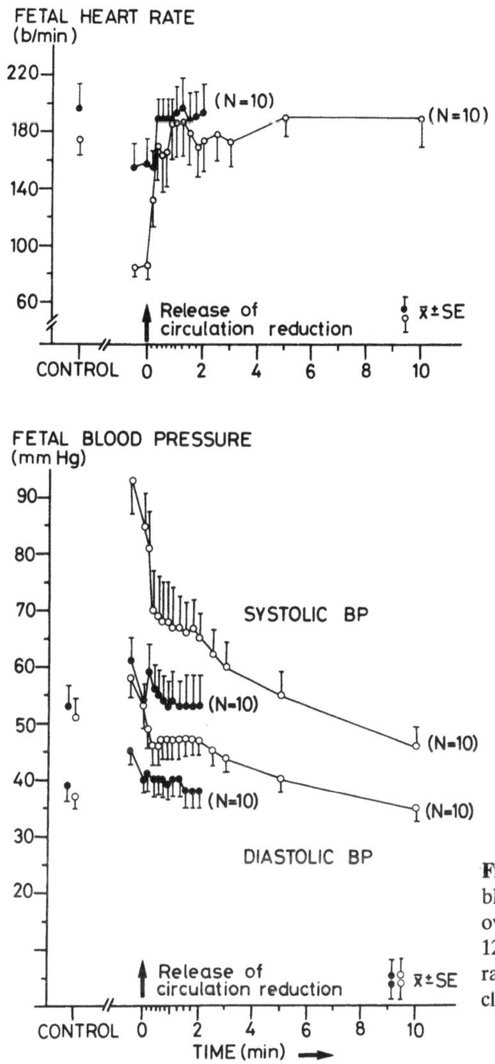

Fig. 8. Fetal heart rate and systolic and diastolic blood pressure following total cord occlusion over less than 10 s *(closed circles)* and over 60–120 s *(open circles)*. Blood pressure and heart rate response related to the time of cord occlusion

Concerning total cord occlusion the following are some thoughts on the physiological mechanism of the first response, i.e., the fall in fetal heart rate and rise in fetal arterial blood pressure following total cord occlusion.

Theoretical Considerations on Total Cord Occlusion

The first cardiovascular response after total cord occlusion is a rise in blood pressure followed by a decrease in fetal heart rate. This initial response of the fetal blood pressure to total cord occlusion depends on the magnitude of umbilical blood flow and fetal arterial blood pressure in the control. During fetal life, cardiac output is

Table 1. Values for mean, standard deviation, and total number for the pH, oxygen saturation (%), mean arterial blood pressure, and umbilical blood flow prior to total cord occlusion

	pH	Oxygen saturation (%)	Mean arterial blood pressure (mmHg)	Umbilical blood flow (ml/kg/min)
Group A (pH, 7.31)				
$\bar{x}$	7.37	61	46	148
SD	0.04	10	7	79
n	12	10	12	10
Group B (pH, 7.21–7.30)				
$\bar{x}$	7.27	54	40	88
SD	0.01	6	6	9
n	8	5	8	5
Group C (pH, <7.20)				
$\bar{x}$	7.18	26	33	51
SD	0.02	13	3	8
n	7	6	7	6

approximately evenly distributed in the fetal tissue and in the placenta (Rudolph and Heymann 1973). The blood pressure in the fetal aorta *(p)* is, according to Eq. (1), dependent on the cardiac output, i.e., tissue blood flow (Q_T) plus umbilical blood flow (Q_{umb}), and vascular resistance of the placental (R_{Pl}) and tissue circulation (R_{Ti}).

$$p = (Q_{umb} + Q_T) \times \frac{R_{Ti} \times R_{Pl}}{R_{Pl} + R_{Ti}} \qquad (1)$$

During fetal deterioration the blood pressure falls, paralleled by a decrease in umbilical blood flow and tissue blood flow and an increase in vascular resistance. The increase in fetal arterial blood pressure (FABP) following total cord occlusion is therefore related to the umbilical blood flow at control. The increase in blood pressure following total cord occlusion (TCO) also depends on the adjustment of cardiac function to the rise in resistance of umbilical circulation and on the redistribution of cardiac output from the placental and fetal tissue.

There is a relationship between umbilical blood flow in the control and the rise in FABP following TCO (Fig. 9). There was maximum response of 15 mmHg to TCO at high umbilical flow rates of more than 150 ml/kg per min. A proportional fall in the BP response occurred if uterine blood flow fell below 100 ml/kg per min. This is not in agreement with the expected rise in BP if the cardiac output remained constant. At high flow rates of 250 ml/kg per min a rise in the BP of about 50 mmHg should occur and decrease in proportion depending on the BP before TCO.

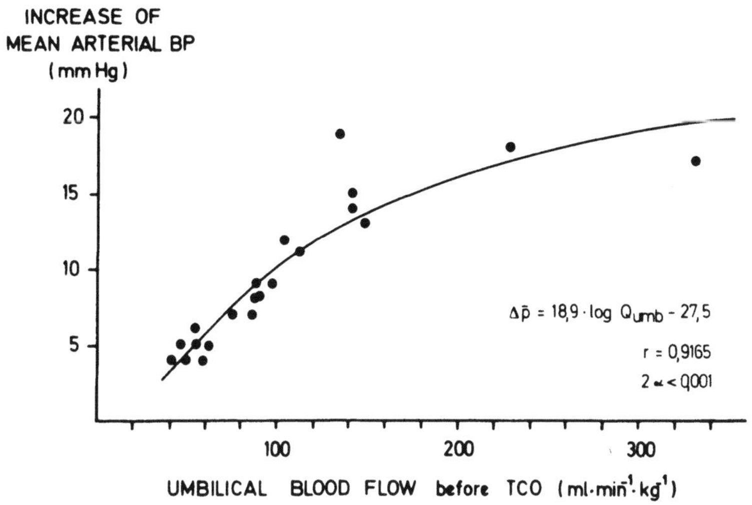

Fig. 9. Increase in mean arterial blood pressure following total cord occlusion *(TCO)* in relation to umbilical blood flow before TCO. At low flow rates increase in BP is low; it increases proportionately at higher flow rates prior to occlusion

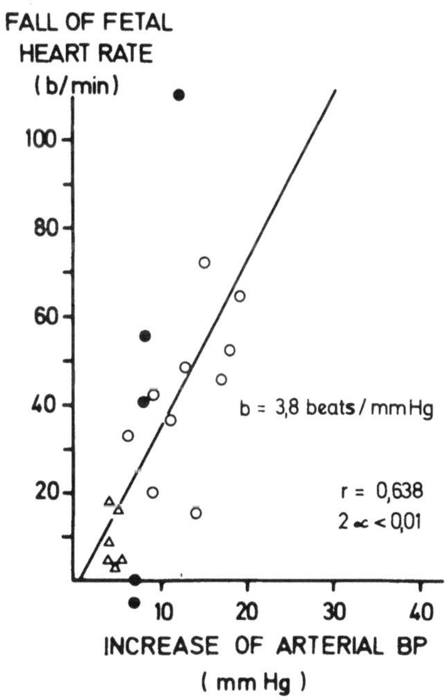

Fig. 10. Relationship between fall in fetal heart rate and rise in systolic blood pressure after 3 s of total cord occlusion. The symbols indicate fetuses with pH >7.31 (○), pH 7.21–7.30 (●), and pH ≤7.20 (△). Severe acidotic fetuses show the slightest response in fetal heart rate deceleration and blood pressure elevation to TCO during the initial seconds

The indefinite rise in placental vascular resistance and the subsequent increase in arterial BP is, however, counteracted by a fall in FHR (Fig. 10). An increase of FABP to 20 mmHg is followed by a fall of 70 beats/min. The fall in fetal heart rate was, however, reduced if the BP increased by only 5 mmHg. This occurred preferentially in the moderate and severe acidotic fetus.

Conclusions

The fetal circulation is protected from uterine contractions and external traumatic influences by the amniotic fluid which surrounds the fetus and the umbilical cord. The loss of amniotic fluid creates the presumption for a disturbed umbilical circulation by either umbilical vein occlusion or umbilical artery compression. In the first case a fall in perfusion pressure across the placenta with subsequent reduction of umbilical blood flow leads to fetal deterioration if a critical flow is reached. Heart rate deceleration is late in onset, similar to that caused by reducing uterine blood flow. In total cord occlusion, however, the first heart rate response during the first few seconds is generated by the baroreceptors, which is followed after 8–10 s by a response now due to the fetal hypoxia. Whether the decelerations are caused by umbilical vein occlusion or by occlusion of the umbilical artery is of less clinical significance. Both are followed by fetal hypoxemia often combined with fetal deterioration and fetal acidosis.

References

Acheson GH, Dawes GS, Mott JC (1957) Oxygen consumption and the arterial oxygen saturation in foetal and newborn lambs. J Physiol (Lond) 135:623

Borell U, Fernstrom J, Ohlsom L, Wiqwist N (1965) Influence of uterine contractions on the utero-placental blood flow at term. Am J Obstet Gynecol 93:44

Greiss FC (1965) The effect of labor on uterine blood flow. Am J Obstet Gynecol 93:917

Künzel W, Mann LI, Bhakthavathsalam A, Airomlooi J, Lin M (1977) The effect of umbilical vein occlusion on fetal oxygenation, cardiovascular parameters and fetal electroencephalogram. Am J Obstet Gynecol 128:201

Künzel W, Mann LI, Bhakthavathsalam A, Airomlooi J (1980) Cardiovascular, metabolic and fetal brain function observation following total cord occlusion. J Perinat Med 8:73

Power GG, Longo LD (1975) Fetal circulation times and their implications for tissue oxygenation. Gynecol Invest 6:342

Rudolph AM, Heymann MA (1973) Control of foetal circulation. In: Comline KS, Cross K, Dawes GS, Nathanielsz PW (eds) Foetal and neonatal physiology. Proceedings of the Sir Barcroft, centenary symposium, 25–27 July 1972. Cambridge University Press, Cambridge

Neurohumoral and Metabolic Response of the Fetus to Hypoxia

Adrenal-Medullary Activity and Cardiovascular Control in the Fetal Sheep

C. T. JONES[1] and G. WEI

Introduction

In adult life the function of the adrenal medulla in eliciting acute cardiovascular responses to stress is probably relatively minor [1, 2], that role being fulfilled by the peripheral sympathetic system. The gland is likely to have longer-term, modulating influences, at least through the secretion of adrenaline [3], and possibly through the production of enkephalin and other peptides [4–6]. Moreover, medullary catecholamines appear to be important in the adult for glucose homeostasis [7].

In the fetus, with incomplete sympathetic innervation [8] and progressive development of the medulla [9, 10], the role of the adrenal and its secretions in cardiovascular control is unclear. The fetal tissues can respond directly to catecholamine stimulation, often with marked sensitivity and at plasma levels comparable to those seen under physiological conditions [11–14]. Also, the fetal adrenal medulla produces peptides like VIP and enkephalin [4–6]. However, the quantitative significance of such secretions is not yet established. Moreover, although the conditions leading to adrenal output are well established for the adult, the fact that the medullary output from the adrenal gland can occur via non-neural as well as neural pathways is indicative of potentially more complex control pathways [15]. One feature of fetal life that is particularly clear is that very high plasma levels of adrenaline and noradrenaline, much above adult values, are detected particularly during birth [16–18] (Fig. 1). Hence, the importance of the fetal medulla is probably high, especially

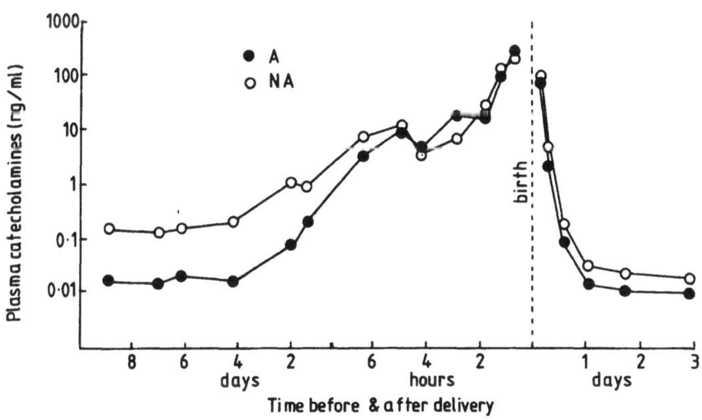

Fig. 1. Changes in plasma adrenaline (●) and noradrenaline (○) concentration in fetal sheep and newborn lambs. Arterial samples were collected daily from one sheep

[1] The Nuffield Institute for Medical Research, Oxford University, GB-Oxford OX3 9DS

Fetal Heart Rate Monitoring
Ed. by W. Künzel

during delivery, although it is notable that sheep fetuses from which the adrenal medulla is removed well before normal term do not appear to have an abnormally high mortality [6, 19; unpublished work].

Control of Catecholamine Output in the Fetus

The majority of studies on adrenal-medullary activity in the fetus rely on the measurement of plasma catecholamine levels [9, 10, 13, 17–21]. Some studies have involved quantification of output from the adrenal gland [22, 23], but in these anaesthesia has been used and this both elevates production substantially and favours noradrenaline output at the expense of adrenaline [24]. Limited work has been done with adrenal cells on the developing mechanism of catecholamine production [10]. Use of plasma catecholamine concentrations, particularly adrenaline, can be a good index of elevated activity in the adrenal medulla, since under conditions such as fetal hypoxia most of the plasma source is adrenal [6, 19; unpublished work]. However, resting plasma levels of noradrenaline appear to be unaffected by adrenal demedullation of fetal sheep [6, 19; unpublished work]. It is possible that the plasma level is not affected only by adrenal output. Turnover is very rapid [20], and clearance across the placenta, presumably by metabolism [20], is almost complete [16] (Table 1). Hence, any redistribution of the fetal circulation that changes the proportion of the cardiac output passing to the placenta [25] could of itself cause changes in the plasma catecholamine level.

If it is accepted that the plasma level, at least of adrenaline, is an adequate reflection of secretion, then medullary activity is elevated to a greater extent in the fetus than in the adult by hypoxia, hypercapnia, hypoglycaemia, haemorrhage, reduced uterine blood flow and pyrogens (Table 2). The pathway develops over the last third of gestation in the fetal sheep in such a way that in response to hypoxia, for instance, there is a progressive increase in adrenaline and noradrenaline response [9, 10, 16,

Table 1. Plasma concentration[a] and placental clearance of catecholamines in 125- to 133-day sheep fetuses

Plasma concentration (pg/ml)	Placental clearance (ng/min per kg fetus)
Adrenaline	
41 ± 20	10.3 ± 3.4
361 ± 129	119 ± 57
1168 ± 655	482 ± 279
Noradrenaline	
157 ± 66	41.3 ± 16.4
743 ± 295	218 ± 79
4239 ± 1766	789 ± 283

[a] Results are means ± SD of four to six experiments

Table 2. Plasma catecholamine concentrations[a] in 120- to 135-day sheep fetuses in different conditions

Condition	Plasma catecholamines (pg/ml)	
	Adrenaline	Noradrenaline
Resting	39 ± 19	216 ± 110
Hypoxia (8.5% O_2)	1241 ± 531	2396 ± 883
Hypoxia (8% O_2) hypercapnia (6% CO_2)	1589 ± 802	4107 ± 1539
Reduced uterine blood flow (30%–50% of normal)	1901 ± 763	8934 ± 4215
Hypoglycaemia (glucose ~0.5 μmol/ml)	367 ± 114	932 ± 278
Haemorrhage (25%)	1432 ± 642	5237 ± 3146

[a] Samples were taken from femoral artery. Results are means ± SD of four to eight experiments. Responses were measured after 30 min of treatment

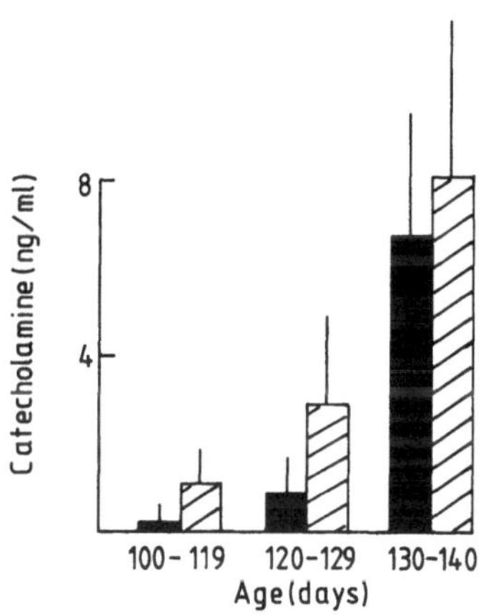

Fig. 2. Changes in plasma adrenaline (■) and noradrenaline (▨), in fetal sheep of different gestational ages, in response to hypoxia induced by maternal breathing of 9% O_2 + 3% CO_2 for 30 min

18, 20, 22, 23] (Fig. 2). Whether this is a change in the capacity of the adrenal to respond or in the sensitivity of afferent pathways influenced by hypoxia is not known. The change in response does correlate with an alteration of catecholamine content of the gland and with sensitivity to splanchnic stimulation [9, 22, 23].

The responses of the adrenal show a positive correlation with changes in pH and pO_2, which suggests the possibility that a major stimulus occurs via chemoreceptors [18, 20] (Fig. 3). The fact that these are enhanced by elevation of pCO_2 (Table 2, Fig. 4) suggests that both central and peripheral chemoreceptors may be involved. Whether the baroreceptors provide an important afferent signal for catecholamine secretion in the fetus is less clear, as stimuli such as haemorrhage could exert their action via chemoreceptors. The proposal that changes in pO_2 have direct effects upon the chromaffin cells of the medulla [9, 20] has not been convincingly proven, and in those early studies such effects were suggested to occur only below a pO_2 of

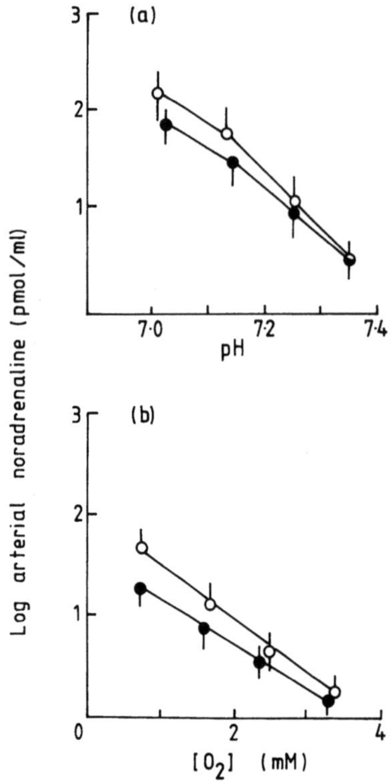

Fig. 3a, b. Relation between changes in plasma adrenaline (●) and noradrenaline (○) concentrations during maternal hypoxia [20] and fetal plasma at different pH (**a**) and [O_2] (**b**) values. The fetuses were at 128–135 days of gestation

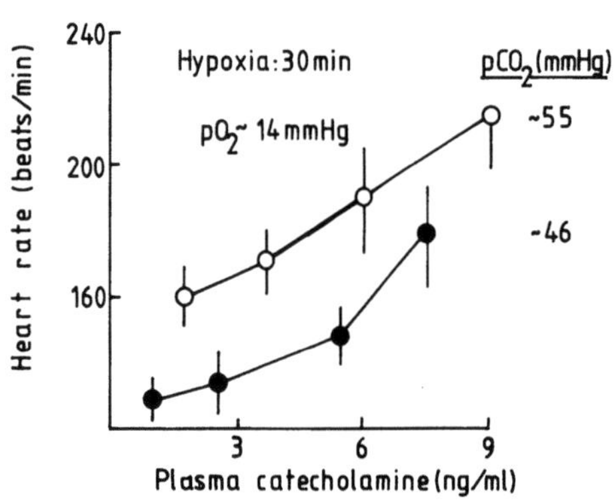

Fig. 4. The relation between fetal heart rate and plasma catecholamine concentration after 30 min of maternal breathing of 9% O_2 + 3% CO_2 (●), or 9% O_2 + 6% CO_2 (○)

about 5 mmHg, a level well below that expected under normal physiological conditions. However, the possible existence of a nonneural pathway of stimulation [16] has to be resolved before the question of direct actions of oxygen.

As hypoxia is a powerful stimulus to catecholamine secretion in the fetus, it is not surprising that a reduction of uterine blood flow to levels that depress fetal arterial pO_2 by about 25%–30% is also a potent stimulus to adrenal-medullary activity (Table 2). This effect is greater than that for hypoxia alone, and although it can in part be explained by the associated hypercapnia other factors must be involved in causing the marked catecholamine secretion in response to reduced uterine blood flow (Table 2). A potential explanation would be diminished placental clearance associated with depressed placental oxygen consumption caused by low maternal-placental blood flow. This stimulus for elevation of the plasma catecholamine level is likely to be important physiologically. If spontaneous depressions of fetal heart rate can be used as an index of fetal hypoxia [26, 27], which in labour at least is caused potentially by uterine contraction [28, 29], then the associated increase in plasma catecholamines in this state (Table 3) could result from periods of reduced uterine blood flow.

Catecholamine responses to hypoglycaemia, a potent stimulator of adrenaline production in the adult [30], are graded and relatively large in the fetus (Fig. 5). This implies that the hypothalamic glucose receptor [30] is well developed in the near-term sheep fetus. However, other mechanisms are operating to regulate this pathway; the newborn lamb, which often has periods of hypoglycaemia, maintains very low plasma levels of adrenaline and noradrenaline (C.T. Jones and P. Johnson, unpublished work).

Table 3. Plasma catecholamine concentrations[a] in fetal sheep during spontaneous falls in heart rate

Heart rate	Plasma catecholamines (pg/ml)	
	Adrenaline	Noradrenaline
Before labour		
Normal heart rate (150–165 beats/min)	36 ± 12	211 ± 86
Spontaneous bradycardia (110–130 beats/min)	93 ± 47	476 ± 152
During labour		
Normal heart rate (155–170 beats/min)	111 ± 57	562 ± 210
Spontaneous bradycardia (115–130 beats/min)	314 ± 126	1143 ± 495

[a] Results are means ± SD measured in arterial samples collected within 1.5–2.5 min of the start of bradycardia in 10–12 separate episodes

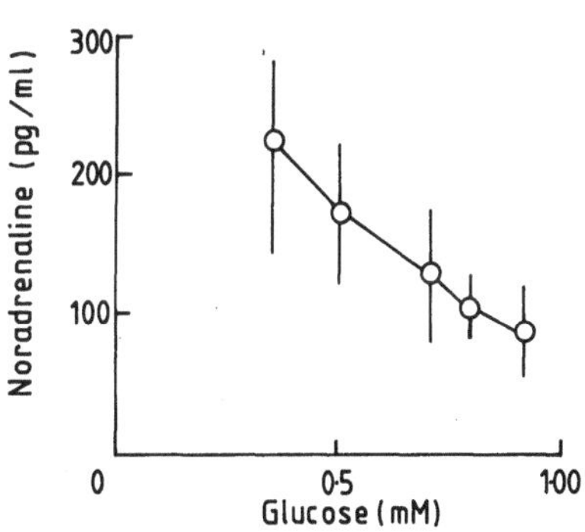

Fig. 5. Relation between plasma noradrenaline and glucose in fetal sheep at 125–135 days of gestation

Of all the fetal conditions leading to marked elevations of plasma catecholamines, birth (Fig. 1) causes the most profound effect, with close to pharmacological levels apparent during the expulsion phase [31]. It is not easy to explain the very high levels solely with reference to any of the mechanisms described above, unless perhaps a progressive deterioration in placental perfusion resulting ultimately in separation causes a substantial decline in the capacity of placental clearance of catecholamines. Compression of the fetal head during delivery could provide a particularly powerful stimulus for secretion. The high plasma catecholamine levels at birth are likely to be required to maintain high cardiac output and perfusion of heart and head, cause reabsorption of lung fluid, stimulate thermogenesis, increase hepatic glycogen breakdown, and enhance mental alertness [8, 9, 11–14, 16, 32–36].

The fetal adrenal medulla produces other factors that are potential regulators of cardiovascular function [4–6]. Thus, adrenal demedullation depresses the relatively high fetal level of met-enkephalin in plasma at least by about 60%. Moreover, stimulation of the splanchnic nerve to the calf adrenal causes a marked adrenal production of met-enkephalin [37].

Control of the Fetal Heart and Catecholamines

During pre- and postnatal development beta-receptor sensitivity in vitro and in vivo increases, since as sympathetic innervation proceeds there is a rise in beta-adrenergic receptor density and adenylate cyclase activity [38–42]. However, the importance of the sympathetic innervation in catecholamine removal means that the fetal heart tends to be apparently more sensitive to exogenous catecholamines than after birth, despite its incompletely developed receptor–adenylate cyclase system [8, 14, 43]. Thus, at the low end of the physiological level of plasma concentration noradrenaline in sheep has the potential to have marked effects upon the fetal heart, whereas in the adult this is not so (Table 4). The significance of such observations is that elevations of plasma catecholamines over the range of concentrations outlined in Table 2 will

Table 4. Relation between plasma catecholamine level and sensitivity of heart to noradrenaline

	Noradrenaline (ng/ml)	
	Fetus	Adult
Plasma level		
Resting	0.15– 0.3	0.03– 0.1
Hypoxia	1 – 10	0.2 – 0.5
Level causing positive ionotropic effect[a]		
Lower limit	0.04– 0.08	0.75– 1.5
50% of maximum response	10 – 20	75 –150
Maximum response	1000 –2000	>2000

[a] [14]

presumably have marked ionotropic, but not necessarily chronotropic [11, 13, 14, 16], effects on the fetal heart. Moreover, these responses are not saturated even at the very high plasma catecholamine levels observed during birth (Fig. 1). Clearly increased vagal activity will reduce the apparent sensitivity to sympathetic stimulation, as it does the heart rate, during hypoxia or noradrenaline infusion [11, 16, 20]. However, during noradrenaline infusion the marked chronotropic effect of noradrenaline leads to a maintenance of cardiac output despite a 25% fall in heart rate [13]. Although the fetal heart appears to have a limited capacity to increase stroke volume [44], it is clear that it has done so under these circumstances and may also do so during hypoxia [24]. The apparent sensitivity of the fetal heart to catecholamines is paradoxical when set against the close relationship between heart rate and cardiac output [44]. Its predominant function may be to maintain cardiac contractility at times when there is marked parasympathetic drive to depress heart rate and hence ensure that cardiac arrest does not occur during labour, for instance.

Such an action may be the mechanism that, when the plasma catecholamine concentration rises, causes first a fall in fetal heart rate and then a rise above resting levels [11], in consideration of the steady-state responses to fetal hypoxia [16] or the biphasic changes during infusion [11, 16]. The latter phase, in which the rate may be elevated, is caused by enhanced sympathetic stimulation overcoming vagal inhibition [16, 45]. The temporal interaction between sympathetic and parasympathetic stimulation in controlling heart rate is shown clearly by the effect of CO_2 (Fig. 4). The responses to catecholamines are enhanced when plasma CO_2 is elevated, and this appears to operate by reducing parasympathetic inhibition of the heart [45]. Thus the fetal responses to reduced uterine blood flow, which are first a reduced and then an

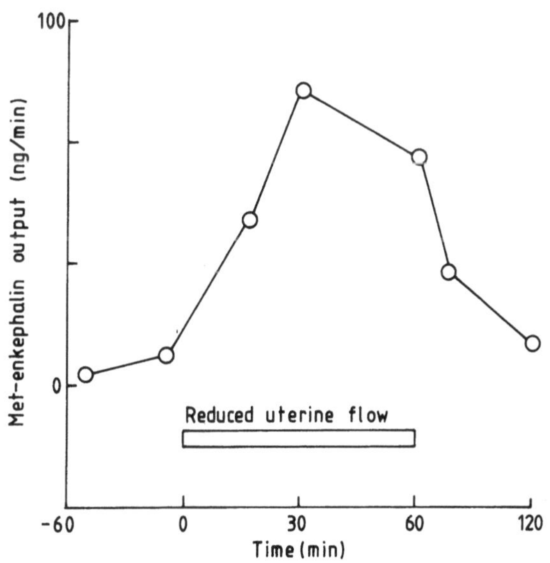

Fig. 6. The output of met-enkephalin from the placenta of a 130-day sheep fetus in response to a 68% reduction of uterine blood flow caused by the inflation of a "cuff" catheter around the uterine artery

enhanced heart rate, can be explained if hypoxia initially stimulates vagal activity and catecholamine output. Then, as the fetal asphyxia progresses, elevated CO_2 reduces vagal activity and the heart responds increasingly to elevated plasma catecholamines. These are important factors to remember when analysing fetal heart rate patterns, and particularly periods of bradycardia. Thus the duration of the fall in heart rate may not be indicative of the total duration of a fetal asphyxia, particularly when high plasma catecholamine levels are likely (Table 3).

Other adrenal-medullary secretions are also potentially capable of influencing or regulating fetal heart rate. The adrenal secretes VIP, enkephalins and NPY [4–6]. The last two at least appear to have cardiovascular effects and hence could be important signals of adrenal activity in the fetus. However, in the fetus the adrenal may not be the only source of such peptides or necessarily the major one under many circumstances. Thus reduction of uterine blood flow, causing asphyxia in the fetal sheep, leads to an enhanced output of enkephalin peptides (Fig. 6). Whether this offers a method of placental-fetal communication [46] important in cardiovascular regulation remains to be established, as does the quantitative significance of such plasma factors irrespective of the origin.

References

1. Celander O (1954) Acta Physiol Scand [Suppl] 116:1
2. Neil E (1975) Am Handbook Physiol Sect 7, Vol VI, p 473
3. Borkowski KR, Quinn P (1983) Br J Pharmacol 80:429
4. Viveros OH, Diliberto EJ, Hazum E, Chang K-J (1979) Mol Pharmacol 16:1101
5. Hexum TD, Barron BA (1984) In: Hanin I (ed) Dynamics of neurotransmitter function. Raven, New York, pp 137–142
6. Jones CT, Roebuck MM, Walker DW (1984) Neurol Neurobiol 8A:121
7. Deibert DC, DeFronzo RA (1980) J Clin Invest 65:717
8. Pappano AJ (1977) Pharmacol Rev 29:3
9. Comline RS, Silver M (1966) Br Med Bull 22:16
10. Jones CT (1979) In: Usdin E, Kopin I, Barchas J (eds) Catecholamines: Basic and clinical frontiers. Pergamon, Oxford, pp 854–856
11. Jones CT, Ritchie JWK (1978) J Physiol 285:381
12. Jones CT, Ritchie JWK (1978) J Physiol 285:395
13. Lorijn RHW, Longo LD (1980) Am J Physiol 239:R115
14. Friedman WF (1972) In: Friedman WF, Lesch M, Sonnenblick EH (eds) Neonatal heart disease. Grune and Stratton, New York, pp 21–49
15. Slotkin TA, Seidler FJ (1984) Neurol Neurobiol 8A:129
16. Jones CT (1980) In: Parvez H, Parvez S (eds) Biogenic amines in development. Elsevier/North-Holland, Amsterdam, pp 63–85
17. Irestedt L, Lagercrantz H, Hjemdahl P, Hagnevik K, Belfrage P (1982) Am J Obstet Gynecol 142:1004
18. Cohen WR, Piasecki GJ, Jackson BT (1982) Am J Physiol 243:R520
19. Johnston BM, Jones CT, Lagercrantz H, Roebuck MM, Walker DW (1984) J Physiol 348:68P
20. Jones CT, Robinson RO (1975) J Physiol 248:15
21. Padbury JF, Roberman B, Oddie TH, Hobel CJ, Fisher DA (1982) Obstet Gynecol 60:607
22. Comline RS, Silver M (1961) J Physiol 156:424
23. Comline RS, Silver IA, Silver M (1965) J Physiol 178:211
24. Jones CT, Rurak D (1976) Q J Exp Physiol 61:287
25. Rudolph AM (1984) J Dev Physiol 6:11
26. Jones CT, Ritchie JWK (1976) Biol Neonate 29:286
27. Harding R, Sigger JN, Wickham PJD (1983) J Dev Physiol 5:267

28. Parer JT, Krueger RT, Harris JL (1980) Am J Obstet Gynecol 136:478
29. Nathanielsz PW, Jansen CAM, Yu HK, Cabalum T (1984) In: Beard RW, Nathanielsz PW (eds) Fetal physiology and medicine, 2nd edn. Dekker, New York, pp 629–653
30. Brown MR, Fisher DA (1980) In: Bloom FE (ed) Peptides: Integrators of cell and tissue function. Raven, New York, pp 81–97
31. Lagercrantz H (1984) Neurol Neurobiol 8A:113
32. Downing SE, Gardner TH, Rocamora JM (1969) Am J Physiol 217:728
33. Moore RE (1963) Fed Proc 22:920
34. Frankenhaeuser M (1971) Brain Res 31:241
35. Lawson EE, Brown ER, Torday JS, Madansky DL, Taeusch HW (1978) Am Rev Respir Dis 118:1023
36. Abdellatif MM, Hollingsworth M (1980) Pediatr Res 14:916
37. Edwards AV, Jones CT, Tindell D (1985) J Physiol (in press)
38. Beck N, Park MK (1981) Dev Pharmacol Ther 3:129
39. Chen FC, Yamamuro HI, Roeske WR (1979) Eur J Pharmacol 58:255
40. Seidler FJ, Slotkin TA (1979) Br J Pharmacol 65:431
41. Wildenthal K (1973) J Clin Invest 52:2250
42. Clark JB, Vinicor F, Carr L, Clark CM (1980) Pediatr Res 14:291
43. Rosen MR, Hordoff AJ, Uvento JP, Danielo P (1977) Circ Res 40:390
44. Rudolph AM, Heymann MA (1974) Annu Rev Physiol 36:187
45. Gu W (1984) DPhil Thesis, Oxford University
46. Jones CT, Gu W, Parer JT, Lafeber HN, Rolph TP, Harding JE (1985) In: Jones CT, Nathanielsz PW (eds) Physiological development of fetus and newborn. Academic, London, pp 11–20

The Dip Area: A Measure of Acid Base Alterations?

W. KÜNZEL[1], E. KASTENDIECK[2], M. HOHMANN[1], and A. JENSEN[1,3]

It is a saying in old textbooks that the fetus, if in danger during parturition, decreases its heart rate to below 100 beats/min and remains at this level during the following contractions of the uterus. Depending on the dilation of the cervix and the stage of the fetal head, cesarean section is performed or a forceps is applied to deliver the baby.

The continuous recording of fetal heart rate (FHR) during labor has made these heart rate alterations detectable. A number of papers have described that not only the slowing of FHR between the consecutive contractions leads to fetal hazard, but also the decelerations that are observed during the contractions. There is a direct relationship between the incidence and the severity of heart decelerations and fetal outcome and the acid base status in the cord blood after birth (reviewed by Fischer et al. 1973).

With an "index of fetal welfare in labor" Tipton and Shelley (1971) put forward using the dip area as a measure of fetal condition during birth. From the assumption that the dip area mirrors the duration of fetal hypoxia it may be concluded that the dip area could also be used to estimate the acid base alterations during labor.

The Dip Area and Acid Base Alterations During Labor in Man

A first approach to estimate this relationship was made 10 years ago (Kastendieck et al. 1974). The dip area and the change in base excess between the fetal scalp and umbilical artery blood were measured. The deceleration area was calculated by planimetry. In calculating the dip area, no differentiation was made between the early, variable, and late deceleration. As a result of these measurements in the human fetus, it could be shown that, if there were no or only small decelerations, no change of base excess in the fetal blood could be measured. With rising dip area, however, there was an increased loss of buffer base in the fetal blood. With a dip area of 300 beats/min · min the change in base excess was about 10 mEq/liter. These data were collected at the end of the second stage of labor.

In a second set of experiments in the human fetus during labor the dip area was measured during the first stage of labor and for comparison also during the second stage of labor (Künzel and Cornely 1976). In this study 39 women during labor were

[1] Frauenklinik und Hebammenlehranstalt der Justus-Liebig-Universität Gießen, Klinikstr. 28, D-6300 Gießen
[2] Universitäts-Frauenklinik, Josef-Schneider-Str. 4, D-8700 Würzburg
[3] University of California, San Francisco School of Medicine, Cardiovascular Research Institute, San Francisco, CA 94143, USA

Fetal Heart Rate Monitoring
Ed. by W. Künzel

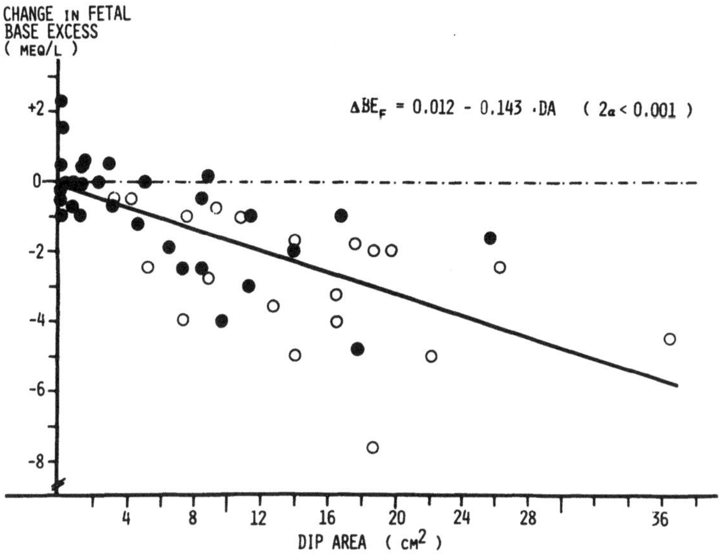

Fig. 1. The relationship between the alteration of base excess in the fetal blood and the dip area of the FHR. The *closed circles* represent measurements during the first stage and the *open circles* measurements during the second stage of labor. The base excess remains unchanged if no heart rate alterations occur; it decreases, however, if deceleration of the FHR takes place. With increasing dip area the deviation of the acid base alterations also rises. (Künzel and Cornely 1976)

investigated (Fig. 1). There is no striking difference in the correlation coefficient of both parameters between the first and second stage of labor.

The dip area was less, however, in the first group (9.9 beats/min · min; SD, 11.9; *N*, 30) than when measured during the second stage of labor (42.8 beats/min · min; SD, 30.6; *N*, 20). The results of the former experiments are in agreement with the second experimental approach. An interesting observation was: if no decelerations are present, no change in base excess takes place. With increasing dip area, however, the increase in base excess was paralleled by an increase in the deviation of acid base alterations. With a dip area of 200 beats/min · min, the fall in base excess ranged from 1.5 to 7 mEq/liter.

The deviation of these metabolic changes during labor for a given cardiovascular alteration in the fetus is certainly influenced by various factors: it may be speculated that:

1. The fetal cardiovascular response to a definite time of hypoxia may vary.
2. At normal fetal oxygenation the production of lactate between the various hypoxic episodes may be smaller than that of the lactate which is generated if the fetus is already under hypoxic stress.
3. The disappearance of lactate from the fetal blood may not only depend on fetal oxygenation after fetal hypoxia has occurred, but also on the concentration gradient that exists for lactate between the mother and fetus across the placenta.

In an experimental model of the sheep fetus the cardiovascular response and the metabolic alterations of the fetus to hypoxia induced by the reduction of uterine blood flow was investigated (Künzel et al. 1981).

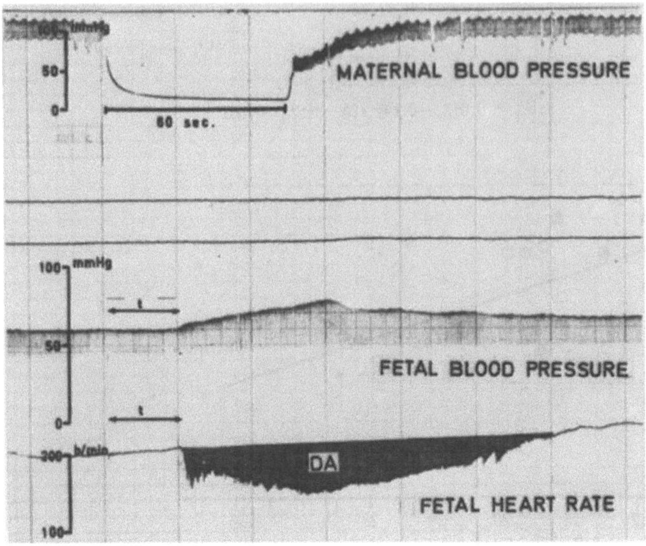

Fig. 2. Maternal and fetal blood pressure and fetal heart rate following the reduction of uterine blood flow for 60 s. The maternal blood pressure was measured distal to the location of occlusion to ensure complete reduction of uterine blood flow

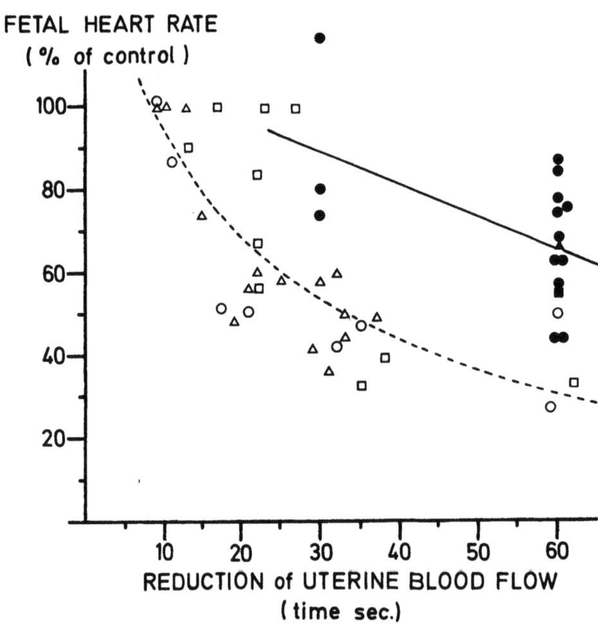

Fig. 3. Fetal heart rate response as a percentage of control related to the time of occlusion of the maternal aorta. The *open symbols* indicate the response in the unanesthetized animal and the *filled symbols* in the anesthetized animal. The *triangles, squares,* and *circles* show the related oxygen saturation in the fetus: ○●, $SO_2 > 50\%$; △▲, SO_2 40%–50%; □■, $SO_2 < 40\%$. There is a good relationship between the fall in fetal heart rate and the time of blood flow reduction in both groups: [FHR_{NA} (% of control) = $179 - 84 \log t$ ($2\alpha < 0.001$; *r,* 0.782; *N,* 33) and FHR_A (% of control) = $114 - 0.79t$($2\alpha < 0.05$; *r,* 0.532; *N,* 16)]. The response of the unanesthetized animal to hypoxia is more pronounced than that of the stressed fetus. (Künzel et al. 1981)

The Cardiovascular Response of the Sheep Fetus to Hypoxia

Experiments were performed on acute and chronic preparations of the sheep fetus. Catheters were placed via the femoral artery into the fetal aorta, one for fetal blood sampling and another for the continuous measurement of fetal heart rate and fetal arterial blood pressure. Uterine blood flow was reduced by an inflatable balloon placed in the maternal aorta. A catheter for blood pressure measurements was placed with its tip below the site of the occlusion to ensure complete reduction of uterine blood flow occurred.

Thirty-three experiments were performed on unanesthetized, and 16 experiments on anesthetized, fetuses. Uterine blood flow was reduced for 10–60 s.

Following complete occlusion of the maternal aorta (Fig. 2), the blood pressure distal to the occlusion fell to about 10 mmHg, with a delay of 10 s. Fetal blood pressure started to rise and fetal heart rate fell, both approachig a maximum response shortly after the release of the aorta occlusion. The maximum response of fetal heart rate deceleration and blood pressure elevation were used for calculation.

Fetal Heart Rate and Deceleration Area

The fall in fetal heart rate (as a percentage of control) was related to the time that uterine blood flow was reduced (Fig. 3). There was no evidence that the fetal cardio-

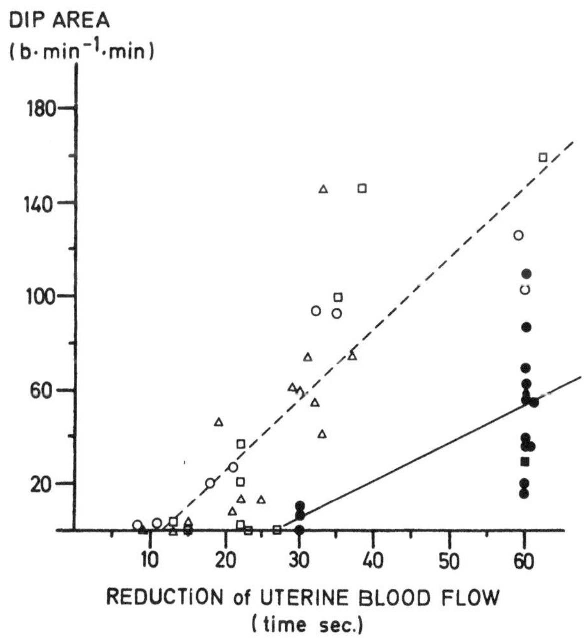

Fig. 4. The dip area (DA) of the FHR in the unanesthetized and anesthetized animal in relation to the time of blood flow reduction. The dip area increases if the time of flow reduction rises, although this is more pronounced in the cases which were not under acute experimental conditions. $DA_{NA} = 0.46t - 5.32$; r, 0.84; $2\alpha < 0.001$; N, 33. $DA_A = 0.23t - 40.8$; r, 0.619; $2\alpha < 0.05$; N, 16. (For symbols see Fig. 3.) (Künzel et al. 1981)

vascular response to hypoxia is related to oxygen saturation at control. The different symbols in Fig. 3 mingle with each other. There is, however, a significant difference in the fall of FHR between the anesthetized fetus as shown by the *filled symbols* and the unanesthetized group of experiments.

The same relationship also exists for the dip area and the duration of blood flow reduction (Fig. 4). As in the human fetus in the sheep the dip area is also scattered over a wide range from 40 to 140 beats/min · min for a definite time of flow reduction of, e.g., 30 s.

The unanesthetized fetus exhibited a different response to hypoxia than the fetus of the anesthetized mother, which might be of importance for the application of sedative drugs during labor. The reduced deceleration area may also be of importance if the fetus is monitored during cesarean section.

Systolic Blood Pressure

During the reduction in uterine blood flow the increase in fetal blood pressure was also related to the time of flow reduction. It was also influenced by anesthesia although not to the extent that the heart rate was. The rate in systolic blood pressure

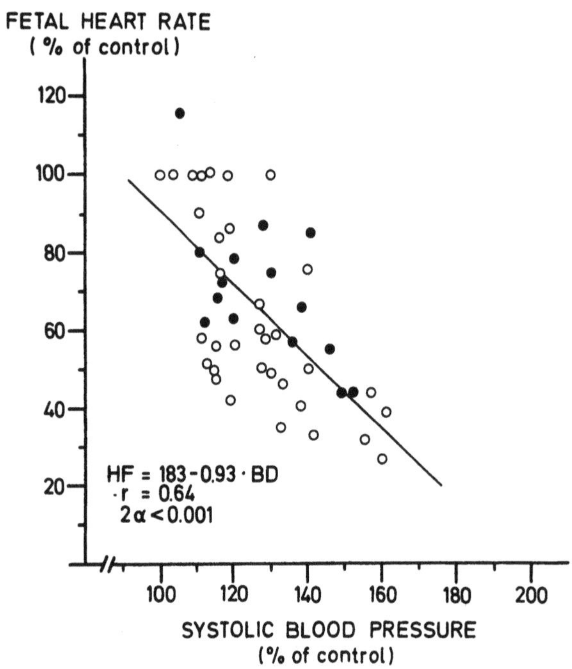

Fig. 5. The relationship between the fall in the FHR and systolic blood pressure (% of control). The fall in heart rate is related to the rise in blood pressure. The measurements in the unanesthetized fetus *(open circles)* mingle with those of the anesthetized fetus *(closed circles)* so that one might assume that the rise in blood pressure and reduced baroreceptor response is the cause of the attenuation of FHR response in the anesthetized sheep fetus. FHR (% of control) = 183 − 0.93 systolic blood pressure (% of control). $2\alpha < 0.001$; *r*, 0.643; *N*, 49. (Künzel et al. 1981)

was less pronounced in the fetus of the anesthesized mother. The blood pressure, however, also exhibited a wide range of response even at a constant time of hypoxia.

The relationship of the maximum response of fetal heart rate and the maximum response of systolic blood pressure to fetal hypoxia is shown in Fig. 5. An increase in blood pressure to 120% of the control is followed by a fall in fetal heart rate to 70% of the control. There is still, however, wide variation in the fetal heart rate response to the increase of fetal systolic blood pressure.

These data of the chronic and acute preparations mingle, suggesting that the different response in both groups is in part due to the varying increase in fetal arterial blood pressure to fetal hypoxia.

From these observations one might speculate that the heart rate response is modulated by:

1. Alterated sensitivity of the chemoreceptors and baroreceptors or both following anesthesia
2. Decreased fetal oxygen consumption during the application of narcotic drugs
3. Altered baroreceptor or chemoreceptor sensitivity by the circulating catecholamines in fetal blood

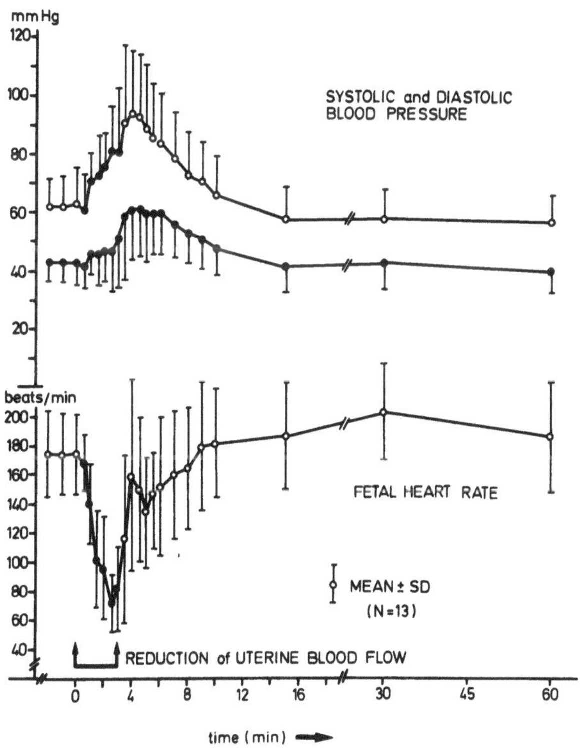

Fig. 6. The alteration in FHR *(bottom)* and systolic blood pressure and diastolic blood pressure *(top)* following reduction of uterine blood flow. Values are given as means and standard deviations *(vertical bars)*; ↑—↑, the time of blood flow reduction (180 s); ○●, values before and after fetal hypoxia. (Künzel et al. 1983)

Metabolic Alterations and Dip Area Following Fetal Hypoxia

The impact of fetal hypoxia on the metabolic alteration in fetal blood following the reduction in uterine blood flow was investigated in 13 experiments on seven near-term pregnant sheep (Künzel et al. 1983). Uterine blood flow was reduced for 3 min.

Fetal heart rate fell within 3–70 s from 175 beats/min to 82 beats/min, mirrored by a rise in fetal systolic and diastolic blood pressure. After the restoration of uterine blood flow fetal heart rate rose again and the blood pressure fell, reaching the control values 15 min later. The alteration of the SO_2 and pCO_2 in the fetal arterial blood was in parallel with the cardiovascular change of the fetus. There was a linear fall of SO_2 and pO_2 following maternal aorta occlusion and a rapid restoration to control values after release of the occlusion. The pCO_2 was still elevated. The alterations in base excess, lactate, and pH were not in parallel with cardiovascular alterations (Fig. 7). The pH fell during fetal hypoxia from 7.31 to 7.16, paralleled by a rise in base deficit from 4.8 to 8.3 mEq/liter and lactate from 5 to 8 mmol/liter. It took more than 60 min until the metabolic alterations were in the control range again. The change of pH with time was measured by planimetry to quantify the metabolic alterations. Deterioration and normalization of pH were dependent on the control

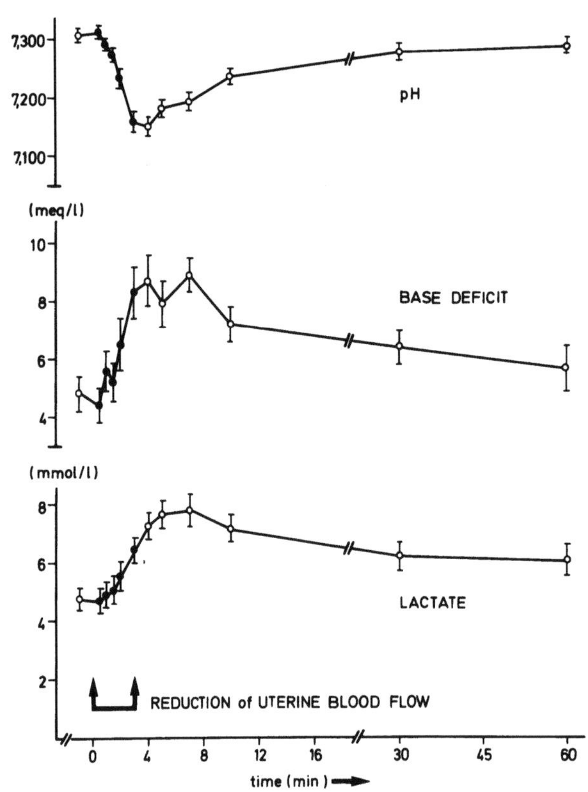

Fig. 7. The metabolic response to fetal hypoxia during and after total reduction of uterine blood flow for 180 s in 13 experiments. The fall in pH was accompanied by an increase in base deficit and a rise in lactate. (Künzel et al. 1983)

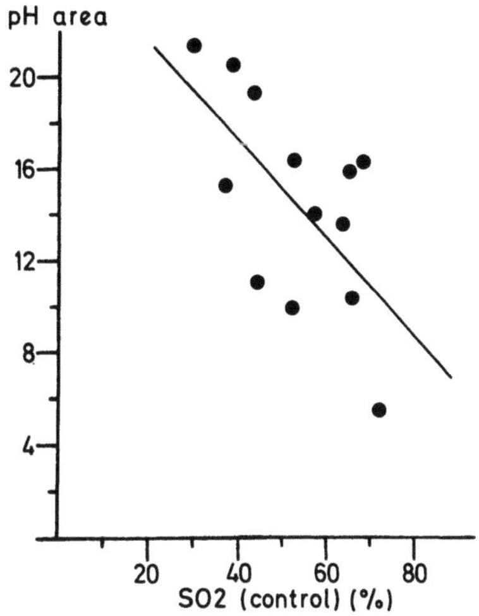

Fig. 8. Relationship between the area of the pH (pH · min · 10^{-3}) during hypoxia and recovery, and the fetal SO_2 at control. The pH area during hypoxia is responsible for 6.5% of the total pH area. The recovery of the pH to the previous value is dependent on the SO_2 at control (pH area, $25.6 - 0.21\,SO_2$; $2\alpha < 0.05$; *r*, 60; *N*, 13). (Künzel et al. 1983)

SO_2 (Fig. 8). With a high control SO_2, the pH area following hypoxia was small, but increased with falling SO_2 at control.

During the same time the dip area of the FHR showed a wide range from 170 to 788 beats/min · min. No correlation could be established between the metabolic alteration in the fetal blood and the deceleration area and no relationship could be found between the control SO_2 and the dip area.

Conclusions

The dip area of FHR deceleration signifies that the fetus suffers from hypoxia. In an initial approach the depth and duration of FHR decelerations were found to mirror the severity and time of hypoxia. If there are no decelerations the base excess of the fetus is usually not altered. The increasing dip area computed during labor is not necessarily paralleled by the rise in fetal base deficit, since fetal oxygenation and placental transfer of lactate have an influence on the fetal base excess. In the presence of decelerations during labor the loss of buffer base from the fetal blood has to be checked therefore, especially in cases such as no impending birth of the child.

References

Fischer WM, Halberstadt E, Rüttgers H, Berg D (1973) Kardiotokographie, Lehrbuch und Atlas. Thieme, Stuttgart

Kastendieck E, Künzel W, Zimmermann P (1974) Quantitative relationship between slowing of fetal heart rate and changes in base excess in the second stage of labor. J Perinat Med 2:106

Künzel W, Cornely M (1976) Dip area in fetal heart rate and its relationship to acid base observations of fetus and mother during labor. J Perinat Med 4:271

Künzel W, Kurz CS, Kastendieck E (1981) Die Variabilität der fetalen Herzfrequenzreaktion auf die Reduktion der uterinen Durchblutung. Z Geburtshilfe Perinatol 185:343

Künzel W, Kastendieck E, Hohmann M (1983) Heart rate and blood pressure response and metabolic changes in the sheep fetus following reduction of uterine blood flow. Gynecol Obstet Invest 15:300

Shelley T, Tipton R (1971) Dip area, a quantitative measure of fetal heart rate patterns. J Obstet Gynecol 78:694

Tipton RH, Shelley T (1971) An index of fetal welfare in labour. Obstet Gynecol 78:702

Fetal Heart Rate and Fetal Deterioration: Clinical and Experimental Observations

A. Jensen[1], W. Künzel, and M. Hohmann

After a prolonged fetal heart rate deceleration induced by maternal aortic occlusion in acute sheep experiments the transcutaneous PO_2 ($tcPO_2$) showed a delayed recovery as compared with arterial oxygen saturation values (Künzel et al. 1979, 1980). An almost identical delayed recovery of the $tcPO_2$ could be demonstrated by injecting norepinephrine into the sheep fetus, thus proving that the delayed response after asphyxia in combination with a fetal heart rate deceleration was probably due to increased sympathetic activity and release of catecholamines. This was the beginning of a series of clinical and experimental trials in which we tried to find out whether fetal heart rate monitoring, as to date the most accepted method of fetal surveillance, could be supplemented by the $tcPO_2$ technique to obtain insights into

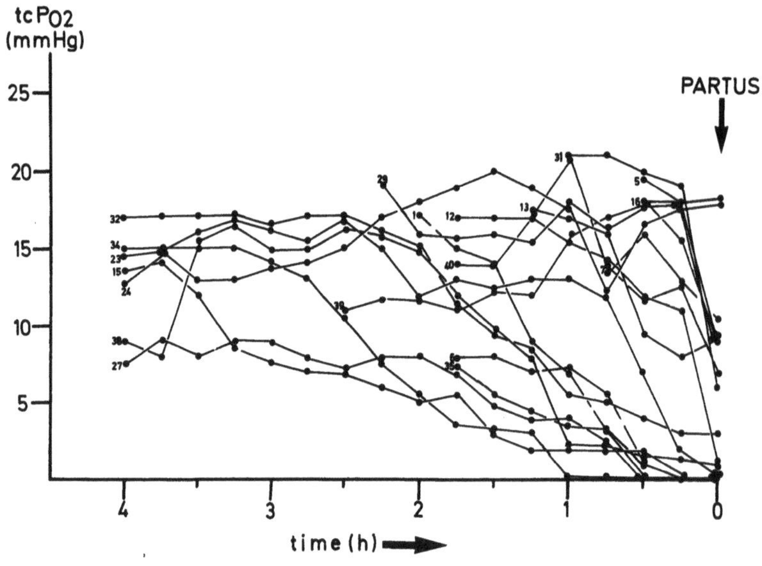

Fig. 1. Transcutaneous PO_2 ($tcPO_2$) recordings from human fetuses 4 h prior to birth. Two simplified groups of measurements can be distinguished. In one group the $tcPO_2$ remains more or less stable and decreases only in the last minutes before parturition to PO_2 values between 6 and 18 mmHg. In the second group of measurements, the $tcPO_2$ decreases as early as 1–2 h antepartum. At the moment of delivery the $tcPO_2$ was approximately zero. In 9 of 19 measurements, in which monitoring could be continued until delivery, the length of the $tcPO_2$ "zero line" recorded antepartum was 2–90 min. (Jensen and Künzel 1980)

[1] Frauenklinik und Hebammenlehranstalt der Justus-Liebig-Universität Gießen, Klinikstr. 28, D-6300 Gießen. At present: Research fellow of the Deutsche Forschungsgemeinschaft (FRG) at the University of California, San Francisco, School of Medicine, Cardiovascular Research Institute, San Francisco, CA 94143, USA

Fetal Heart Rate Monitoring
Ed. by W. Künzel

cardiovascular changes during asphyxial impairment of the human fetus during parturition.

Fetal Deterioration in the Human Fetus

To investigate the clinical validity of the $tcPO_2$ method we measured fetal $tcPO_2$ continuously during labor and checked the PO_2 by simultaneous micro blood sampling (Fig. 1).

In 40 measurements, from which 20 were conducted until the fetal head protruded, we found cases with primarily high $tcPO_2$ values that showed a decrease to about 11 mmHg only during the very last minutes of the second stage of labor. The other group of measurements was characterized by a primarily low $tcPO_2$ that decreased to almost zero mmHg during the course of labor (Jensen and Künzel 1980). Comparing the $tcPO_2$ values with 42 simultaneous PO_2 micro blood measurements from the scalp of 20 fetuses, an increasing discrepancy between both variables toward low $tcPO_2$ values was evident (Fig. 2). To find an explanation for this transcutaneous-arterial PO_2 difference we evaluated the fetal heart rate by a score. There was a linear relation between reduced heart rate scores on the basis of pathologic fetal heart rate pattern and low $tcPO_2$ values. Measurements of low $tcPO_2$ values

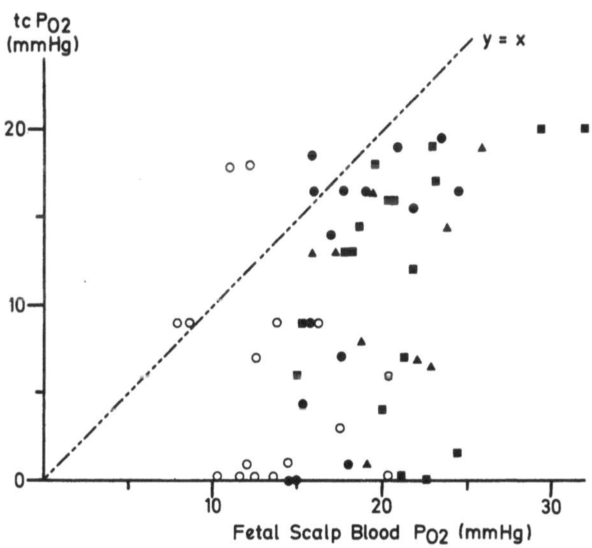

Fig. 2. The relation between the $tcPO_2$ and PO_2 in the arterialized (Finalgon, Anasco, FRG) capillary blood of the fetal scalp (●, ■, ▲) and the umbilical artery (○) blood of human fetuses, respectively. The different *solid symbols* indicate the various times before delivery at which the micro blood samples were taken (■, 2 h; ▲, 2–4 h; ●, 4 h). The *dashed line* (—-—-—-— y = x) represents the line of identity, reflecting the theoretical relationship between both variables when the $tcPO_2$ and the PO_2 in the scalp blood and umbilical arterial blood were equal. The $tcPO_2$ values neither correlate with the arterial scalp PO_2 nor with the umbilical artery PO_2. At a transcutaneous PO_2 of 0 mmHg, the PO_2 in the scalp blood is between 14.5 and 22.5 mmHg, and between 10 and 20.5 mmHg in the umbilical artery blood. (Jensen and Künzel 1980)

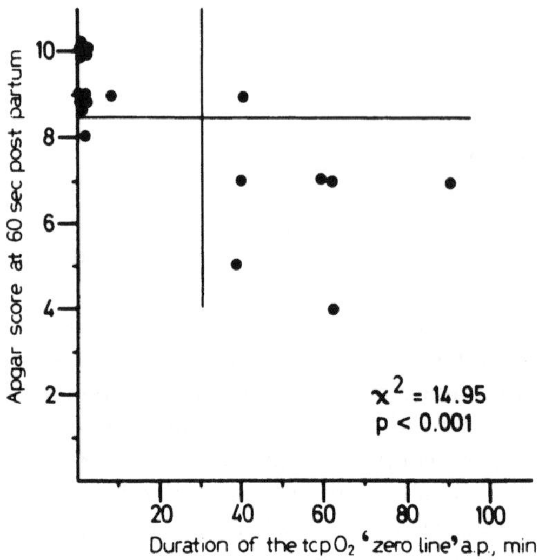

Fig. 3. The relation between the Apgar score evaluated in 20 newborns 60 s after birth and the length of the $tcPO_2$ "zero line" monitored before delivery (a.p.). These two variables correlate well ($P<0.001$). When the $tcPO_2$ antepartum remained at approximately 0 mm Hg for more than 30 min, the Apgar score at 60 s decreased significantly. (Jensen and Künzel 1980)

during parturition showed more and deeper fetal heart rate decelerations, a loss of the beat-to-beat variation, and an increased baseline heart rate. Some fetuses showed prolonged $tcPO_2$ readings of almost zero, which were related to the clinical state of the fetus at birth (Fig. 3). The fetal outcome, quantified by the Apgar score at 1 min postpartum, was plotted against the length of the "zero-line" of the $tcPO_2$ before parturition. There was a significant decrease of the 1-min Apgar score, when this "zero-line" exceeded 30 min. These findings suggested that the difference between the $tcPO_2$ and the central arterial PO_2 is indicative of a fetal circulatory shock syndrome. Hence, elevated plasma catecholamine concentrations were to be expected. On the basis of this concept we tried to mimic repeated asphyxia that might occur during labor by the following experimental protocol in acutely instrumented sheep fetuses.

Fetal Deterioration After Repeated Asphyxia in Sheep Experiments

In 15 experiments under general anesthesia of the ewe we exposed the fetuses to arrest of uterine blood flow by 11 repeated maternal aortic occlusions of 30-, 60-, or 90-s duration within 33 min. Fetal heart rate, blood pressure, continuous O_2 saturation, relative local skin flow, and $tcPO_2$ were measured. The plasma catecholamine concentrations were estimated by radio enzymatic assay (Jensen et al. 1981).

An original tracing, deriving from an experiment with repeated asphyxia of 60-s duration, is shown in Fig. 4. All variables including the $tcPO_2$ show a rapid fall during asphyxia, and immediate recovery after uterine blood flow was restored. This holds particularly true for the $tcPO_2$. The rapid changes of the skin vasomotor response

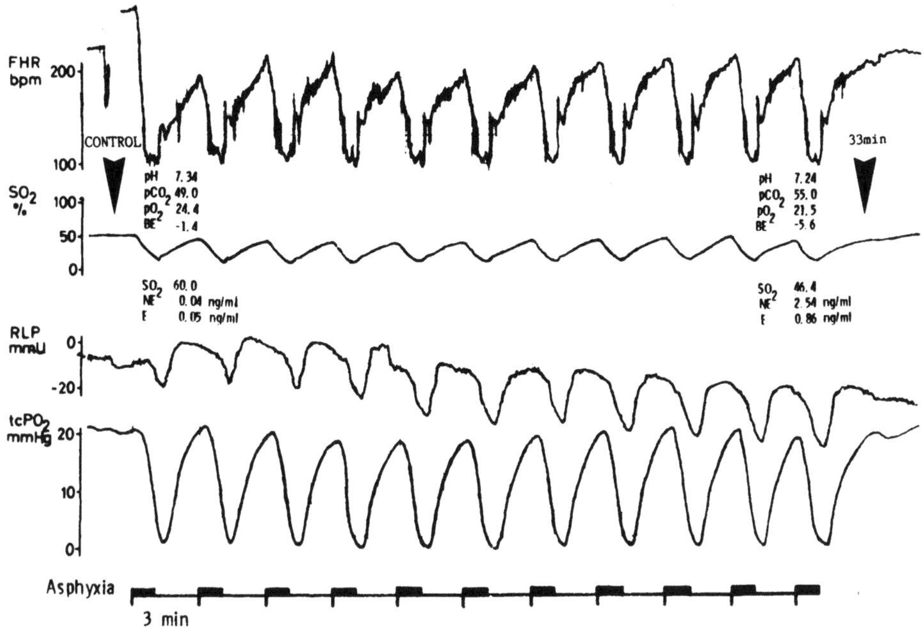

Fig. 4. 60 s episodes of asphyxia. Original recording of fetal heart rate *(FHR)*, oxygen saturation *(SO_2)*, skin perfusion *(RLP)*, and *$tcPO_2$*. The acutely instrumented fetus at 140-days gestation (147 days is term) was exposed to 11 asphyxial episodes within 33 min each of 60-s duration (■■■). Asphyxia was caused by arrest of uterine blood flow. All variables fall during asphyxia and show almost total recovery after uterine blood flow is restored. Repeated asphyxia caused an increase in plasma norepinephrine (NE, 2.54 ng/ml) and epinephrine (E, 0.86 ng/ml) concentrations and mild acidemia (pH, 7.24). Note the rapid vasomotor response *(RLP)* during each episode with progressively delayed recovery and a slight baseline decrease of the flow tracing throughout the experiment. (Jensen et al. 1983)

during asphyxia, generated by sympathetic nervous activity and norepinephrine release, showed a remarkably rapid reversibility, so that only slight changes of the mean skin flow values were measured in this well-oxygenated fetus. However, the area of the relative local skin perfusion tracing, produced by each asphyxial episode, progressively increased with the number of maternal aortic occlusions—a phenomenon that might be related to prolonged adrenoreceptor stimulation by impaired norepinephrine uptake mechanisms in the synaptic gap.

Prolongation of asphyxia from 60 to 90 s (Fig. 5a, b) was followed by a more pronounced fetal heart rate deceleration area, accompanied by a decrease of the fetal skin perfusion, a rapid fall of the $tcPO_2$ to zero, and severe acidemia. In contrast to the previous experiment, in which uterine blood flow was arrested for 60 s, the $tcPO_2$ did not recover, despite the fact that the oxygen saturation values had already reached control values. A transcutaneous-arterial PO_2 difference had developed and the progressive decrease of the mean skin blood flow was accompanied by increasing plasma catecholamine concentrations.

The mean relative local skin perfusion of each experiment as a percentage of the control was related to the norepinephrine and epinephrine concentrations of the

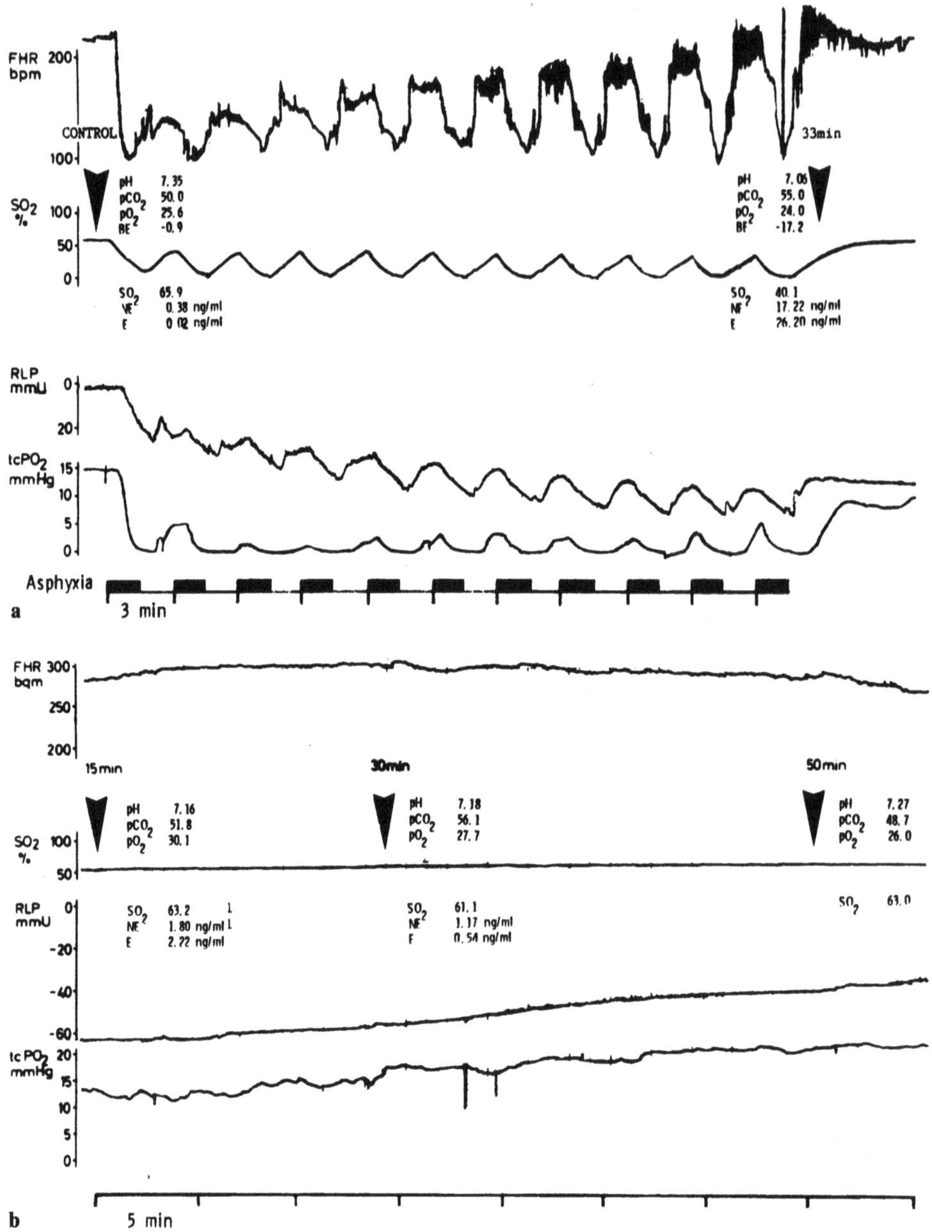

Fig. 5a. 90 s episodes of asphyxia. Original recording of fetal heart rate *(FHR)*, oxygen saturation *(SO_2)*, skin perfusion *(RLP)*, and *$tcPO_2$*. The acutely instrumented fetus at 140-days gestation (term is 147 days) was exposed to 11 asphyxial episodes within 33 min each of 90-s duration (■■■). Asphyxia was caused by arrest of uterine blood flow. This severe repetitive asphyxia was followed by a large heart rate deceleration area, low skin perfusion, and a rapid fall of the transcutaneous PO_2 to zero. Note: In contrast to asphyxia of 60-s duration (see Fig. 4), $tcPO_2$ does not recover intermittently, although the fetal O_2 saturation returns to normal. A transcutaneous-arterial PO_2 difference developed, accompanied by high norepinephrine (NE, 17.22 ng/ml) and epinephrine (E, 26.2 ng/ml) concentrations as well as severe acidemia (pH, 7.06). (Jensen et al. 1983)

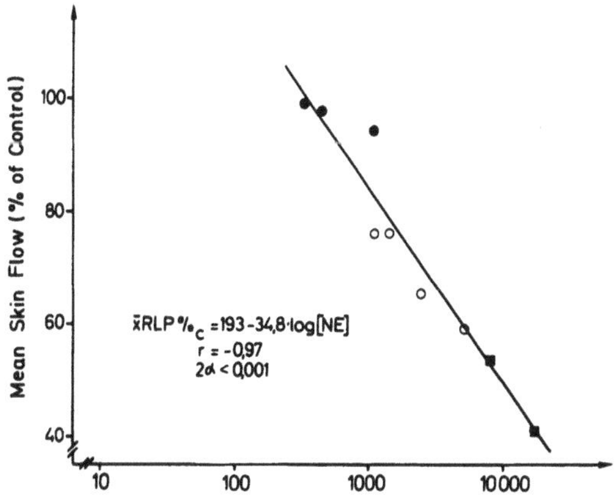

a

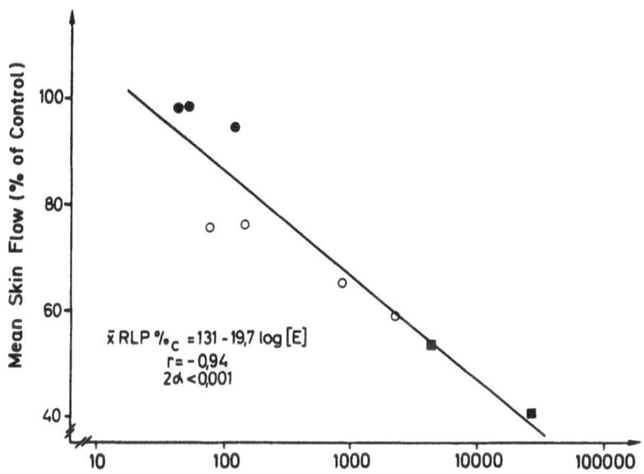

b

Fig. 6. Relationship between fetal plasma norepinephrine (**a**) and epinephrine (**b**) concentrations after the experiment (33 min) and mean relative local skin perfusion *($\bar{x}$ RLP)* as a percentage of control in acutely instrumented fetuses at 125–145-days gestation (term is 147 days). The fetuses were exposed to repeated arrest of uterine blood flow within 33 min by 11 maternal aortic occlusions of 30-s (●), 60-s (○), and 90-s (■) duration. There is a close log-linear relationship between increasing catecholamine concentrations and reduced skin blood flow of the fetus during repeated asphyxia. (Jensen et al. 1983)

◄

Fig. 5b. Recovery after episodes of 90 s of asphyxia. Original recording of fetal heart rate *(FHR)*, oxygen saturation *(SO_2)*, skin perfusion *(RLP)*, and *$tcPO_2$* during the recovery period after exposure of the acutely instrumented fetus at 140-days gestation to 11 asphyxial episodes, each of 90-s duration (see Fig. 5a). The traces start 15 min after the last episode and show a marked posthypoxic tachycardia (300 bpm) and a reduced beat-to-beat variation of the heart rate. The O_2 saturation has already recovered to normal (60%), while skin perfusion is still low (−62 mmU) and the $tcPO_2$ is about 12 mmHg. Within 15 min recovery the catecholamine concentration decreased rapidly from 17.2 to 1.8 ng/ml norepinephrine and from 26.2 ng/ml to 2.2 ng/ml epinephrine (see Fig. 5a). In the further course of the recovery period the heart rate tended to normalize, O_2 saturation remained constant, and the skin perfusion recovered accompanied by increasing transcutaneous PO_2 values. The dependence of the $tcPO_2$ on skin flow is conspicuous. The difference between cutaneous and arterial PO_2 decreased from 15 mmHg (at 30 min) to 5 mmHg (at 50 min) paralleled by declining catecholamine concentrations and a normalization of the acid base balance. (Jensen et al. 1983)

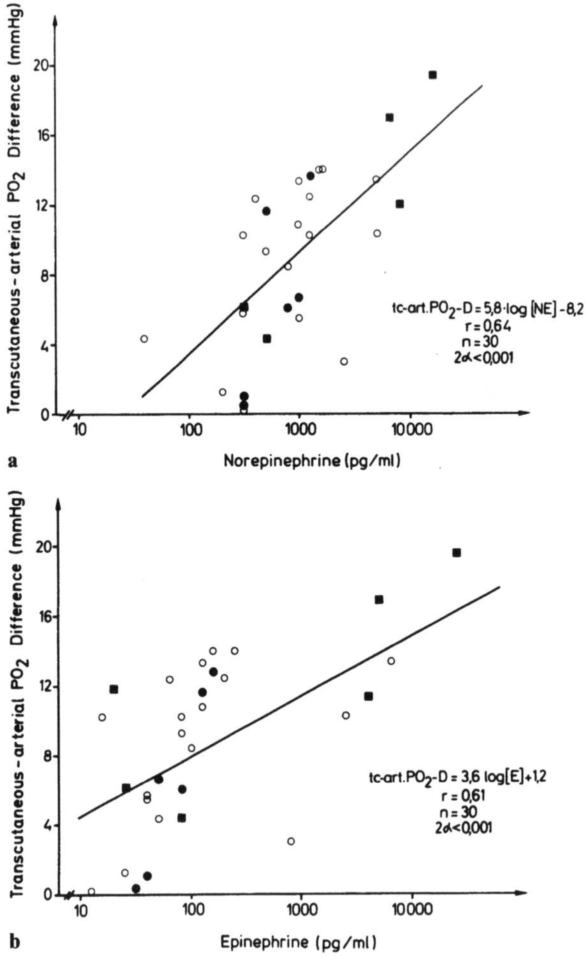

Fig. 7. Relationship between fetal plasma norepinephrine (**a**) and epinephrine (**b**) concentrations and the difference between fetal abdominal aortic PO_2 and $tcPO_2$ (tc-art. PO_2-D) in acutely instrumented fetuses at 125–145 days' gestation (term is 147 days). The fetuses were subjected to repeated arrest of uterine blood flow within 33 min by 11 maternal aortic occlusions of 30-s (●), 60-s (○), and 90-s (■) duration. With logarithmically rising catecholamine concentrations the difference between cutaneous PO_2 and arterial PO_2 increased. (Jensen et al. 1983)

fetal blood at 33 min ($2\alpha < 0.001$) (Fig. 6). This reduced skin perfusion on the strength of sympathetic stimulation was reflected by an increase in the difference between $tcPO_2$ and arterial PO_2 of the fetus. Indeed, both vasoconstrictive hormones exhibited a log-linear relationship to the transcutaneous-arterial PO_2 difference (Fig. 7).

Fetal Organ Blood Flow Redistribution After Repeated Asphyxia

As repeated asphyxia of 90-s duration yielded the most pronounced changes in catecholamine concentrations and relative local skin flow, the next experiment tried

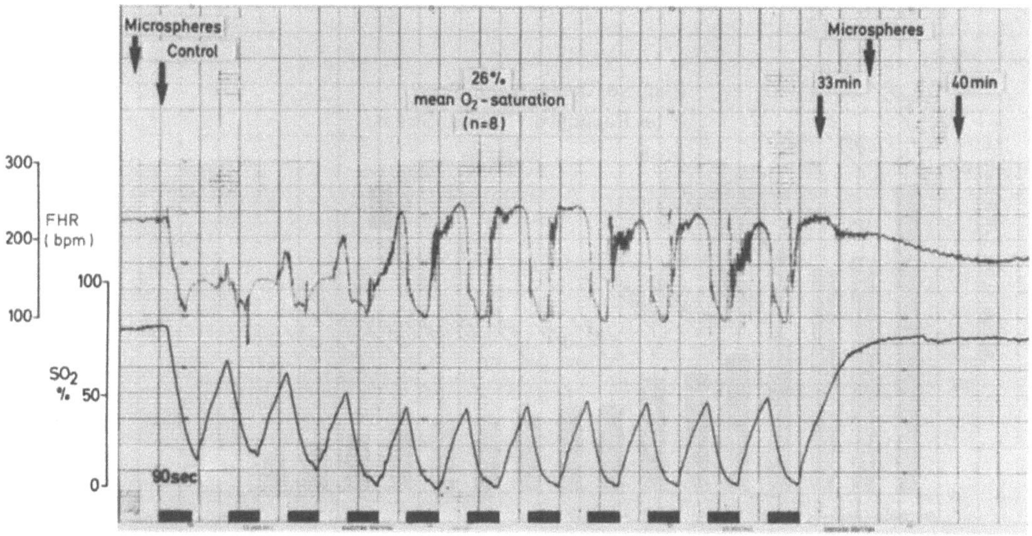

Fig. 8. Experimental protocol to investigate the redistribution of fetal organ blood flow after 11 asphyxial episodes of 90-s duration within 33 min in eight acutely instrumented fetuses at 125–135-days gestation (term is 147 days). Original recording of fetal heart rate *(FHR)* and oxygen saturation *(SO_2)*. Organ blood flow was measured by injection of radioactive labeled microspheres (15 μm) at control and after the experiment. The mean fetal O_2 saturation was reduced to 26% during the experiments. (Jensen et al. 1982)

Table 1. Changes in mean arterial pH, oxygen saturation (SO_2), base excess (BE), norepinephrine (NE), and epinephrine (E) concentrations before and after 11 repeated asphyxial episodes of 90-s duration in eight acutely instrumented fetal sheep at 125–135-days gestation (147 days is term). (Jensen et al. 1982)

	Blood flow redistribution				
	Control $\bar{x}$ (±SE) $n=8$		33 min $\bar{x}$ (±SE) $n=8$		Wilcoxon-rank test P
pH	7.26	(0.02)	7.02	(0.03)	<0.001
SO_2	54.9	(4.39)	44.4	(6.85)	>0.05 NS
BE	−6.1	(0.7)	−18.2	(1.2)	<0.001
NE (pg/ml)	203.3	(65.5)	1899.5	(803.5)	<0.01
E (pg/ml)	13.4	(3.6)	1260.9	(597.9)	<0.001

to investigate the redistribution of fetal organ blood flow under these experimental conditions. Figure 8 demonstrates fetal heart rate and oxygen saturation changes during repeated asphyxia of 90-s duration. Differently labeled radioactive microspheres (15 μm) were injected into eight acutely instrumented fetal sheep at control and after the experiment, using the method developed by Heymann and Rudolph (Heymann et al. 1977; Jensen et al. 1982).

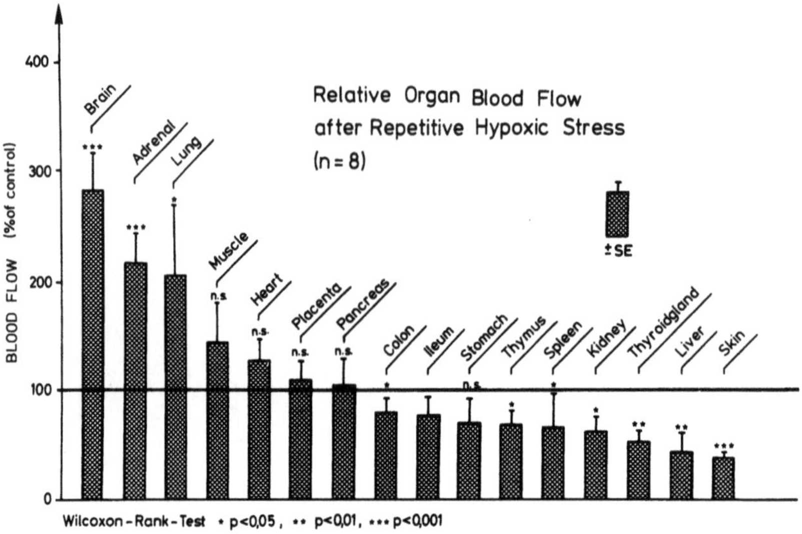

Fig. 9. Relative fetal organ blood flow as a percentage of control (———) after asphyxia of 90-s duration ($n = 8$; $\bar{x} \pm SE$) caused by repeated arrest of uterine blood flow in acutely instrumented fetuses at days 125–135 of gestation (term is 147 days). Blood flow measurements were performed by injection of radioactive labeled microspheres before and after 11 asphyxial episodes. There is an organ blood flow redistribution after the experiments in favor of the brain, adrenal glands, and lungs at the expense of the guts, spleen, thyroid gland, liver, and particularly the skin. (Jensen et al. 1983a)

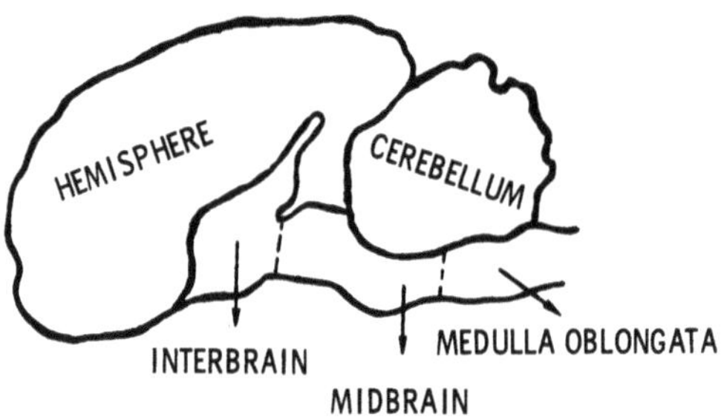

Fig. 10. Schematic drawing of the fetal brain parts dissected for separate brain blood flow measurements. (Jensen et al. 1983a)

During the experiment the mean oxygen saturation of all animals was lowered to 26%, pH dropped from 7.26 to 7.02, and norepinephrine and epinephrine concentrations increased to 1900 and 1260 pg/ml, respectively (Table 1). The organ blood flow changes after repeated asphyxia are shown in Fig. 9. A marked increase in fetal blood flow to the brain and adrenals occurred after asphyxial stress. The increase in blood flow to the heart was not significant. On the other hand the blood flow to the thymus, spleen, kidneys, thyroid gland, liver, and particularly to the skin decreased significantly. In the latter organ, blood flow was reduced to 38% of control values.

The next question was, whether the blood flow to the brain, which was increased to 280% of control after repeated asphyxia, was evenly distributed or showed preferential flow to particular parts of the brain (Fig. 10). For separate blood flow

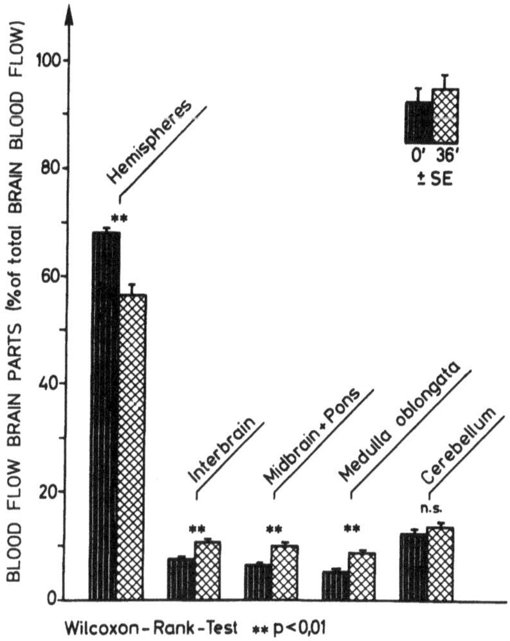

Fig. 11. Relative blood flow of the different brain parts at control and after repeated asphyxia as a percentage of total brain blood flow ($n = 8$; $\bar{x} \pm SE$). These results derive from acutely instrumented fetuses at 125–135-days gestation (term is 147 days). Note: a redistribution of total brain blood flow in favor of the brain stem areas and at the expense of the cerebral hemispheres is evident. (Jensen et al. 1983b)

measurements the brain was cut into five pieces: hemispheres, cerebellum, and brain stem, which was further dissected into interbrain, midbrain and pons, and medulla oblongata. In fact the brain blood flow showed a redistribution toward the brain stem areas (Fig. 11). There was a significant decrease in the cortex blood flow from 70% to 56% of the total brain blood flow. The relative blood flow proportion to the brain stem, however, increased tremendously during asphyxia. The blood flow to the cerebellum did not change.

The results so far raised the question whether the skin flow, as the only organ blood flow that is accessible in the human fetus during parturition, reflects the blood flow redistribution process during asphyxia in the whole fetal circulation. The correlation between the skin blood flow as a percentage of control and the kidney blood flow as a percentage of control was significant (Fig. 12). According to Fig. 12 the skin blood flow of the fetus had to be reduced to about 60% of control values until the kidney blood flow started to decline. We then tried to correlate the skin blood flow with the blood flow of different brain parts. This was neither possible with the hemispheres nor with the cerebellum. Only the brain stem parts showed a linear increase in blood flow as skin flow decreased (Fig. 13). This was particularly true for skin flows that exceeded 30% of control. In two experiments, which showed skin flow values below 30% of control, the expected flow rate to the interbrain was not reached. These two animals died during the recovery period.

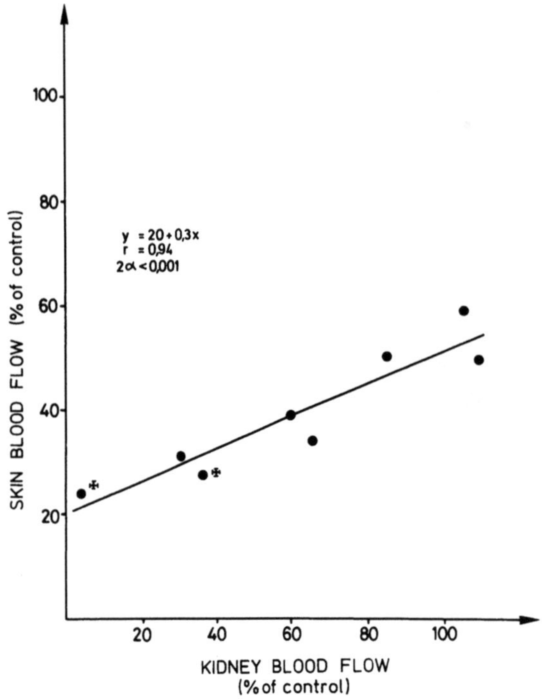
y = 20 + 0,3x
r = 0,94
2α < 0,001
SKIN BLOOD FLOW (% of control)
KIDNEY BLOOD FLOW (% of control)
20
40
60
80
100

Fig. 12

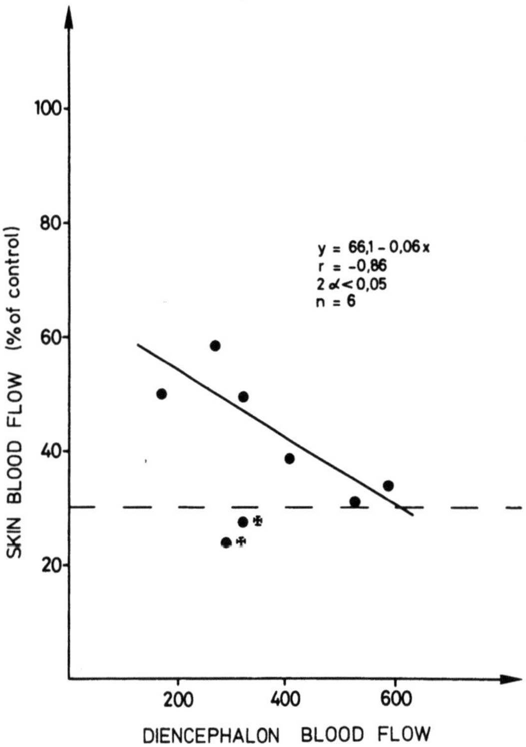
y = 66,1 - 0,06x
r = -0,86
2α < 0,05
n = 6
SKIN BLOOD FLOW (% of control)
DIENCEPHALON BLOOD FLOW (% of control)
20
40
60
80
100
200
400
600

Fig. 13

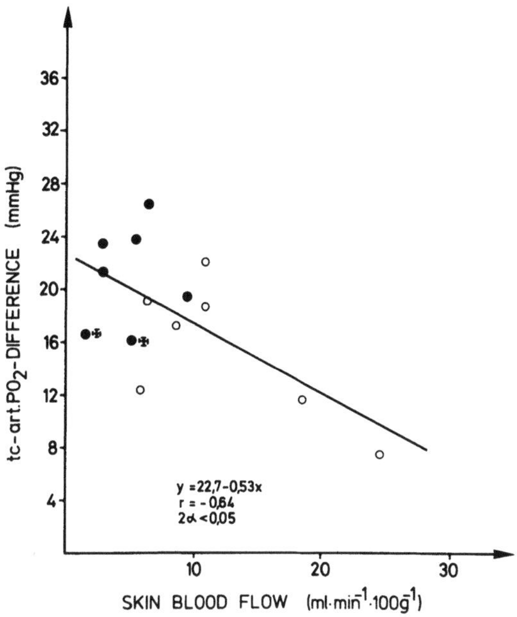

Fig. 14. Relationship between skin blood flow (ml/min/100 g) and the transcutaneous-arterial PO_2 difference (mmHg) in acutely instrumented sheep fetuses at 125–135-days gestation (term is 147 days). Two animals died in the recovery period (✱), showing a comparatively low difference between the transcutaneous and the arterial PO_2. Skin blood flow was minimal and the transcutaneous PO_2 approached zero; however, the difference between arterial and cutaneous PO_2 decreased on the basis of a prefinal fall of central arterial PO_2 values. (Jensen et al. 1983b)

To verify the validity of the transcutaneous-arterial PO_2 difference as an index of fetal skin flow during parturition the skin blood flow was plotted against the transcutaneous-arterial PO_2 difference (Fig. 14). Both variables showed a linear relation, thus providing evidence of close interrelations between fetal asphyxia, catecholamine release, reduced skin blood flow, and increased transcutaneous-arterial PO_2 difference.

Fig. 12. Relationship between the kidney blood flow as a percentage of control and the skin blood flow as a percentage of control in acutely instrumented sheep fetuses at 125–135-days gestation (term is 147 days). Two animals died in the recovery period (✱). Both variables correlate well ($2\alpha < 0.001$). Note: skin blood flow was reduced to 60% of the control value before the kidney blood flow started to decrease linearly. (Jensen, Künzel, and Hohmann 1983, unpublished)

Fig. 13. Relationship between diencephalic blood flow as a percentage of control and skin blood flow as a percentage of control in acutely instrumented sheep fetuses at 125–135-days gestation (term is 147 days). Both variables correlate when the skin blood flow is higher than 30% of the control value ($2\alpha < 0.05$). In two cases the skin flow decreased below 30% and the brain stem blood flow did not reach the expected values. These two animals died in the recovery period (✱). (Jensen, Künzel, and Hohmann 1983, unpublished)

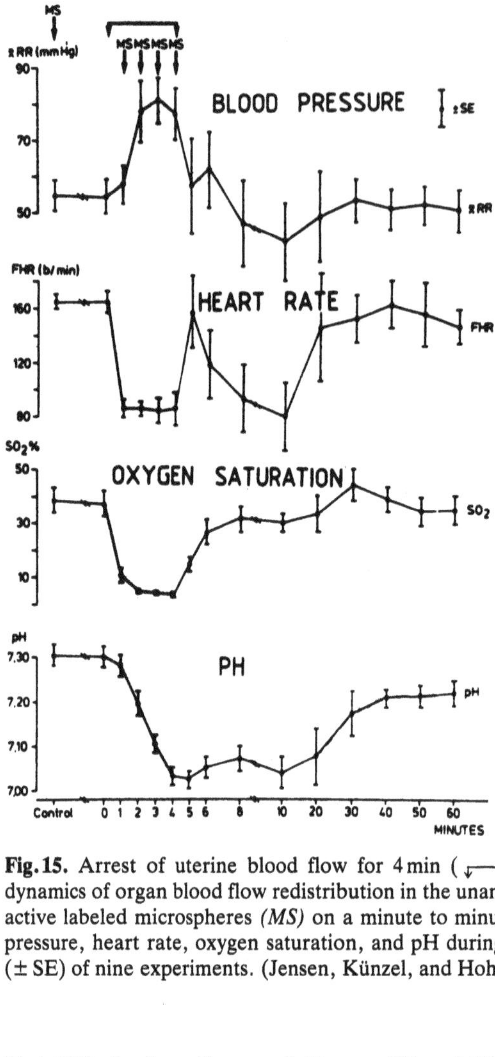

Fig. 15. Arrest of uterine blood flow for 4 min ( ). Experimental protocol to study the dynamics of organ blood flow redistribution in the unanesthetized sheep fetus by injections of radioactive labeled microspheres *(MS)* on a minute to minute basis. The changes of fetal arterial blood pressure, heart rate, oxygen saturation, and pH during severe asphyxia are shown in mean values (± SE) of nine experiments. (Jensen, Künzel, and Hohmann 1983, unpublished)

Fetal Deterioration and Organ Blood Flow Redistribution During One Severe Fetal Heart Rate Deceleration Due to Arrest of Uterine Blood Flow

Our latest experiments were designed to investigate the dynamics of the fetal circulatory centralization during asphyxia, generated by prolonged arrest of uterine blood flow (Fig. 15). In nine unanesthetized fetal sheep in five chronic and four acute experiments, uterine blood flow was arrested for 4 min. Organ blood flow measurements were performed by injections of microspheres at control and after 1, 2, 3, and 4 min of asphyxia. Again fetal heart rate, blood pressure, oxygen saturation, acid base balance, and blood gas tensions were measured. During asphyxia the pH dropped from 7.30 to 7.02 and arterial oxygen saturation decreased from about 40% to 3%. Five animals died in the recovery period of these experiments (Table 2). The

Table 2. Changes in mean arterial pH, oxygen saturation (SO_2), base excess (BE), fetal heart rate (FHR), and arterial blood pressure ($\bar{x}$ RR) during one severe asphyxial episode of 4-min duration are given as mean values ± SE ($n = 9$). The experiments were performed on nine unanaesthetized fetal sheep in five chronic and four acute preparations at days 125–135 of pregnancy. (Jensen, Künzel, and Hohmann 1983, unpublished)

	Dynamics of centralization		
	Control $\bar{x}$ (±SE) $n=9$	4 min $\bar{x}$ (±SE) $n=9$	Wilcoxon-rank test P
pH	7.31 (0.03)	7.03 (0.02)	<0.001
SO_2	38.6 (5.2)	3.5 (0.5)	<0.001
BE	−2.7 (2.1)	−12.2 (1.8)	<0.01
FHR	164.9 (4.9)	86.9 (12.7)	<0.001
$\bar{x}$ RR	53.1 (3.1)	66.6 (5.1)	<0.05

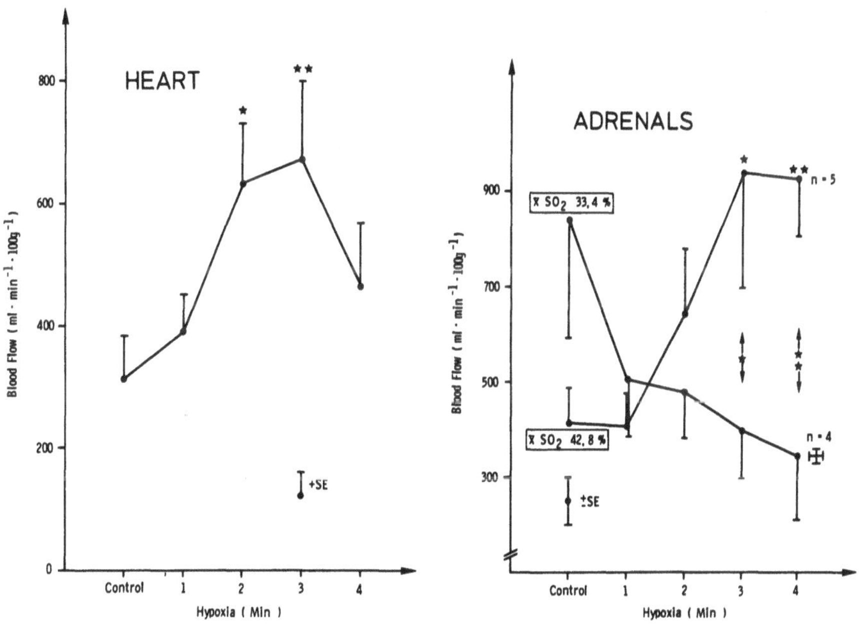

a b

Fig. 16. Dynamics of blood flow changes of the fetal heart (**a**) and the adrenals (**b**) during 4 min of asphyxia in nine unanesthetized sheep fetuses at days 125–135 of pregnancy. The blood flow values are given as means ± SE ($n = 9$). The blood flow to the heart increased progressively, reaching mean peak values of 650 ml/min per 100 g of tissue at 3 min of asphyxia. Adrenal blood flow changes were variable. Fetuses with high O_2 saturation and low blood flow control values showed a progressive rise during asphyxia, while there was a decrease of adrenal blood flow in fetuses with low oxygen saturation and high adrenal blood flow at control. The latter group of animals died in the recovery period. (Jensen, Künzel, and Hohmann 1983, unpublished)

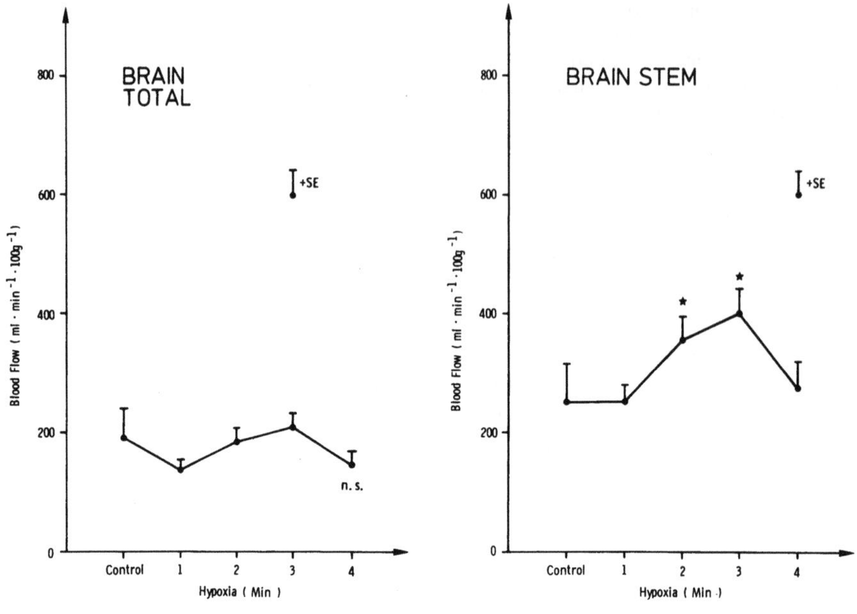

a b

Fig. 17a, b. Dynamics of fetal blood flow changes of the total brain and the brain stem during 4 min of asphyxia, investigated in nine unanesthetized fetal sheep at days 125–135 of pregnancy. Blood flow values are given as means ± SE. The total brain blood flow does not change during acute asphyxia, while the blood flow to the brain stem areas progressively increases. (Jensen, Künzel, and Hohmann 1983, unpublished)

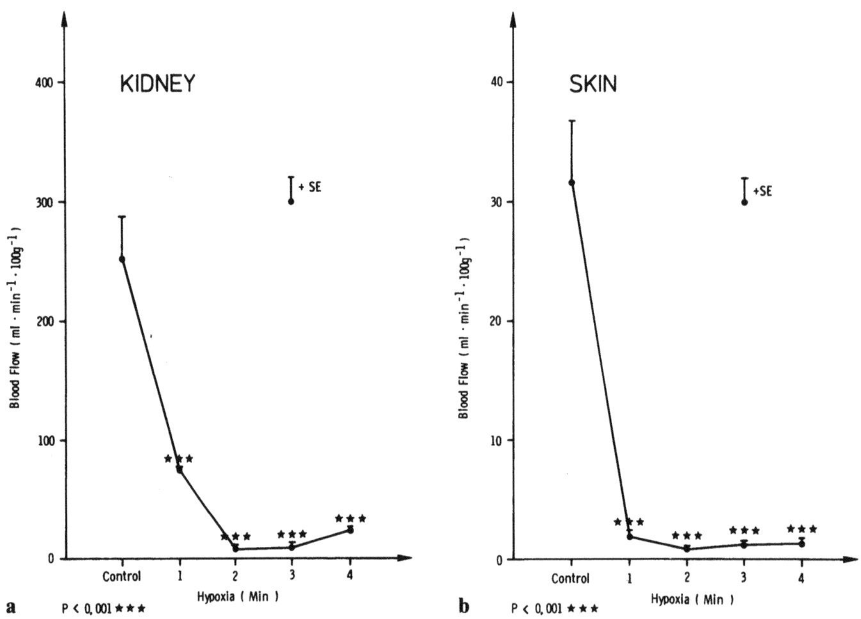

a b

Fig. 18

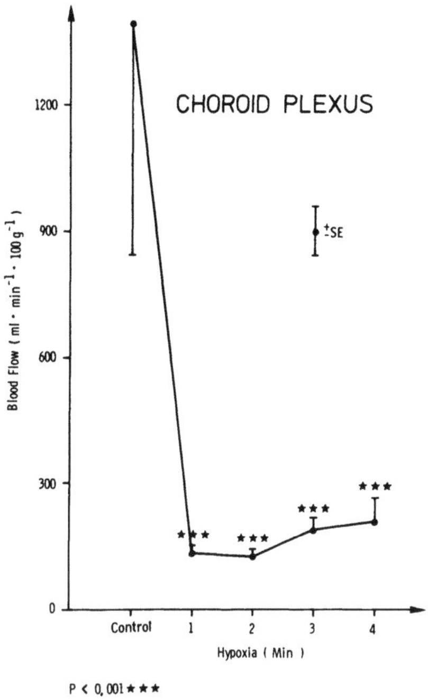

Fig. 19. Dynamics of fetal blood flow changes of the chorioid plexus during 4 min of asphyxia, investigated in nine unanesthetized fetal sheep at days 125–135 of pregnancy. Blood flow values are given as means ± SE. The fetal choroid plexus is highly perfused during normoxia and shows a tremendous vasoconstriction during the first minute of asphyxia, almost like the skin vasculature. Accumulative effects of anoxia, acidemia, and vasoconstriction may well damage the plexus endothelium with consequent capillary leaks and plexus or intraventricular hemorrhages of the fetus. (Jensen, Künzel, and Hohmann 1983, unpublished)

dynamics of blood flow changes in the heart and adrenal glands during asphyxia are shown in Fig. 16. The blood flow to the heart increased progressively during oxygen deprivation, while the response of the adrenal blood flow was variable: five experiments showed a decrease and the other four an increase in blood flow. All animals died in the group, which showed high mean adrenal flow rates at control and a decrease of the adrenal blood flow during asphyxia. Thus, fetal deterioration seems to be inevitable when sympathoadrenal-compensating mechanisms operate above capacity.

The blood flow pattern during asphyxia in the fetal brain was different in the various brain parts (Fig. 17). There were no significant changes in total brain blood flow during asphyxia, whereas the blood flow to the brain stem areas increased progressively with time, with peak values of 400 ml/min per 100 g. The kidney blood flow decreased rapidly and reached 10% of the control values after 2 min of asphyxia (Fig. 18). The skin flow reacted most sensitively and decreased to almost 10% of control values after only 1 min of arrest of uterine blood flow.

One of the most interesting findings of the experiments is illustrated in Fig. 19. In contrast to the brain stem areas, which showed an increase in blood flow during

Fig. 18a, b. Dynamics of fetal blood flow changes of the kidneys and the skin during 4 min of asphyxia, investigated in nine unanesthetized fetal sheep at days 125–135 of pregnancy. Blood flow values are given as means ± SE. Both organs show a rapid decrease of organ blood flow during asphyxia. The kidney and the skin blood flows fell to 30% and below 10% of their control values, respectively. Fetal skin blood flow indicates the process of circulatory centralization most sensitively. (Jensen, Künzel, and Hohmann 1983, unpublished) asphyxia, the chorioid plexus demonstrated a steep and rapid decrease of blood flow almost like the skin. The combination of maximum blood flow supply during normal circulatory conditions and the tremendous vasoconstriction during asphyxia may lead to hypoxical damage of the endothelial layer of the plexus vasculature and may be responsible for capillary leaks and consequent ventricular hemorrhage of the fetus.

Summary and Conclusions

Fetal heart rate decelerations and concomitant oxygen deprivation during parturition are accompanied by increased sympathetic activity with circulatory centralization of the fetus. This is most sensitively indicated by skin blood flow changes. Since indirect assessment of the fetal organ blood flow redistribution is possible by transcutaneous PO_2 measurements in the human, polygraphic monitoring of the transcutaneous PO_2 and relative skin flow together with the fetal heart rate seem to predict fetal deterioration more effectively.

Acknowledgements. We would like to thank Mrs. S. Jelinek for her invaluable technical assistance and Dr. R. Dietz and Dr. A. Schömig, Department of Pharmacology, University of Heidelberg (FRG), for their catecholamine analyses. We are further gratefully indebted to Dr. B. Winkler and Prof. Dr. W. Schaper, Max Planck Institute for Heart Research, Bad Nauheim (FRG), and Prof. Dr. Sattler and Dr. Lewe, Zentrale Abteilung Strahlenzentrum, Giessen University (FRG), for their help with our blood flow measurements.

References

Heymann MA, Payne BP, Hoffmann JIE, Rudolph AM (1977) Blood flow measurements with radionuclide-labeled particles. Prog Cardiovasc Dis 20:55–79

Jensen A, Künzel W (1980) The difference between fetal transcutaneous PO_2 and arterial PO_2 during labour. Gynecol Obstet Invest 11:249–264

Jensen A, Künzel W, Kastendieck E (1981) Catecholamine release and transcutaneous PO_2 in the sheep fetus following hypoxic stress: 28th Annual meeting of the society for gynecologic investigation, March 1981, St. Louis, Missouri, USA. Scientific Abstracts no. 42, p 24

Jensen A, Künzel W, Hohmann M (1982) Fetal organ blood flow (FOBF) and its redistribution after repetitive hypoxic stress: Pflügers Arch [Suppl] 394:20 (Abstract)

Jensen A, Künzel W, Kastendieck E (1983) Transcutaneous PO_2 and norepinephrine release in the fetal sheep after repetitive reduction of uterine blood flow. In: Huch R, Huch A (eds) Continuous transcutaneous blood gas monitoring. Reproductive medicine series, vol 5, no. 8. Marcel Dekker, New York, pp 591–602

Jensen A, Hohmann M, Künzel W (1983a) Änderung der Organdurchblutung des Feten nach rezidivierenden Hypoxien. Wissenschaftliche Information 9(4):255–259

Jensen A, Hohmann M, Künzel W (1983b) Änderung der Organdurchblutung und des transkutanen PO_2 des Feten nach rezidivierenden Hypoxien. Arch Gynecol 235(1–4):646–647

Künzel W, Kastendieck E, Kurz CS (1979) A comparative study of continuous intravascular O_2 saturation and transcutaneous PO_2 measurements in the sheep fetus following the reduction of uterine blood flow. In: Huch A, Huch R, Lucey JF (eds) Continuous transcutaneous blood gas monitoring. Birth Defects 15(4):591–597

Künzel W, Kastendieck E, Kurz CS, Paulick R (1980) Transcutaneous PO_2 and cardiovascular observations in the sheep fetus following the reduction of uterine blood flow. J Perinat Med 8:85

Kinetics of Lactic Acid Accumulation and Removal in the Fetus

W. Moll[1] and E. Kastendieck[2]

Fetal hypoxia is one of the causes of fetal heart rate alterations, certainly the most important one clinically. Fetal hypoxia, on the other hand, is reflected by accumulation of lactic acid in the fetal body. The rise in fetal lactate concentration provides information on the hypoxic component of fetal heart rate alterations. Thus we can consider the use of the plasma lactate concentration in the fetus as a quantitative indicator of fetal hypoxia. This paper will describe the quantitative relationship between fetal lactate concentration and hypoxia. What is the hypoxic threshold for the increase in lactate concentration? How is the rise in lactate concentration related to the degree of fetal hypoxia? What is the rate of net lactate production and the maximum anaerobic metabolic rate in lactate production? Which processes remove fetal lactate in posthypoxic periods? How fast is the removal, i.e., how long does the "lactate signal" of hypoxic periods last?

Lactic acid production and removal can be studied conveniently on a specially prepared anesthetized guinea pig (Fig. 1). In this experimental arrangement the carotid artery is connected with the dilated part of a placental artery via an electromagnetic flowmeter and a clamp. Uteroplacental blood flow and, thereby, fetal arterial O_2 saturation can be adjusted in a wide range around the physiological value. When maternal placental blood flow has a normal value of 15 ml/min/100 g fetal weight, fetal O_2 saturation is about 60% and pH is 7.33 in this preparation (Girard et al. 1983). The O_2 uptake of the fetal-placental unit can be obtained from the uterine arteriovenous O_2 concentration difference and the uterine blood flow. Fetal arterial concentrations of O_2 and lactate as well as pH can be measured in samples obtained from the fetal carotid artery. The fetus can be rapidly removed for a whole body analysis. A drawback of the preparation is the need for anesthesia; an advantage is the presence of a hemochorial placenta which seems to differ from the epitheliochorial placenta of the sheep in functional aspects.

Threshold for Fetal Lactic Acid Production

When uterine blood flow is reduced in this preparation, fetal arterial O_2 saturation and O_2 concentration fall and lactic acid is finally produced. Where is the threshold for the lactic acid production? By successively drawing blood samples from the fetal carotid artery the change of lactate in fetal plasma can be followed and related to the simultaneously measured blood oxygen concentration. In Fig. 2, the rise of lactate concentration in fetal arterial plasma is plotted against the O_2 concentration in the

[1] Universität Regensburg, Institut für Physiologie, Universitätsstr. 31, D-8400 Regensburg
[2] Universitäts-Frauenklinik, Josef-Schneider-Str. 4, D-8700 Würzburg

Fetal Heart Rate Monitoring
Ed. by W. Künzel

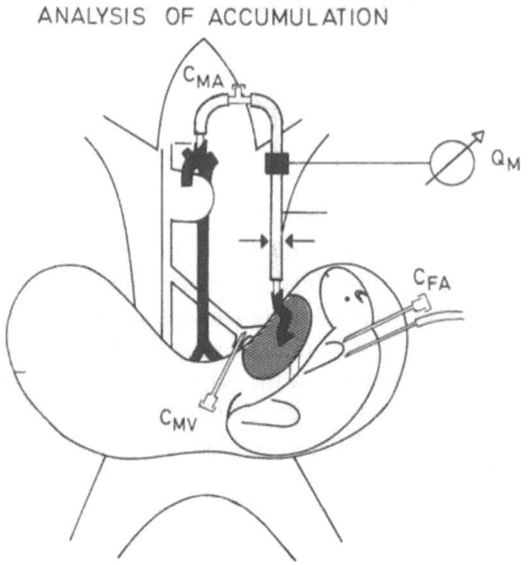

Fig. 1. Preparation of the pregnant guinea pig. The maternal carotid artery of the anesthetized animal was connected with the final, dilated part of an uteroplacental artery via a silastic tube and an electromagnetic flowmeter as described by Herberger and Moll (1976). The other uteroplacental arteries were tied. An additional catheter was inserted into the maternal uterine vein. After making a 3-cm incision in the uterus and the fetal membranes the fetal head was partially exposed, fixed to the uterine muscle by suture, and covered with thin plastic sheets. The fetal carotid artery and the jugular vein were cannulated with small polyvinyl tubes. Blood samples of a maximum of 200–300 µl were drawn from the fetus; the blood was replaced by maternal arterial blood. The preparation enables one to measure maternal placental flow (Q_M) and to obtain samples to determine the concentrations in maternal arterial, maternal uterovenous and fetal arterial blood (C_{MA}, C_{MV}, C_{FA}). (Moll and Kastendieck 1978)

fetal arterial blood. The rise in lactate concentration is proportional to the rise in base deficit; it is lactic acid which accumulates in the blood. The diagram enables us to define the threshold of lactic acid production in this animal and in these conditions: lactic acid begins to accumulate when the oxygen concentration falls below 5 ml_{STPD}/100 ml, i.e., when the oxygen saturation falls below 25%.

This threshold may be true only for this species and the present conditions, and a more general definition for the threshold for a rise in lactic acid concentration is wanted. In Fig. 3, the O_2 uptake of the fetal-placental unit is related to the fetal arterial O_2 saturation under the same experimental conditions as above. It can be seen that at 25% oxygen saturation (SO_2), i.e., at the threshold of lactic acid accumulation in fetal plasma, O_2 uptake falls steeply with O_2 saturation. Thus, we may state more generally that lactate concentration rises when O_2 supply to fetal tissue falls short of O_2 need. This is in accordance with other data on the guinea pig fetus (Girard et al. 1983). Blood flow through fetal tissues is about 20 ml/min/100 g for normal conditions of O_2 supply in the guinea pig. For the same rate of blood flow the mean O_2 supply to fetal tissue is around 1 ml_{STPD}/min/100 g fetal weight when O_2 saturation is 25%. Thus, in the situation where lactic acid production starts, the mean O_2 supply to fetal tissue approaches the mean oxygen consumption of tissues

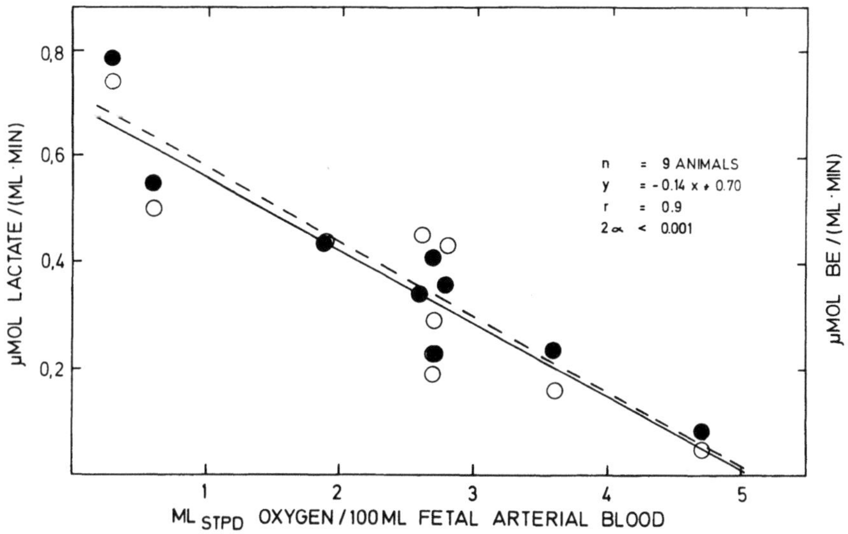

Fig. 2. Rise in lactate concentration in fetal arterial plasma *(solid line, closed circles)* and the base deficit in the extracellular space *(broken line, open circles)* related to the oxygen concentration in fetal arterial blood ($n = 9$). (Moll and Kastendieck 1978)

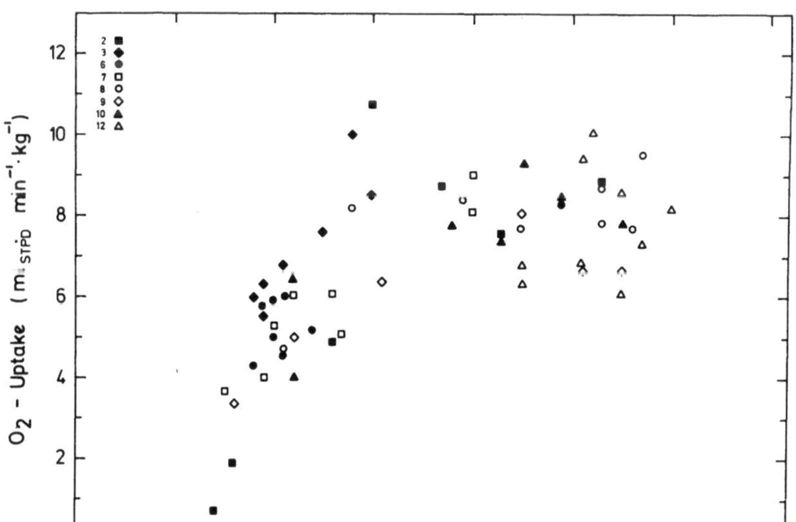

Fig. 3. Oxygen uptake of the anesthetized guinea pig fetus and its placenta related to the O_2 saturation in fetal arterial blood

in normal conditions and anoxia probably occurs in unfavorably located parts of the tissue.

Very roughly, the threshold for lactic acid production found in the guinea pig coincides with the threshold for deceleration of the fetal heart rate in the rhesus monkey. According to Myers et al. (1973) minor decreases in fetal heart rate occur as the saturation of the hemoglobin of fetal arterial blood falls below 35%. Marked late deceleration occurs when hemoglobin saturation with oxygen falls below 20%.

Acceleration of Lactic Acid Accumulation with Decrease in Fetal O_2 Concentration

As Fig. 2 shows, the rise in lactic acid concentration in fetal arterial blood is accelerated when the O_2 concentration in fetal arterial blood falls. The *rate* of lactate accumulation is therefore a measure of the degree of hypoxia. The plasma lactate acid concentration itself reflects the product of time and degree of fetal hypoxia.

The rise in lactate concentration reaches a maximum value of 0.5–1.0 m*M*/min when fetal arterial O_2 concentration is virtually zero. A similar maximum speed of lactic acid accumulation in fetal plasma has been found in lambs, according to data of Dawes et al. (1959). The rise in base deficit after clamping the umbilical cord in human and rhesus monkey fetuses is also in this range [1.0 m*M*/min according to Paterson (1971) and Myers (1977)].

Rate of Net Lactate Production in the Fetal Body During Hypoxia

When the anesthetized guinea pig fetus is rapidly removed from the uterus and homogenized, mean whole body lactate concentration can be measured with the appropriate methods (Moll and Kastendieck 1978). Mean whole body lactate concentration in µmol/g is about 60% of the lactate concentration in fetal plasma in µmol/ml (Fig. 4). Thus, there is a lactate space in the fetal body which amounts to about 60% of the fetal body weight. From the rise in lactate concentration in the fetal plasma the total accumulation of lactate in the fetal body can be evaluated.

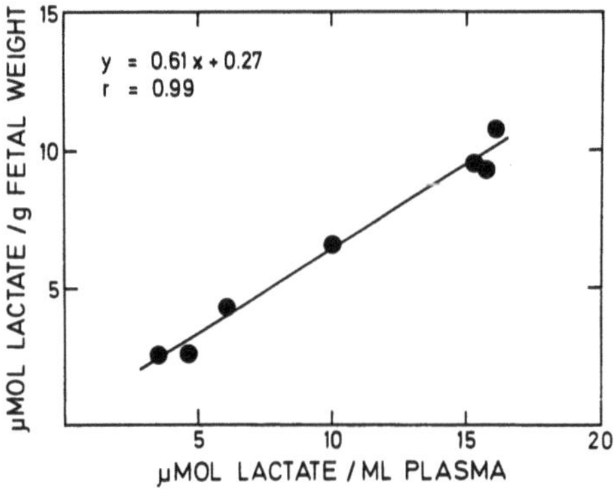

Fig. 4. Mean fetal body lactate concentration in the fetal body related to the plasma concentration. (Moll and Kastendieck 1978)

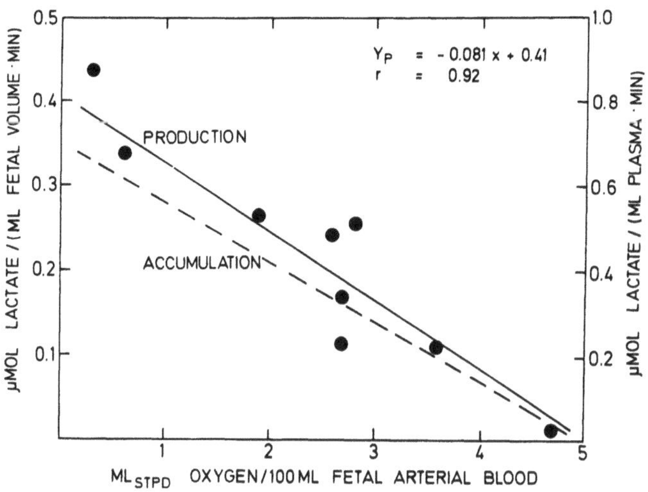

Fig. 5. Lactate production *(closed circles, solid line)* and lactate accumulation *(broken line)* in the fetal body related to the oxygen concentration in fetal arterial blood. The distance between the two lines indicates the placental transfer ($n = 9$). (Moll and Kastendieck 1978)

Measurements of uteroplacental blood flow and arteriovenous differences of lactate show that some 15% of the lactate produced in the fetus is transferred to the mother across the placenta. By adding up the accumulation in the fetal body and the placental transfer, the rate of net lactic acid production can be obtained for the fetus:

Net production = accumulation + placental transfer

As Fig. 5 shows, net lactate production in the fetal body rises with the degree of hypoxia and reaches a maximum value of about 0.5 μmol/g/min during complete anoxia. The maximum rate of net lactate production is similar to the maximal O_2 uptake of the fetal placental unit (8 ml_{STPD}/min/kg = 0.4 μmol/g/min). Since the ATP production per mole of lactate is one-sixth of the ATP production per mole of O_2 we may conclude that the maximum anaerobic metabolic rate that is based on lactate production is about 20% of the maximum aerobic metabolic rate. Only a small fraction of the normal metabolic rate can be maintained by lactate production.

Removal of Fetal Lactic Acid

How fast does the lactic acid which is accumulated in the fetus disappear during a hypoxic period, when the fetus is normally oxygenized again? How long is the "lactate signal" indicating a hypoxic period in the past? In the preparation described above, O_2 saturation in fetal arterial blood usually rises rapidly to the previous value when the placental ischemia is released. As measurements in fetal arterial plasma show, fetal plasma lactate concentration falls in an exponential way toward the concentration in maternal plasma. In Fig. 6 the single value of the rate of lactate concentration changes are related to fetal oxygen concentration. There is a highly

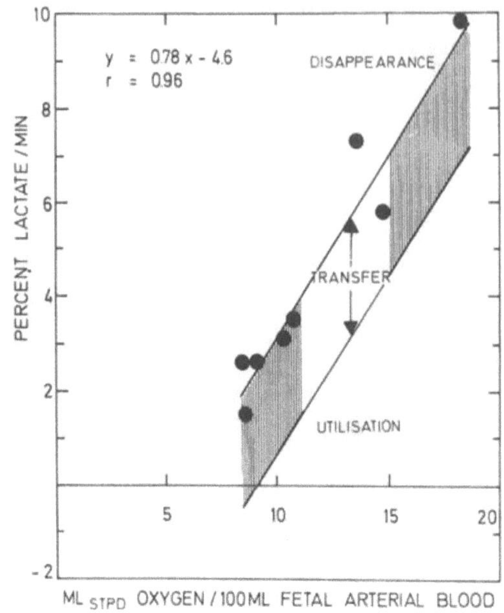

Fig. 6. Disappearance rate of lactate *(closed circles, solid line)* after a hypoxic period related to the oxygen concentration in fetal arterial blood. The disappearance rate is calculated as rate of change of the lactate concentration per concentration difference between the fetal and maternal arterial plasma. According to the placental clearance the rate of lactate removal by placental transfer is 2.5%/min. The rate of removal by utilization *(broken line)* is obtained by subtracting these 2.5%/min from the disappearance rate. (Moll and Kastendieck 1978)

significant correlation between the rate of lactate concentration fall and O_2 concentration in fetal arterial blood. The rate of lactate removal seems to reach a maximum value of 10%/min at an extraordinary high O_2 concentration in fetal arterial blood.

The removal of fetal lactate is based on two processes: placental lactic acid transfer and lactic acid utilization by fetal and placental metabolism.

Removal of Lactic Acid by Placental Transfer

The hemochorial placenta of the guinea pig seems to be remarkably permeable for lactic acid. Figure 7 shows the placental permeability for lactate per placental weight for the hemochorial placenta of the guinea pig and for the epitheliochorial placenta of the sheep. In the guinea pig the placental permeability for lactate per placental mass is about 20 times higher than the placental lactate permeability in the sheep. The high placental permeability for lactate in the guinea pig seems to be based on a specific transport system in the placenta. Placental lactate transfer exhibits saturation kinetics as shown in Fig. 8. Stereospecificity of lactate transport was also demonstrated for the guinea pig placenta (Moll et al. 1980; Leichtweiss and Schröder 1981) and recently also for the human placenta (Carstensen et al. 1983). There is evidence that lactate ions and protons which are produced simultaneously in the placenta. In

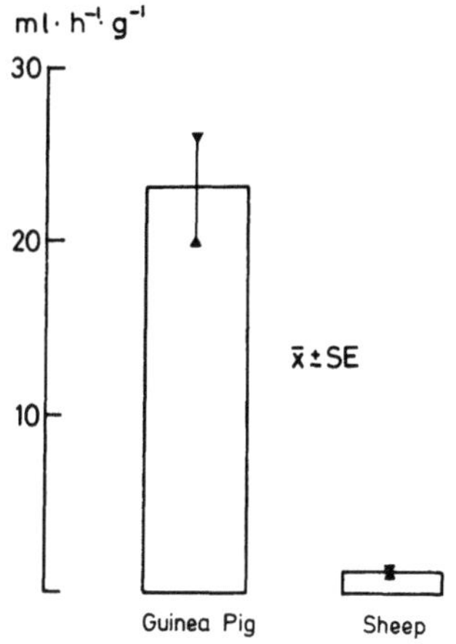

Fig. 7. Placental permeability for lactate per gram of placental weight in guinea pigs and sheep (according to data of Kastendieck and Moll 1977; Kastendieck et al. 1979)

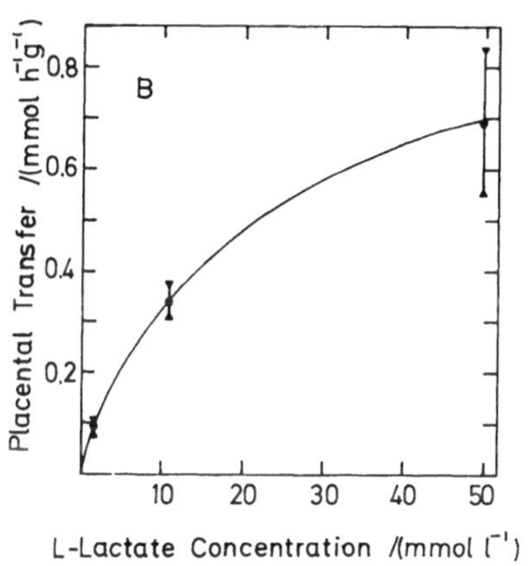

Fig. 8. Fetal maternal transfer of lactate in the guinea pig placenta related to the fetal lactate concentration. The transfer exhibits saturation kinetics. (Moll et al. 1980)

guinea pigs, protons affect the placental lactate transfer and lactate ions affect the placental proton transfer (Moll et al. 1980). Partial correlation analysis of data of lactate concentrations and pH indicate a coupling between lactate and proton transfer also for the human placenta (Haberey et al. 1981a). Evidently, there seems to be a placental transfer mechanism for lactic acid.

In the guinea pig, the placental lactate transfer per concentration difference between fetal and maternal arterial plasma (the placental diffusional clearance) is 15 ml/min/kg fetal weight (Kastendieck and Moll 1977). According to Haberey et al. (1981a) the placental diffusional clearance in human is also in this range. (Maternal-fetal transfer is calculated to be 34 µmol/min and the arterial lactate concentration difference to be 0.82 µmol/min. The placental diffusional clearance is therefore 41 ml/min or 13 ml/min/kg fetal weight.) Thus, about 10–15 ml/min of fetal fluid seems to be cleared per min and per kg of fetal weight by the hemochorial placenta. A major portion of lactate removal occurs by placental transfer in species with a hemochorial placenta.

Maternal Lactate in Fetal Plasma

In view of the high placental permeability, lactate of maternal origin is expected to enter the fetal circulation when maternal plasma lactate concentration is higher than the fetal plasma lactate concentration. On the basis of the observed correlation between maternal and fetal lactate concentration during birth, Derom (1964) concluded that the increase in lactate in cord blood is probably of maternal origin. However, the correlation between maternal and fetal plasma lactate concentration is mostly weak and fetal plasma lactate concentration is usually higher than maternal plasma concentration (see Haberey et al. 1981b). This indicates that placental lactate flux is usually directed toward the mother.

Lactic Acid Removal by Utlization in the Fetal-Placental Unit

In Fig. 6 the lactate removal by placental transfer, derived from the diffusional placental clearance and the maternal-fetal arterial concentration difference, is subtracted from the total lactate disappearance in order to calculate the lactate utilization by fetal and placental metabolism:

Utilization = removal − placental transfer

It is evident that, under the above conditions and in the above species, lactate utilization starts when fetal arterial oxygen saturation exceeds 10 ml_{STPD}/100 ml, i.e., when the O_2 concentration exceeds 50% under these conditions. The rate of utilization rises with the oxygen concentration in fetal blood. At the normal O_2 saturation of 60% (O_2 concentration of 12 ml_{STPD}/100 ml) the lactate utilization is 2.5%/min. A similar value for lactate utlization (2.2%/min) has been found in sheep applying a different method (Kastendieck et al. 1980). In the guinea pig at the normal O_2 saturation of 60%, lactate is removed at an equal rate by placental transfer and fetal utilization. At lower oxygen concentrations the transfer plays the dominant role; at higher concentrations the utilization is dominant.

Overall Rate of Lactic Acid Removal

At the normal O_2 saturation of 60%, the overall rate of lactate removal is 5%/min in the guinea pig under the above conditions. This means that the lactate signal has faded to one-half of its original value in about 15 min. For the anesthetized sheep, Kastendieck et al. (1980) calculated a half-time for lactic acid removal of 30 min. We may conclude that lactic acid which has accumulated in hypoxic periods is removed with a half-time of about 30 min or less. Thus, the fetal lactate concentration gives a summary of hypoxic periods in the preceding 30 min before sampling and even earlier hypoxic periods if there is no time interval of improved oxygenation.

Conclusions

Lactate is produced in the fetal body at a significant rate when fetal arterial O_2 saturation falls below a certain level (25% in the anesthetized guinea pig fetus) where, as indicated by the decreased O_2 uptake of the fetal-placental unit, O_2 supply to fetal tissue falls short of O_2 need. The rate of lactate accumulation rises with falling O_2 saturation of fetal arterial blood; fetal lactate concentration is related to duration and degree of fetal hypoxia. Maximum anaerobic metabolic rate is only a small fraction of maximum aerobic metabolism. Removal of fetal lactic acid occurs, during normoxic periods, by placental transfer and fetal-placental utilization. For the above conditions in the guinea pig, the half-time for lactate removal at a normal fetal oxygenation is about 20 min. The fetal lactate concentration presents a medium-term history of duration and degree of fetal hypoxic periods.

References

Carstensen MH, Leichtweiss HP, Schröder H (1983) Lactate carriers in the artificially perfused human term placenta. Placenta 4:165–174

Dawes GS, Mott JC, Shelley HJ (1959) The importance of cardiac glycogen for the maintenance of life in foetal lambs and new-born animals during anoxia. J Physiol (Lond) 146:516–538

Derom R (1964) Anaerobic metabolism in the human fetus. Am J Obstet Gynecol 89:241–251

Girard H, Klappstein S, Bartag I, Moll W (1983) Blood circulation and oxygen transport in the fetal guinea pig. J Dev Physiol 5:181–193

Haberey P, Piquard F, Hsiung R, Schaefer A, Lazarus S, Dellenbach P (1981a) Mécanisme du transfert foeto-maternel et métabolisme placentaire du lactate dans l'espèce humaine. Rev Fr Gynecol Obstet 76:813–828

Haberey P, Piquard F, Hsiung R, Schaefer A, Dellenbach P (1981b) Etude critique de l'acidose transmise. Rev Fr Gynecol Obstet 76:877–888

Herberger J, Moll W (1976) The flow resistance of the maternal placental vascular bed of anesthetized guinea pigs. Z Geburtshilfe Perinatol 180:61–66

Kastendieck E, Moll W (1977) The placental transfer of lactate and bicarbonate in the guinea-pig. Pflügers Arch 370:165–171

Kastendieck E, Künzel W, Kurz CS (1979) Placental clearance of lactate and bicarbonate in sheep. Gynecol Obstet Invest 10:9–22

Kastendieck E, Künzel W, Kurz CS (1980) Utilization of lactic acid and cardiovascular response in the sheep fetus receiving an infusion of lactic acid. Arch Gynecol 230:21–32

Leichtweiss HP, Schröder H (1981) L-lactate and D-lactate carriers on the fetal and the maternal side of the trophoblast in the isolated guinea-pig placenta. Pflügers Arch 390:80–85

Moll W, Kastendieck E (1978) Accumulation and disappearance of lactate in a fetus with a hemochorial placenta. The role of placental transfer and fetal metabolism. J Perinat Med 6:246–254

Moll W, Girard H, Gros G (1980) Facilitated diffusion of lactic acid across the guinea-pig placenta. Pflügers Arch 385:229–238

Myers RE (1977) Experimental models of perinatal brain damage: relevance to human pathology. In: Gluck L (ed) Intrauterine asphyxia and the developing fetal brain. Year Book Medical, New York, pp 37–97

Myers RE, Mueller-Heubach E, Adamsons K (1973) Predictability of the state of fetal oxygenation from a quantitative analysis of the components of late deceleration. Am J Obstet Gynecol 115:1083–1094

Paterson PJ (1971) The effect of asphyxia on the mid gestation human fetus. Biol Neonate 17:285–291

Pharmacological Aspects of Fetal Heart Rate Regulation During Hypoxia

C. B. Martin, Jr.[1]

Introduction

Reduction in the level of fetal oxygenation can produce a variety of changes in the fetal heart rate (FHR). In addition to the degree and duration of the lack of oxygen, other factors which can influence the FHR response to hypoxia include the age of the fetus, its condition at the onset of the hypoxic stress, and the presence and degree of hypercapnia and acidemia accompanying the hypoxia. Hypoxia can affect the FHR by reflex mechanisms involving both major divisions of the autonomic nervous system, by stimulating the release of catecholamines from the adrenal medulla and by direct depression of myocardial rhythmicity. The FHR can be influenced indirectly by hypoxia-induced changes in brain activity state, breathing, and somatic movements.

The FHR response to hypoxia has been examined pharmacologically, chiefly by the use of autonomic blocking agents. Although it is unlikely that this examination has been complete, at least some conclusions can be drawn from the available results as to the mechanisms and pathways involved.

Fetal Heart Rate Response to Hypoxia

The response of the FHR to isocapnic hypoxia has been studied most extensively in the fetal sheep and fetal rhesus monkeys. In both species after about 120 days' gestational age, the most typical response of a chronically instrumented, unanesthetized fetus to an acute reduction in p_aO_2 is an initial slowing of the FHR accompanied by an increase in FHR variability (Boddy et al. 1974; Jones and Robinson 1975; Dalton et al. 1977; Ikenoue et al. 1981; Parer et al. 1979, 1980a).

The decrease in FHR is accompanied by arterial hypertension. With prolongation of the hypoxic stress, the heart rate of fetal sheep begins to recover after a variable period and may reach or even exceed the baseline level while hypoxia is still present (Boddy et al. 1974; Dalton et al. 1977). FHR variability, on the other hand, remains elevated until extreme levels of acidosis are reached (Dalton et al. 1977).

Effect of Autonomic Blockade on the Fetal Heart Rate Response to Hypoxia

The influence of autonomic blockade on the average FHR during moderate hypoxia (mean p_aO_2 values usually 1.6 kPa or lower) has been studied by a number of investi-

[1] 7612 Hillcrest Ave., Middleton, WI 53562, USA

Fetal Heart Rate Monitoring
Ed. by W. Künzel

gators. Atropine will prevent or reverse the initial bradycardia during hypoxia (Berman et al. 1976; Cohn et al. 1978; Ikenoue et al. 1981; Parer 1979), and the FHR increase after atropine is greater during hypoxia than in normoxia (Cohn et al. 1978; Parer 1979). These observations demonstrate (1) the reflex nature of the initial fetal bradycardia during hypoxia and (2) an increased level of cardioaccelerator tone during hypoxia, which is usually obscured by the reflex bradycardia.

There is much additional evidence for increased beta-adrenergic effects on the fetal heart during hypoxia. Both adrenaline and noradrenaline are released from the fetal adrenal medulla during even mild hypoxemia in sheep (Jones and Robinson 1975). The pre-ejection period of the fetal cardiac cycle is shortened during hypoxia, in spite of the elevation in diastolic blood pressure which should produce the opposite effect; and the shortening can be prevented by beta-adrenergic blockade with propranolol (Evers et al. 1981b).

Beta-adrenergic blockade impairs the ability of the fetus to withstand hypoxemia, resulting in an exaggerated fall in FHR, a decrease in cardiac output and umbilical blood flow, and a reduction in myocardial blood flow (Cohn et al. 1978, 1982; Court et al. 1983). The tendency of the FHR to return toward control levels during hypoxia is related to plasma catecholamine levels (Jones and Robinson 1975; Jones and Ritchie 1983) and can be prevented by propranolol (Jones and Ritchie 1983).

Alpha-adrenergic mechanisms are also importantly involved in the fetal cardiovascular response to hypoxia, although their role with regard to the FHR response is probably indirect. Both reflex and neurohumoral mechanisms are involved. Stimulation of the aortic chemoreceptors produces vasoconstriction in the hind limb of the fetal sheep (Dawes et al. 1968), and sinoaortic denervation prevents hypoxia-induced vasoconstriction in the carcass, gut, and kidneys (Itskovitz et al. 1983). As noted earlier, hypoxia stimulates the release of adrenaline and noradrenaline from the fetal adrenal medulla (Jones and Robinson 1975). Infusion of noradrenaline or adrenaline into fetal sheep to produce levels equivalent to those found during hypoxia reproduces the FHR changes of hypoxia (Dalton et al. 1977; Jones and Ritchie 1978). Druzin et al. (1979) also pointed out similarities between the FHR response to hypoxia and those following bolus injections of noradrenaline, adrenaline, or metariminol into chronically prepared fetal rhesus monkeys. In both instances, the FHR changes could be blocked by phentolamine. The importance of adrenal catecholamines in the fetal cardiovascular response to hypoxia is further shown by the observation that fetal sheep subjected to chemical peripheral sympathectomy (6-hydroxy dopamine) retain their ability to respond to hypoxia with hypertension and bradycardia (Lewis et al. 1983). Alpha-adrenergic blockade (phentolamine or phenoxybenzamine) instituted during hypoxia reverses the selective vasoconstriction in the gut, spleen, liver, and lungs and results in tachycardia and relative hypotension. Vascular resistance in the carcass is reduced, but not to normoxic levels (Reuss et al. 1982).

The autonomic mechanisms involved most directly in the FHR response to acute hypoxia or asphyxia can be summarized as follows: stimulation of peripheral chemoreceptors increases the activity of the peripheral sympathetic nervous system producing selective vasoconstriction, redistribution of the cardiac output, and usually some degree of arterial hypertension. Simultaneously adrenaline and noradrenaline are released from the adrenal medulla. These circulating catecholamines reinforce the effects of peripheral sympathetic nervous activity and further exert positive chronotropic and ionotropic effects on the fetal heart. The positive chronotropism is, however, initially antagonized by increased vagal cardiodecelerator activity resulting principally from activation of the chemo- and baroreflexes. With time, increasing levels of plasma catecholamines cause the heart rate to increase toward or even above the level prior to the hypoxic stress. Suppression of vagal activity, or adaptation or resetting of the baroreflex, may also contribute to the recovery of heart rate in the face of continuing arterial hypertension. The increased FHR variability probably reflects increased oscillations in the cardiovascular control systems associated with greater levels of input from chemoreceptors and baroreceptors and with the redistribution of cardiac output.

Fetal Heart Rate Response to Mild Asphyxia

Fetal hypoxia occurring during clinical fetal stress or distress is not usually isocapnic. Moreover, differences between the FHR and fetal plasma catecholamine responses to isocapnic hypoxia, hypercapnic hypoxia induced by alteration of the maternal inspired gas mixture, and asphyxia produced by reducing uterine blood flow have recently been reported for the fetal sheep (C. T. Jones, this volume). We studied the FHR response produced by partial occlusion of the uterine blood supply for 30 min to produce mild asphyxia in nine experiments on seven fetal sheep between 114 and 140 days' gestation (Table 1) (Martin et al. 1979a). During asphyxia the mean FHR decreased by an average of 19 bpm in six experiments (four fetuses) and increased by 7, 11, and 17 bpm in three other fetuses. Both the long-term irregularity (LTI) index of FHR oscillations (De Haan et al. 1971) and the interval difference (ID) index of beat-to-beat variability (Jongsma et al. 1978) increased substantially (Table 1). The mild degree of asphyxia produced in these experiments probably accounts for the inconsistency of the change in mean FHR; nonetheless, the most frequent pattern was slowing and all fetuses showed increases in the variability indices.

Effect of Autonomic Blockade on the Fetal Heart Rate Response to Mild Asphyxia

The effect of autonomic blocking agents on the FHR response to mild asphyxia was also studied in the fetuses described above (Martin et al. 1979b). After a 30-min control period, blockade was induced by means of atropine, 0.5–1.7 mg/kg estimated fetal weight (EFW), propranolol, 1 mg/kg EFW, or phentolamine, 1–4 mg/kg EFW. Following a 30-min observation period with blockade, the uterine blood supply was partially occluded for a further 30-min period. The adequacy of the block was tested initially, before the start of the occlusion, and after the release of the occlusion with the appropriate agonist: acetylcholine, isoprenaline, or norepinephrine.

The results of these experiments are given in Tables 2–4. Muscarinic cholinergic blockade with atropine (Table 2) produced the expected increase in heart rate (decrease in R-R interval) and in beat-to-beat variability (ID index). FHR fluctua-

Table 1. Changes in fetal arterial blood gas values, FHR, and blood pressure during 30 min of partial occlusion of the maternal common internal iliac artery in nine experiments in seven sheep. Values are means (SD) except for LTI and ID which are medians (Q_1–Q_3). *, $2P<0.05$; **, $2P<0.01$

	pO_2 (kPa)	pCO_2 (kPa)	pH	R-R (ms)	BP (mm Hg)	LTI	ID
Control	3.6 (1.0)	4.8 (0.6)	7.37 (0.03)	399 (60)	46 (5)	8.4 (6.3, 10.4)	8.5 (6.3, 14.0)
	**	*	*			*	*
Occlusion	2.3 (0.6)	5.9 (1.2)	7.30 (0.09)	423 (61)	47 (6)	13.7 (11.2, 27.2)	17.1 (15.1, 33.7)

Table 2. Changes in fetal arterial blood gas values, FHR, and blood pressure during a 30-min period of muscarinic cholinergic blockade with atropine, followed by 30 min of partial occlusion of the uterine blood supply. Values are means (SD) except for LTI and ID which are medians (range). *, $2P<0.05$; *N*, 5 unless otherwise specified

	p_aO_2 (kPa)	pCO_2 (kPa)	pHa	R-R (ms)	BP (mm Hg)	LTI	ID
Control	3.7	5.4	7.38 (0.02)	410 (54)	44 (2)	8.4 (5.1, 15.6)	10.4 (6.7, 30.4)
	(*N*, 3)	(*N*, 3)	(*N*, 4)	*			*
Block	2.8 (1.0)	5.1 (0.4)	7.38 (0.04)	326 (46)	46 (3)	7.4 (2.7, 18.0)	4.6 (3.8, 5.6)
	*						
Block plus occlusion	2.2 (0.6)	5.7 (1.9)	7.32 (0.10)	314 (26)	48 (3)	5.2 (2.7, 17.3)	7.1 (3.2, 22.8)

Table 3. Changes in fetal arterial blood gas values, FHR, and blood pressure during a 30-min period of β-adrenergic blockade with propranolol, followed by 30 min of partial occlusion of the uterine blood supply. Values as in Table 2. *N*, 4

	p_aO_2 (kPa)	pCO_2 (kPa)	pHa	R-R (ms)	BP (mm Hg)	LTI	ID
Control	2.8 (0.2)	5.4 (0.2)	7.33 (0.03)	427 (37)	53 (8)	11.4 (7.8, 16.3)	8.6 (3.6, 11.6)
Block	3.1 (0.4)	5.5 (0.1)	7.34 (0.04)	436 (41)	53 (9)	8.1 (4.9, 10.2)	9.4 (2.9, 16.7)
Block plus occlusion	2.2 (0.1)	5.9 (0.4)	7.42 (0.03)	433 (26)	50 (8)	10.6 (6.9, 13.7)	11.6 (3.0, 18.0)

Table 4. Changes in fetal arterial blood gas values, FHR, and blood pressure during a 30-min period of alpha-adrenergic blockade with phentolamine, followed by 30 min of partial occlusion of the uterine blood supply. Values as in Table 2. *N*, 5 unless otherwise specified. *, $2P < 0.05$

	p_aO_2 (kPa)	pCO_2 (kPa)	pHa	R-R (ms)	BP (mm Hg)	LTI	ID
Control	2.8 (0.8)	5.5 (0.2)	7.38 (0.04)	387 (56)	44 (9)	9.1 (7.4, 9.8)	12.9 (6.9, 15.6)
	*				(*N*, 4)	*	*
Block	2.5 (0.8)	5.5 (0.4)	7.38 (0.03)	336 (42)	40	16.4 (9.6, 18.7)	23.7 (14.2, 33.5)
	*				(*N*, 3)		
Block plus occlusion	2.0 (0.5)	6.0 (0.9)	7.29 (0.10)	341 (55)	49 (10)	14.1 (8.1, 16.9)	22.4 (13.6, 35.5)

tions (LTI index) were not affected. Mild asphyxia during atropine blockade resulted in an insignificant further shortening of RR interval, no increase in FHR fluctuations, and only a small average increase in beat-to-beat variability, most of which was contributed by one fetus which also demonstrated an incomplete block at the end of the occlusion period.

This same experiment was attempted six times with beta-adrenergic blockade with propranolol; however, on two occasions the protocol could not be completed because of marked fetal bradycardia in response to the asphyxial stress. In the four remaining fetuses, propranol produced an insignificant prolongation of the average R-R interval, a consistent but modest reduction in the LTI index, and no consistent change in beat-to-beat variability (Table 3). During asphyxial stress, average heart rate did not change, FHR fluctuations increased in three and beat-to-beat variability rose in two of the four fetuses. Both indices of FHR variability remained below the levels observed in unblocked fetuses at an approximately equal level of asphyxial stress (Table 1).

The effect of alpha-adrenergic blockade with phentolamine was studied in five experiments on five fetuses (Table 4). Phentolamine alone produced an increase in the FHR in four of the five fetuses and consistent increases in both the LTI and ID indices equivalent to those observed during asphyxia in the unblocked fetuses. It should be noted, however, that the fetal p_aO_2 decreased significantly after the administration of phentolamine with no consistent change in p_aO_2 or pH. During the period of reduced uterine blood flow, FHR and the variability indices changed inconsistently but remained generally in the range present during alpha blockade prior to asphyxia.

The changes in average FHR with asphyxia in these experiments were small, both in the presence and absence of autonomic blockade. Since we were primarily interested in effects on FHR variability, we kept the degree of asphyxia in the unblocked fetuses mild so as to avoid marked fetal bradycardias, and a similar degree of asphyxia was intended in the experiments during blockade. The changes in fetal blood pressure were also small and statistically insignificant. Nonetheless, both FHR fluctuations and bcat-to-bcat variability incrcased substantially in the unblocked fetuses, whereas the increases in both components of FHR variability were considerably blunted during either cholinergic or beta-adrenergic blockade with similar degrees of asphyxia. This indicates that both of these automatic divisions are involved in producing the increased FHR variability during asphyxia, since blockade of either of them reduces the increase in variability.

The increase in FHR variability during alpha-adrenergic blockade with phentolamine is difficult to interpret because of the simultaneous fall in fetal p_aO_2. We have no explanation for this decrease, which was not accompanied by any changes in p_aCO_2 or pH. The increased FHR variability may thus have been a response to mild hypoxemia, but there was no further increase with the additional fall in p_aO_2 during asphyxia. Another possibility is that, with the vasomotor limb of the baroreflex paralyzed, the activity of the cardiac limb increased, resulting in the greater FHR variability; however, blood pressure fluctuations, measured as the standard deviation of mean blood pressure of the individual fetuses, showed no consistent change between the control and blockade periods.

Pharmacological Influences on the Fetal Heart Rate Response to Phasic Asphyxia

This discussion has so far been restricted to "stable" hypoxia or asphyxia produced by the administration of low O_2 gas mixtures or reduction of uterine blood flow for periods of many minutes to a few hours. Fetal hypoxia or asphyxia during labor has a prominent phasic character resulting from intermittent reduction of uterine blood flow or umbilical cord compression by uterine contractions.

We studied the effects of intermittent total occlusion of the maternal common iliac artery, the major source of the uteroplacental blood supply, in chronically instrumented fetal sheep at 122–144 days' gestation (Martin et al. 1979a). The occlusion was maintained for 30–60 s and was repeated at intervals of 2.5 min. Fetal p_aO_2 (abdominal aorta) was 2.1 ± 0.6 kPa ($x \pm SD$) at the beginning of the experiments, but fell to 1.4 ± 0.3 kPa 1 min after the series of five to ten repetitive occlusions. We observed wide V- or U-shaped FHR decelerations beginning 15–25 s after the start of the occlusion, accompanied by transient hypertension (Fig. 1).

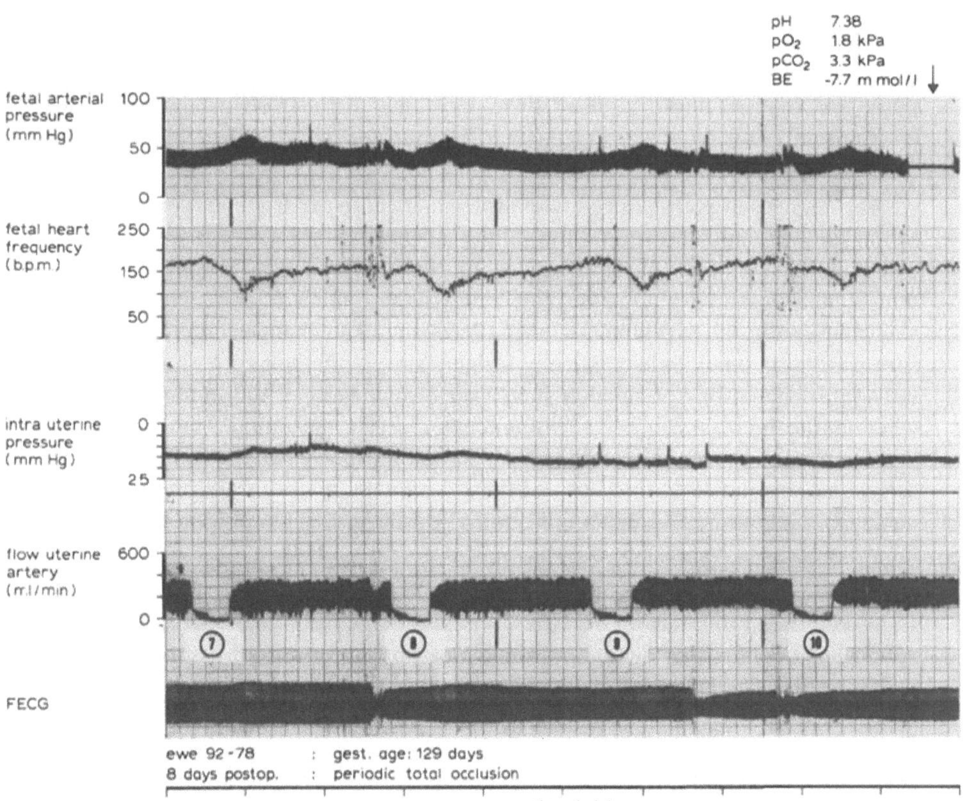

Fig. 1. Periodic FHR decelerations and hypertension in response to periodic occlusion of the maternal common hypogastric artery in a fetal lamb. (Martin et al. 1979a)

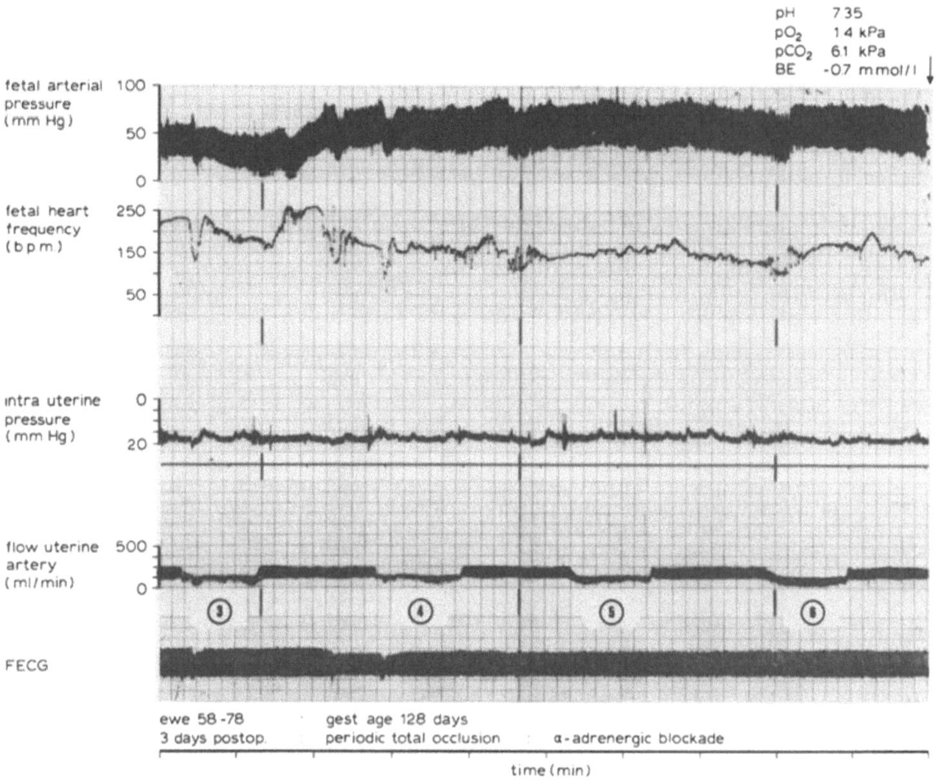

Fig. 2. Modification of the fetal response pattern following alpha-adrenergic blockade with phentolamine. The phasic fetal hypertension is absent. A V-shaped deceleration occurred with fetal movement during occlusion 3, and brief decelerations occurred after occlusion 4 and during occlusion 6. (Martin et al. 1979a)

Alpha-adrenergic blockade (phentolamine) eliminated both the phasic hypertension and the greatest part of the FHR decelerations (Fig. 2). Atropine converted the FHR decelerations into accelerations (Fig. 3), and the addition of beta-adrenergic blockade suppressed these (Fig. 4). We concluded that, in nonacidemic fetal lamb, the FHR decelerations produced by periodic occlusion of uteroplacental blood flow are reflex in origin, representing mainly a baroreflex-induced cardiac slowing in response to chemoreflex-induced hypertension. Since the FHR slowing not infrequently began before the onset of the hypertension, we proposed also that the chemoreflex could initiate the cardiac slowing in some instances.

When one fetus was made progressively acidotic by repeated total occlusions superimposed on continuous partial occlusion of the uterine blood supply, the hypertensive response was reduced (Fig. 5) and eventually replaced by hypotension (Fig. 6). We inferred that this indicated direct depression of cardiac chronotropism by the hypoxia. Administration of atropine to the severely acidotic fetus resulted in elevation of heart rate, demonstrating that tonic vagal activity had still been present, but no change in the amplitude of the decelerations (Fig. 6).

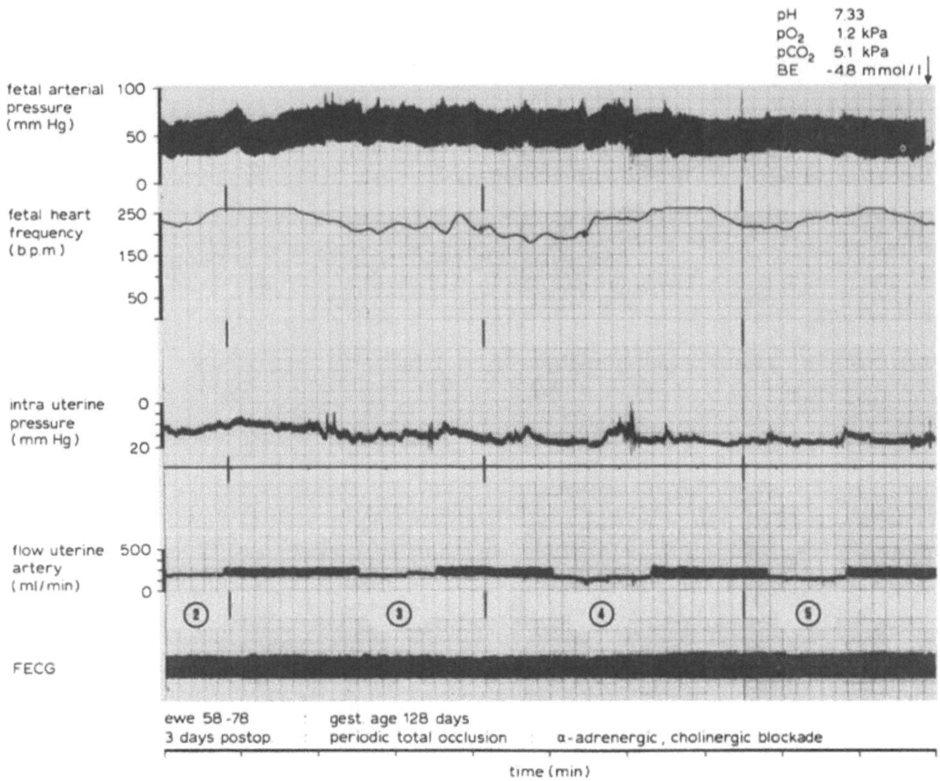

Fig. 3. Combined alpha-adrenergic and cholinergic blockade in the same fetus shown in Fig. 2. The FHR now responds to the occlusions with periodic acceleration. (Martin et al. 1979a)

Our conclusions as to the mechanisms involved in late decelerations of the FHR, based on these observations, are shown schematically in Fig. 7.

Subsequently Parer and co-workers (Parer et al. 1980b; Harris et al. 1981, 1982) and Itskovitz et al. (1982) have also analyzed the mechanisms involved in late FHR decelerations. They interrupted uteroplacental blood flow by inflating a balloon-tipped catheter in the abdominal aorta of the ewes for periods of 10–20 s. Their findings differ from those described above chiefly on one point. In normoxic fetuses (x p_aO_2, 2.8–3.9 kPa), the FHR decelerations resulting from 20-s occlusions were not accompanied by significant fetal hypertension; and these decelerations were not altered by alpha-adrenergic blockade (Harris et al. 1981). Hypertension did occur in hypoxemic fetuses (x p_aO_2, 1.3–1.6 kPa), but not until the recovery phase of the decelerations. These investigators concluded that late decelerations in nonacidemic fetuses are initiated via the chemoreflex. Harris et al. (1982) further demonstrated the occurrence of direct hypoxic depression of the FHR in nonacidemic fetuses first made hypoxic by administration of a low O_2 gas mixture to the ewe, then further subjected to 20-s interruptions of uteroplacental blood flow. Both groups observed FHR accelerations in response to transient occlusion of the uteroplacental blood flow in normoxic fetuses pretreated with atropine.

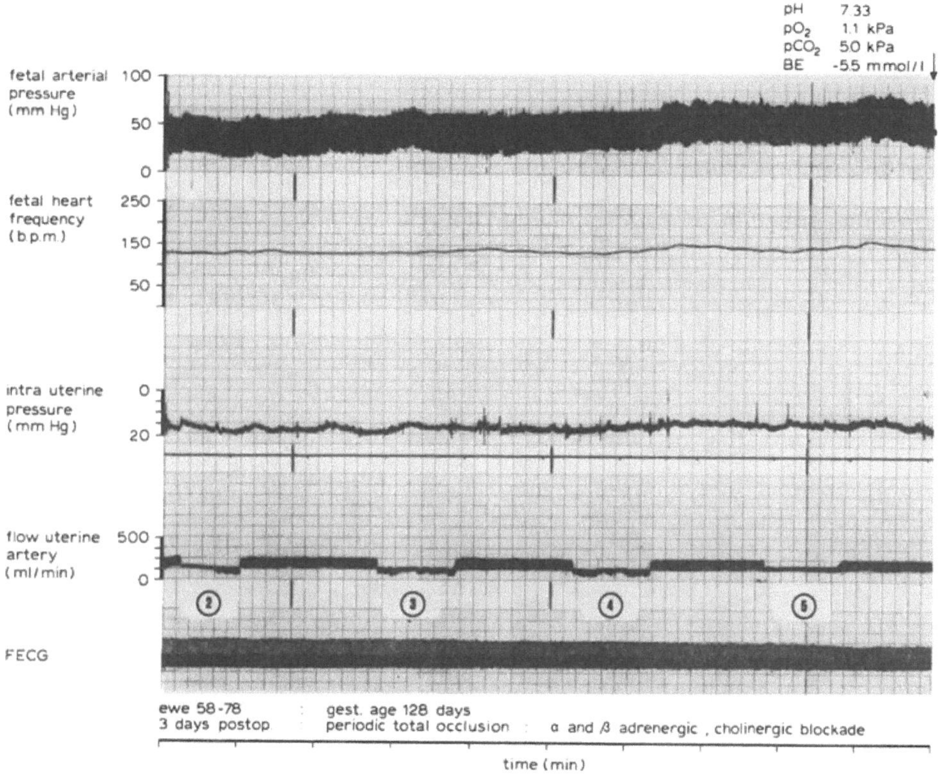

Fig. 4. Fetal response to periodic occlusion of the maternal common hypogastric artery trunk in the presence of combined alpha- and beta-adrenergic and cholinergic blockade. There remains a slight FHR acceleration during the occlusion and a small hypertensive response following some of them, probably reflecting incomplete blockade

Thus the relative importance of the various pathways shown in Fig. 7, and the sequence in which they are activated, varies with the epxerimental (and clinical) circumstances. The basic validity of this pharmacologic dissection of late FHR decelerations, however, appears to remain intact.

Studies with autonomic blocking agents during umbilical cord compression have led to the diagram of mechanisms shown in Fig. 8. The observation of Barcroft (1946) of the difference in the FHR response to cord occlusion before and after vagotomy established early the role of vagal reflexes in the immediate FHR slowing. This has been substantiated since by many investigators using pharmacologic blockade with atropine. Evers et al. (1981a) demonstrated the presence of both alpha- and beta-adrenergic influences on the heart and circulation after about 10–15 s of umbilical cord occlusion. This corresponds roughly to the time at which increased chemoreceptor discharge begins (Blanco et al. 1982). At this point Evers et al. (1981a) often found a second, progressive increase in fetal blood pressure which could be blocked by phentolamine. When this secondary hypertension was eliminated, a shortening of the pre-ejection period suggesting increased adrenergic influence on

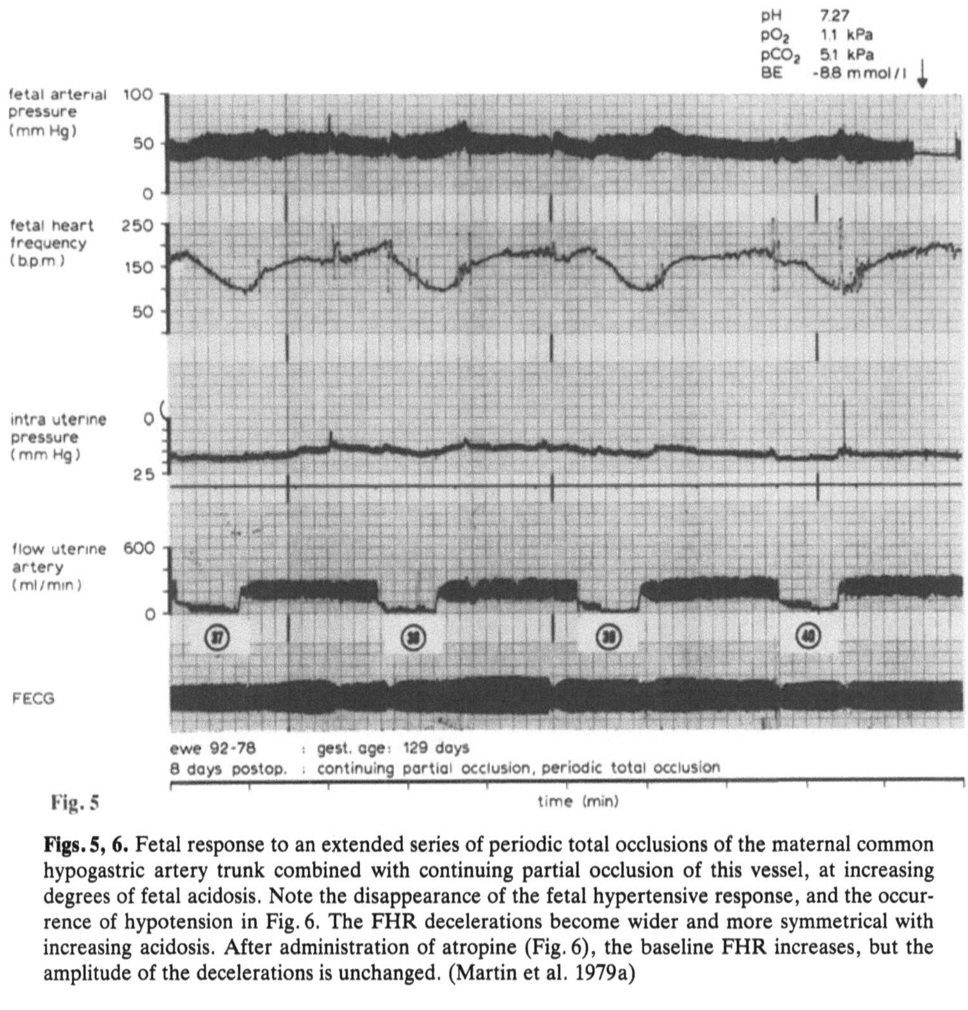

Fig. 5

Figs. 5, 6. Fetal response to an extended series of periodic total occlusions of the maternal common hypogastric artery trunk combined with continuing partial occlusion of this vessel, at increasing degrees of fetal acidosis. Note the disappearance of the fetal hypertensive response, and the occurrence of hypotension in Fig. 6. The FHR decelerations become wider and more symmetrical with increasing acidosis. After administration of atropine (Fig. 6), the baseline FHR increases, but the amplitude of the decelerations is unchanged. (Martin et al. 1979a)

the myocardium could be identified. After pretreatment with propranolol, shortening of the cardiac pre-ejection period was not observed, either during or after cord occlusion, and both heart rate and blood pressure fell markedly toward the end of the 30-s occlusion period. Increased beta-adrenergic activity appears to be necessary during umbilical cord compression to oppose the strong vagal activity and perhaps also to sustain myocardial contractility during hypoxia.

Central Nervous System Influences During Hypoxia

Although it has been demonstrated that in fetal sheep hypoxia exerts a number of effects on the central nervous system including alterations in the proportion of high- and low-voltage electrocortical activity (Boddy et al. 1974; Clewlow et al. 1983) and active suppression of fetal breathing movements (Dawes et al. 1980) and multi-

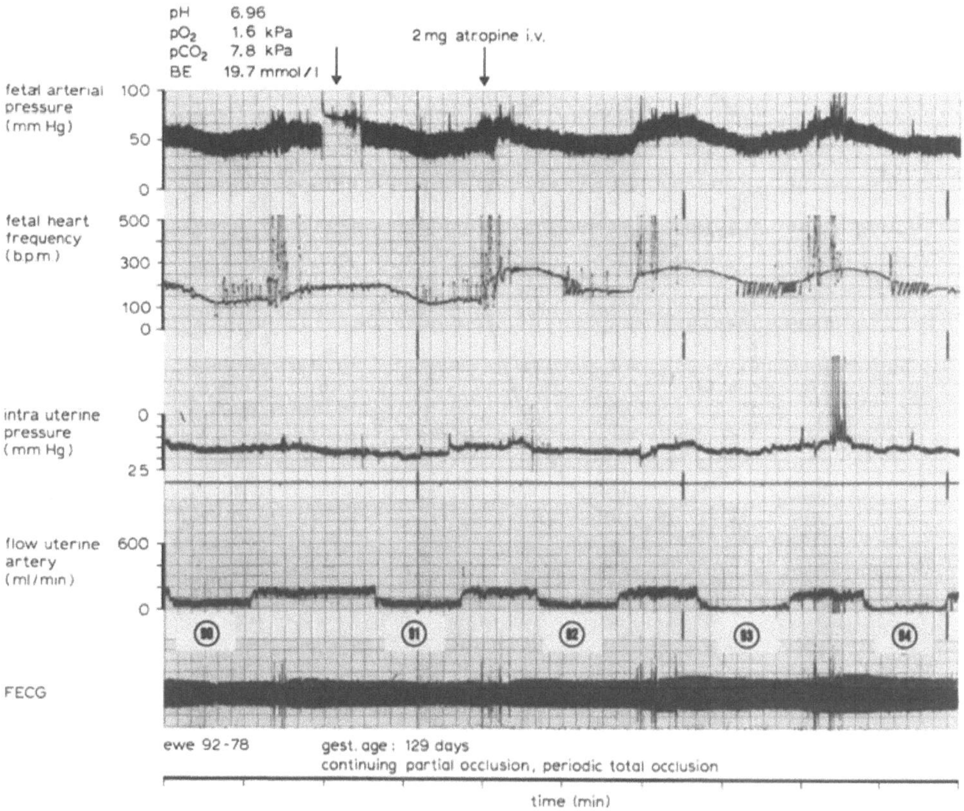

Fig. 6

neuronal limb reflexes (Blanco and Walker 1982), all of which can potentially influence the FHR (Van Der Wildt 1982), there has been little investigation into the pharmacologic basis of these effects. Recently, however, Stark et al. (1982) have demonstrated that beta-endorphin is released during hypoxia in fetal sheep. LaGamma et al. (1982) found that opiate receptor antagonism with naloxone exaggerates the fetal bradycardia during hypoxia, and leads to a slowly undulating FHR pattern. These effects on the FHR could be blocked with atropine, suggesting that the opiate (beta-endorphin) effect might be to modulate parasympathetic tone. Together with the ionotropic effect of the increased plasma catecholamines, this mechanism might explain the gradual conversion of fetal bradycardia to tachycardia during protracted hypoxia.

Vasopressin levels are increased in fetal sheep during hypoxia (Rurak 1978), the neurohormone being released in parallel with beta-endorphine (Stark et al. 1982). Infusion of vasopressin into fetal sheep produces hypertension, bradycardia, and redistribution of the cardiac output similar to that observed during hypoxia (Iwamoto et al. 1979). In the absence of studies with blockers of vasopressin activity, however, the importance of this neurohormone in the fetal response to hypoxia remains uncertain.

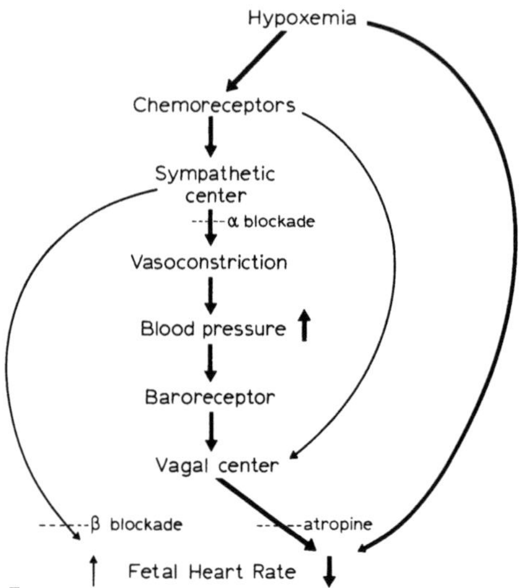

7

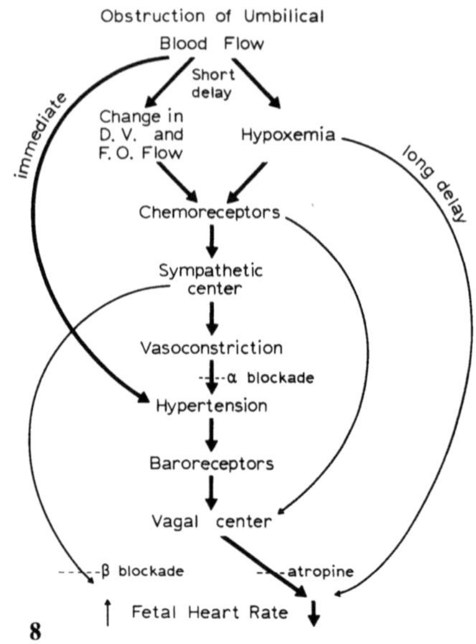

8

Fig. 7. Schematic diagram of the mechanisms presumed to be involved in the production of late decelerations

Fig. 8. Schematic diagram of the mechanisms presumed to be involved in the production of variable decelerations

It is clear, however, that many factors other than activity of the parasympathetic and sympathoadrenal systems are involved in the fetal cardiovascular responses to hypoxia, and their elucidation will undoubtedly occupy perinatal researchers for some years into the future.

References

Barcroft J (1946) Researches on prenatal life. Blackwell, Oxford

Berman W, Goodlin RC, Heymann MA, Rudolph MA (1976) Relationship between pressure and flow in the umbilical and uterine circulations of the sheep. Circ Res 38:262

Blanco CE, Walker DW (1982) Effect of hypoxaemia on hind limb reflexes in unanesthetized fetal and newborn lambs. J Physiol 320:125

Blanco CE, Dawes GS, Hanson M, McCooke HB (1982) The arterial chemoreceptors in fetal sheep and newborn lambs. J Physiol 330:38

Boddy K, Dawes GS, Fisher R, Pinter S, Robinson JS (1974) Fetal respiratory movements, electrocortical and cardiovascular responses to hypoxaemia and hypercapnia in sheep. J Physiol 243:599

Clewlow F, Dawes GS, Johnston BM, Walker DW (1983) Changes in breathing, electrocortical and muscle activity in unanaesthetized fetal lambs with age. J Physiol 341:463

Cohn HE, Piasecki GJ, Jackson BT (1978) The role of autonomic nervous control in the fetal cardiovascular response to hypoxemia. In: Longo LD, Reneau DD (eds) Fetal and newborn cardiovascular physiology, vol 2. Garland STPM, New York, p 249

Cohn HE, Piasecki GJ, Jackson BT (1982) The effect of β-adrenergic stimulation on fetal cardiovascular function during hypoxemia. Am J Obstet Gynecol 144:810

Court DJ, Block BS, Llanos AJ, Parer JT (1983) The effects of propranolol on blood flow redistribution in hypoxemic fetal sheep. Society for Gynecologic Investigation (Abstracts), p 126

Dalton KJ, Dawes GS, Patrick JE (1977) Diurnal, respiratory and other rhythms of fetal heart rate in lambs. Am J Obstet Gynecol 127:414

Dawes GS, Lewis BV, Milligan JE, Roach ML, Talner NS (1968) Vasomotor responses in the hind limbs of foetal and newborn lambs to asphyxia and aortic chemoreceptor stimulation. J Physiol 195:55

De Haan J, Van Bemmel JH, Versteeg B, Veth AFL, Stolte LAM, Janssens J, Eskes TKAB (1971) Quantitative evaluation of fetal heart rate patterns. I. Processing methods. Eur J Obstet Gynecol Reprod Biol 1:95

Druzin ML, Ikenoue T, Murata Y, Socol M, Martin CB (1979) A possible mechanism for the increase in fetal heart rate variability following hypoxemia. Society for Gynecologic Investigation (Abstracts), p 91

Evers JLH, De Haan J, Jongsma HW, Crevels J, Arts THM, Martin CB (1981a) The preejection period of the fetal cardiac cycle. 1. Umbilical cord occlusions. Eur J Obstet Gynecol Reprod Biol 11:401

Evers JLH, De Haan J, Jongsma HW, Crevels J, Arts THM, Martin CB (1981b) The preejection period of the fetal cardiac cycle. 2. Maternal common internal iliac artery occlusions. Eur J Obstet Gynecol Reprod Biol 11:419

Harris JL, Krueger TR, Parer JT (1979) Effects of parasympathetic and β-adrenergic blockade on the umbilical circulation in the unanesthetized fetal sheep. Gynecol Obstet Invest 10:306

Harris JL, Krueger TR, Parer JT (1981) Mechanism of late decelerations: effect of alpha-adrenergic blockade. Society for Gynecologic Investigation (Abstracts), p 164

Harris JL, Krueger TR, Parer JT (1982) Mechanisms of late decelerations of the fetal heart rate during hypoxia. Am J Obstet Gynecol 144:491

Ikenoue T, Martin CB, Murata Y, Ettinger BB, Lu PS (1981) Effect of acute hypoxemia and respiratory acidosis on the fetal heart rate in monkeys. Am J Obstet Gynecol 141:797

Itskovitz J, Goetzman BW, Rudolph AM (1982) The mechanism of late deceleration of the heart rate and its relationship to oxygenation in normoxemic and chronically hypoxemic fetal lambs. Am J Obstet Gynecol 142:66

Itskovitz J, La Gamma EF, Bristow J, Rudolph AM (1983) Role of arterial chemoreflex in fetal circulatory response to acute hypoxemia. Society for Gynecologic Investigation (Abstracts), p 126

Iwamoto HS, Rudolph AM, Keil LC, Heymann MA (1979) Hemodynamic responses of the sheep fetus to vasopressin infusion. Circ Res 44:430

Jones CT, Ritchie JWK (1978) The cardiovascular effects of circulating catecholamines in fetal sheep. J Physiol 285:381

Jones CT, Ritchie JWK (1983) The effects of adrenergic blockade on fetal response to hypoxia. J Dev Physiol 5:211

Jones CT, Robinson RO (1975) Plasma catecholamines in foetal and adult sheep. J Physiol 248:15

La Gamma EL, Itskovitz J, Rudolph AM (1982) Effects of naloxone on fetal circulatory responses to hypoxia. Am J Obstet Gynecol 143:933

Lewis AB, Wolf WJ, Sischo W (1983) Fetal cardiovascular and catecholamine responses to hypoxia after chemical sympathectomy. Pediatr Res 17:136

Martin CB Jr, De Haan J, Van Der Wildt B, Jongsma HW, Dieleman A, Arts THM (1979a) Mechanisms of late decelerations in the fetal heart rate. A study with autonomic blocking agents in fetal lambs. Eur J Obstet Gynecol Reprod Biol 9:361–373

Martin CB, De Haan J, Jongsma HW, Van Der Wildt B, Evers JLH, Dieleman A, Arts THM (1979b) Quantitative investigation of the effect of hypoxemia on FHR variability indices in fetal lambs. Society for Gynecologic Investigation (Abstracts), p 193

Parer JT (1979) Effect of atropine on heart rate and oxygen consumption of the hypoxic fetus. Gynecol Invest 8:50

Parer JT, Laros RK, Heilbron DC, Krueger TR, Rubsamen RM, Wong WS (1979) The effect of acute hypoxia hypercarbia on fetal heart rate variability in awake monkeys. Society for Gynecologic Investigation (Abstracts), p 93

Parer JT, Dijkstra HR, Vredebregt PPM, Harris JL, Krueger TR, Reuss ML (1980a) Increased fetal heart rate variability with acute hypoxia in chronically instrumented sheep. Eur J Obstet Gynecol Reprod Biol 10:393

Parer JT, Krueger TR, Harris JL (1980b) Fetal oxygen consumption and mechanisms of heart rate response during artificially produced late decelerations of fetal heart rate in sheep. Am J Obstet Gynecol 136:478

Reuss ML, Parer JT, Harris JL, Krueger TR (1982) Hemodynamic effects of alpha-adrenergic blockade during hypoxia in fetal sheep. Am J Obstet Gynecol 142:410

Rurak DW (1978) Plasma vasopressin levels during hypoxemia and the cardiovascular effects of exogenous vasopressin in foetal and adult sheep. J Physiol 277:341

Stark RL, Wardlaw SL, Daniel SS, Husain MK, Sanocka UM, James LS, Van De Wiele RL (1982) Vasopressin secretion induced by hypoxia in sheep: developmental changes and relationship to β-endorphin release. Am J Obstet Gynecol 143:204

Van Der Wildt B (1982) Heart rate, breathing movements and brain activity in fetal lambs. Doctoral thesis, Catholic University, Nijmegen, The Netherlands

Pathophysiology of Fetal Heart Rate Variability and Base Line Fetal Heart Rate

The Control of Fetal Heart Rate and Its Variability in Lambs

G. S. Dawes[1]

For more than 200 years obstetricians have recognized that slowing of the fetal heart in labour may be a sinister sign. For a much shorter period of time, since methods became available for recording fetal heart rate at the bedside, it has been suspected that a substantial decrease in heart rate variability also is sinister. So it is reasonable to ask what light animal experiments have thrown on the subject, and what are the physiological mechanisms which control the heart rate and its variation near term.

The basic facts are well known. Most experimental work has been done on sheep in which, although precocial (i.e. mature at birth), autonomic control of the heart is not established until more than halfway through normal gestation. Up to 110-days gestation (0.75 of term) the primary response to moderate isocapnic hypoxia (a fall in PaO_2 from 23 down to 15 mmHg) is a rise in heart rate and a small fall in arterial pressure (Table 1). The heart rate continues to rise over 60 min. With increasing age after 110 days' gestation a primary fall of heart rate and rise of arterial pressure during hypoxia becomes evident. Bilateral vagotomy, which interrupts both the parasympathetic efferent nerves to the heart and the afferent nerves from the aortic bodies, abolishes both the initial fall of heart rate during hypoxia and also the rise of arterial pressure. The rise of arterial pressure during hypoxia of this degree is therefore attributed to stimulation of the aortic chemoreceptors. The primary fall in heart rate is also probably due to chemoreceptor stimulation, either peripheral or central. It is unlikely to be due to baroreceptor excitation, because an increase in arterial pressure of 5–8 mmHg by expanding an aortic balloon causes an insignificant change

Table 1. Changes during isocapnic hypoxia in unanaesthetized fetal lambs at different ages in utero. (G. S. Dawes, K. Koike, and R. Phibbs, unpublished observations)

			Gestational age (days)					
			95–110 (9)		119–129 (25)		130–139 (30)	
Hypoxia (min)	Fetal PaO_2	Fetal pH	Blood pressure (mmHg)	Heart rate (beats/min)	Blood pressure (mmHg)	Heart rate (beats/min)	Blood pressure (mmHg)	Heart rate (beats/min)
0	22.6	7.35	41 ± 2.5	193 ± 4	48 ± 2	178 ± 7	48 ± 1	162 ± 3
10	14.7	7.34	40 ± 3.1	203 ± 16	48 ± 4	153 ± 11	54 ± 3	132 ± 8
60	14.7	7.30	44 ± 3.3	221 ± 14	51 ± 6	169 ± 6	52 ± 2	166 ± 10

Number of experiments in parentheses; mean values ± SE

[1] University of Oxford, Nuffield Institute for Medical Research, Headley Way, Headlington, Oxford OX3 9DS, Great Britain

Fetal Heart Rate Monitoring
Ed. by W. Künzel

in heart rate in fetal lambs. It is also worth comment that infusion of adrenaline into mature fetal lambs also causes a fall in heart rate initially.

This degree of isocapnic hypoxia has little effect on the fetal electrocorticogram, but arrests breathing movements, eye movements and movements of the neck, trunk and limbs by a complex set of central mechanisms involving suprapontine and medullary centres. These effects are independent of the peripheral arterial chemoreceptors. They are accompanied by a large rise in plasma catecholamines, vasopressin and adrenocorticotropic hormone. There is maintenance of the output of the two ventricles and of blood flow to the placenta. Otherwise cardiac output is redistributed, flow to the heart and brain being substantially increased at the expense of all the other organs, including the lungs, kidneys and especially the skeletal musculature.

I have not so far referred to the carotid chemoreceptors, which play an important part in short-term stabilization of the circulation and respiration postnatally. Recent experiments on fetal lambs have shown that they respond to hypoxia or hypercapnia as early as 0.7 of term. The part they play, if any, in prenatal physiological control is uncertain. They must adapt soon after birth to the changed environment, with the large elevation of PaO_2 and fall in $PaCO_2$.

More severe and more prolonged hypoxia, with a rising blood lactate and severe metabolic acidaemia (base excess < -12 mEq/litre), induces a prolonged fall of heart rate due partly to a local cardiac action with, ultimately, evidence of cardiac failure.

Now let us turn to heart rate variations. With increasing gestational age, in sheep (Dalton et al. 1977) and in man, the mean heart rate falls and variability becomes greater. The fetal heart is subject to modulation in association with many physiological variables, such as fetal breathing, movements of the trunk, neck and limbs, singly or in episodes, over minutes, hours and diurnally. In both species there is a linear relation between the standard deviation of pulse intervals and the logarithm of time. This implies that there is a large range of influences which modulate the heart rate with increasing time. We can define, if we so wish, shorter or longer term variations as experimental tools, but we must recognize that the choice of time selected is arbitrary and may not be appropriate for discriminating between normal and pathological phenomena. The choice of beat-to-beat variation and so-called long-term variability, restricted to visual inspection over a few minutes, has been an empirical decision.

It is only in the past 7 years that the importance of episodic behavioural variations has been appreciated. In the sheep they are related to episodic changes in electrocortical activity attributed to cyclical activity in a midbrain centre. In man they probably have a similar origin, though of this there is no direct evidence. It is also worth noting that while this episodic behaviour is readily manipulated by the action of a variety of drugs in sheep (including prostaglandin E_2 and inhibitors of prostaglandin synthesis, 5-hydroxytryptophane derivatives, atropine or physostigmine, opiates such as morphine, and gamma-aminobutyric acid agonists or antagonists) it is not readily disturbed by handling the fetus or by other sensory stimuli, other than perhaps cold.

In fetal lambs near term β-sympathetic blockade with propranolol caused a considerable fall in heart rate, but hardly affected its variability (measured beat-by-beat or as the SD over 2 min). Parasympathetic blockade with atropine sulphate caused an increase in heart rate but reduced its variation. Even after double blockade (with both propranolol and atropine) some 35%–40% of the original heart rate variation remained, suggesting there is a substantial non-neural component (Dalton et al. 1983). Administration of phentolamine to cause α-sympathetic blockade caused a small fall of arterial pressure, a large rise in heart rate and an increase in variability by about 50%, consistent with an increase in plasma catecholamine concentration (Dalton et al. 1977). Hence we conclude that fetal heart rate variation is dependent on several immediate mechanisms.

This can be illustrated in another way. During experiments on transection of the fetal brain stem near term we have sometimes accidentally caused total loss of the brain above the cervical cord. Such fetuses have an exceptionally flat heart-rate trace; in hypoxia there is only a gradual rise in heart rate of slow onset. In fetal lambs with suprapontine transection of the brain stem, heart rate variation appears normal (Dawes et al. 1983). Fetal lambs show brief accelerations in heart rate in association with fetal movements, qualitatively similar to those in man. Neuromuscular blockade of the fetus abolishes the movements but not the accelerations, suggesting that they arise independently from medullary or pontine activity (F. Clewlow, unpublished observations).

Finally let us consider the effects of hypoxia, hypercapnia and metabolic acidaemia on fetal heart rate variation in sheep. Isocapnic hypoxia over 1 h (with a fall in mean p_aO_2 from 20 to 12 mm Hg, and in pH from 7.33 to 7.26) was associated with a substantial *increase* in heart rate variation, by more than 80% on average (Dalton et al. 1977). Hypercapnia also caused an increase in heart rate variation. These animal experiments demonstrated that moderate changes in fetal behaviour and a gross redistribution of cardiac output (yet not beyond the bounds of fetal adaptation) do not reproduce the clinical picture which is so generally accepted as characteristic of fetal asphyxia.

Two points arise. First, is there a species difference, perhaps quantitatively? The latter seems unlikely, since even severe asphyxia over many hours did not reproduce the picture. It seems more probable that the loss of variability sometimes seen in association with multiple prolonged decelerations in labour is a secondary metabolic consequence, at the level of the pons or medulla or indeed on the heart itself. We have not made an extended attempt to reproduce it experimentally.

Secondly the results suggest caution in assigning the low heart rate variation of some small-for-dates human infants to a respiratory cause.

It is evident from these animal experiments that the control of heart rate and its variation changes with age during the last quarter of gestation. It is unusual for account to be taken of age when human fetal heart rate traces are examined, although there is now clear evidence that in man also they change quantitatively. In sheep there is an episodic change in behaviour which also develops during the last quarter of gestation. The evidence that a comparable process occurs in man is very suggestive, but incomplete because we cannot record the electrocorticogram in utero. The significance of these episodic changes in behaviour, in the fetal heart rate as in other variables, for the identification of human pathological processes is still uncertain.

Finally I would make the point that in three respects recent advances have changed our views about the control of breathing and movements before birth. First, section of the brain stem through the pons or inferior colliculus prevents the arrest of breathing during isocapnic hypoxia, i.e. there must be a higher centre, rostral to the inferior colliculus but caudal to the hypothalamus, which is sensitive to small changes in fetal PaO_2 (Dawes et al. 1983). Second, spinal reflexes are controlled by a medullary centre, equally sensitive to fetal PaO_2 (Blanco et al. 1983). Third, contrary to previous work, it has proved possible to record from carotid and aortic chemoreceptors, as well as baroreceptors, in fetal lambs at 0.7 of term (Blanco et al. 1982). Yet there is good evidence that they do not normally cause reflex effects in response to changes in fetal blood gases or arterial pressure, respectively, presumably through central inhibition. Evidently there are more possibilities still to consider in relation to the nervous control of fetal heart rate.

References

Blanco CE, Dawes GS, Hanson MA, McCooke HE (1982) The arterial chemoreceptors in fetal sheep and newborn lambs. J Physiol (Lond) 330:88

Blanco CE, Dawes GS, Walker DW (1983) Effect of hypoxia on polysynaptic hindlimb reflexes of unanaesthetized fetal and newborn lambs. J Physiol (Lond) 339:453–466

Dalton KJ, Dawes GS, Patrick JE (1977) Diurnal, respiratory and other rhythms of fetal heart rate in lambs. Am J Obstet Gynecol 127:414–424

Dalton KJ, Dawes GS, Patrick JE (1983) The autonomic nervous system and fetal heart rate variability. Am J Obstet Gynecol 146:456–462

Dawes GS, Gardner WN, Johnston BM, Walker DW (1983) Breathing in fetal lambs: the effect of brain stem section. J Physiol (Lond) 335:535–553

Short- and Long-Term Variability in Fetal Heart Rate Pattern and Its Relation to Basal Heart Frequency

J. DE HAAN[1]

Introduction

Since the introduction of cardiotocography, variability within the fetal heart rate pattern has received attention. The significance of this phenomenon with respect to the assessment of fetal condition and later on with respect to the analysis of fetal activity states has been studied extensively (Hammacher et al. 1968, 1974). Detailed and/or quantitative analysis of this variability presents, however, a number of problems due to technical and scaling factors and definition problems (de Haan 1973a, b). This means that, especially in research concerning this parameter, its correct definition and quantification is necessary.

Definitions and Quantification of Variability

In our studies we have defined the phenomena in fetal heart rate patterns in the following way:

Short-term variability is the beat-to-beat differences between consecutive heart beats. We have quantified this parameter by the "short-term irregularity index."

Long-term variability is the variations in interval length over a certain number of R-R intervals, clinically expressed as the number of zero crossings, the bandwidth, or the amplitude of frequency changes.

Periodic changes are large positive or negative deviations from the estimated mean frequency, clinically described as accelerations and decelerations.

Visual analysis detects primarily long-term variability and not short-term variability. Especially the short-term variability, but in fact also the long-term variability, needs quantification in case of detailed analysis.

Since we developed a method of quantitating these phenomena (de Haan and van Bemmel 1970; de Haan et al. 1971a), several other methods have been proposed. These methods correspond rather well as far as they concern the quantification of short-term variability and if they make use of the difference between two consecutive R-R intervals in their calculation. The differences between the several methods of quantification of the long-term variability are greater, however (Laros et al. 1977; Organ et al. 1978; Parer et al. 1984).

The principle of these quantifications is: based on a certain calculation, a parameter is obtained from the original R-R intervals which has a certain distribution during the epoch under study. From such a distribution an index is obtained on a

[1] Rijksuniversiteit Limburg, Faculty of Medicine, Ziekenhuis St. Annadal, Afdeling Obstetrie en Gynaecologie, NL-6201 BX Maastricht

Fetal Heart Rate Monitoring
Ed. by W. Künzel

statistical basis: for example, the interquartile range of a histogram or the standard deviation. This calculated index is the quantitative measure for the variability under study.

We have used the so-called second-order joint interval distribution to obtain parameters and indices for the short- and long-term variability. In this distribution consecutive intervals are plotted against each other in a two-dimensional system. The angle (argument) is a measure of the short-term variability and the distance between the origin and the point determined by T_i, T_{i-1} (modulus) is a measure of the long-term variability. Histograms of the argument and the modulus are constructed, and the widths of the interquartile range of these histograms are the short- and long-term irregularity indexes, over a distinct number of R-R intervals (epoch) (de Haan et al. 1971a, b).

Several studies showed that variability indices are subject to random sampling fluctuations, when computed over a finite number of cardiac cycles (Wheeler et al. 1979; Detweiler et al. 1980). Using the interquartile range diminishes this effect, however, to a large extent.

The short- and long-term variability indices, as defined by us, show almost no interdependency, especially not the LTI, as shown by ourselves (Jongsma et al. 1978a) and others (Laros et al. 1977; Parer et al. 1984).

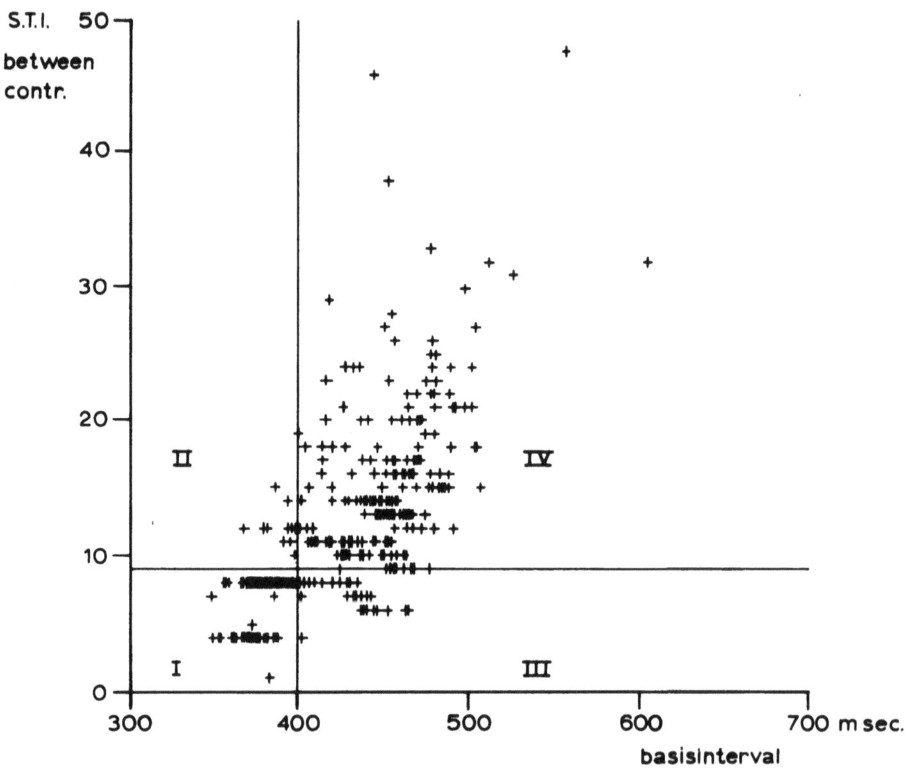

Fig. 1. Relation between short-term variability *(STI)* and the basal heart frequency before administration of sedatives to the mother

In our original studies fetal heart rate patterns were analyzed during labor in between and during contractions. We found a close correlation between short-term variability as defined by the STI index and the mean heart rate: the short-term variability decreased by increasing the heart rate and vice versa. This correlation was completely disrupted following the administration of analgetics and/or sedatives to the mother (de Haan et al. 1971b, 1973) (Figs. 1, 2). The same correlation was found later on in neonatal heart rate patterns during different behavioral states (van Geyn et al. 1980a).

Our conclusion at that time was, that for an optimal comparison of short-term variability in between certain parts of heart rate tracings or in between different fetuses correction was necessary for the basal heart frequency. Moreover, if variability is studied, no drugs should be administered to the mother for several days. Seven years later Jongsma et al. analyzed the relation between the short-term irregularity index and the R-R interval length in detail, during different activity states in the neonate (Jongsma et al. 1978b; van Geyn et al. 1980b). For each 12.5 ms in the second-order interval distribution, the interquartile range of the interval differences was plotted against the mean interval length, which shows the dependency of the dispersion of the interval differences on heart rate (Fig. 3). By mathematical description of this line the original STI index was corrected in the following way: the interval difference is divided by the mean interval diminished by a constant time of 320 ms

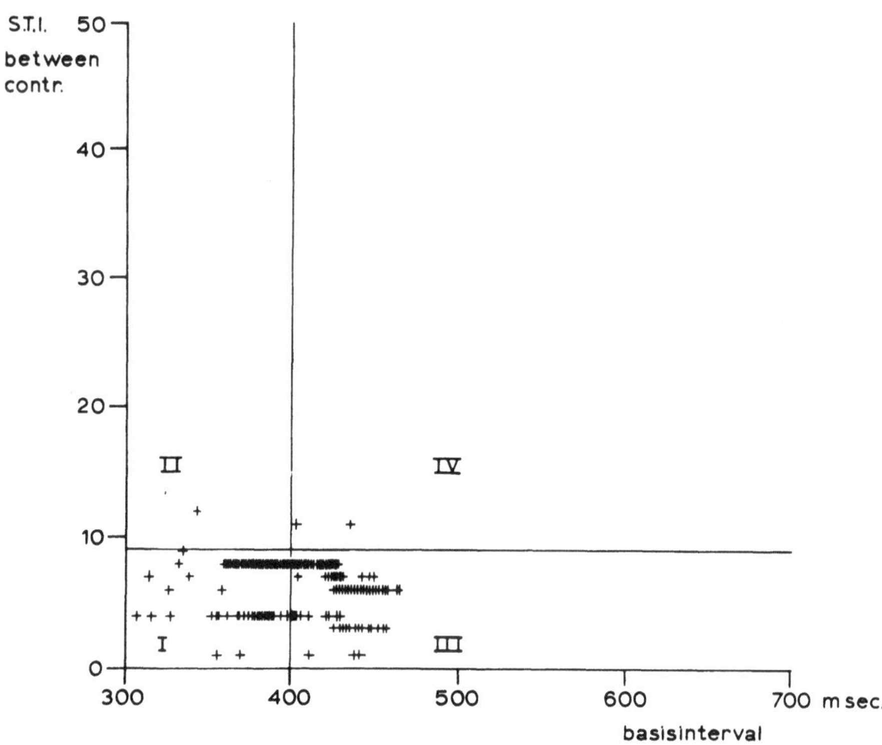

Fig. 2. Relation between short-term variability *(STI)* and basal heart frequency following administration of sedatives to the mother

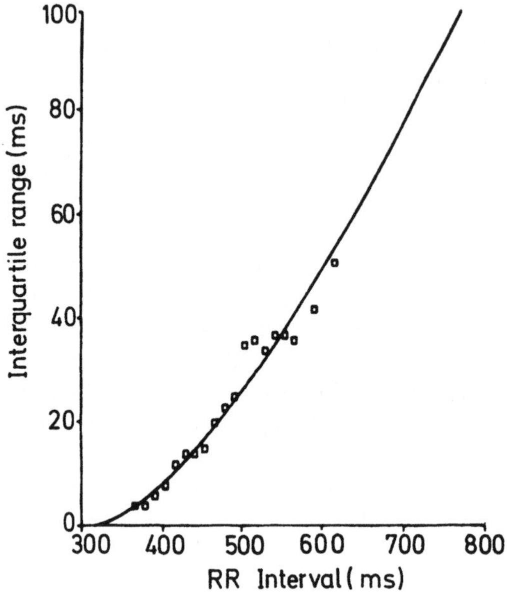

Fig. 3. Dispersion in second-order interval distribution in the neonate. $N=19$, $R=0.98$. (Jongsma et al. 1978b)

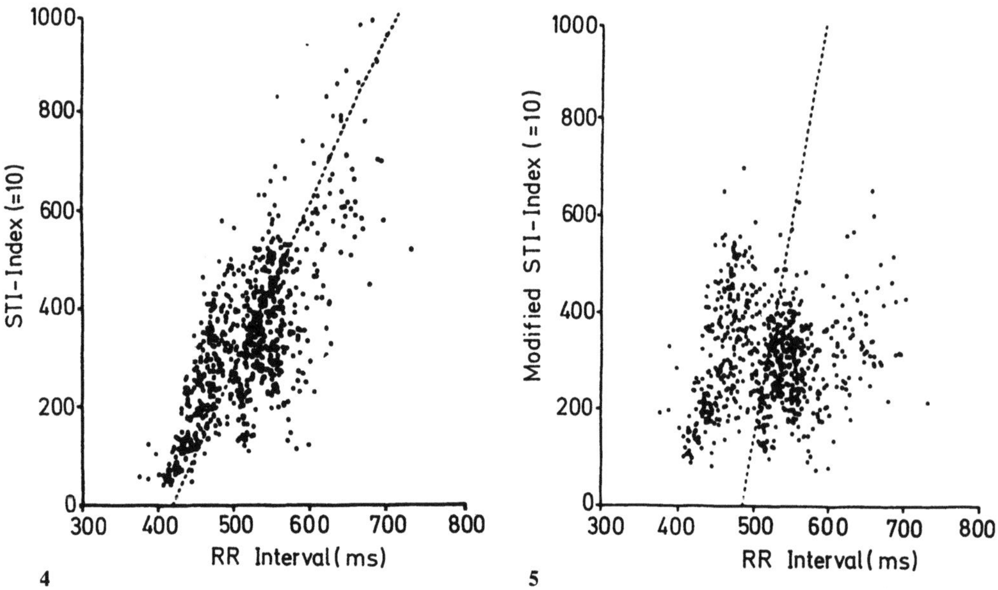

Fig. 4. Relation between RR-interval length and short-term variability index (STI index) in the neonate. $N=740$, $R=0.73$, $P\ (R=0)<0.001$. (Jongsma et al. 1978b)

Fig. 5. Relation between RR-interval length and modified short-term variability index (modified STI index) in the neonate. $N=745$, $R=0.13$, $P\ (R=0)=0.0005$. (Jongsma et al. 1978b) instead of by the mean interval only. In order to estimate the beat-to-beat variability independently from heart rate its value was normalized arbitrarily at 500 ms. For different basal heart frequencies the calculated variability must be multiplied by a certain number according to the fitted line. In Figs. 4 and 5 the independency of the modified index from R-R interval length is shown.

The foregoing shows clearly that confusion in this field can easily arise between different centres; this is mainly due to:

1. Definitions and properties of the indices used
2. Length of the studied epoch in the fetal heart rate pattern
3. Conditions during which the studies have been performed (animals, human beings, activity state, fetal breathing, different basal heart frequencies, maternal drug administration)

Relation Between Short- and Long-Term Variability and Basal Heart Rate Frequency

The relation between short-term variability and basal heart frequency is obviously very complex. Among other factors this is due to different types of variability with different time constants, caused by several physiological processes (swallowing, behavioral state, changes in blood pressure, changes in venous return). Besides these physiological events a number of pathological mechanisms can interfere with such a relationship, for example hypoxemia. Three mechanisms will be discussed in more detail:

1. Relation between the basal heart rate and variability and gestational age
2. Changes in basal fetal heart rate and variability during behavioral state changes
3. Changes in basal heart rate frequency and variability during fetal hypoxemia

1. In men the basal heart frequency decreases during the course of pregnancy (Ibarro Polo et al. 1972; Wladimiroff and Seelen 1972). The same phenomenon was observed in fetal sheep (Boddy et al. 1974; Dalton et al. 1977). Variability increases during the same time course in man, both long-term and short-term variability (Wheeler et al. 1979). This means in daily obstetrical practice that the gestational age has to be taken into account when estimating the fetal condition by the variability in the heart rate pattern.

2. Concerning the relationship between the changes in basal fetal heart frequency and variability, and fetal (neonatal) activity states, data are available from research in human fetuses as well as in animals (mainly chronic sheep experiments). This paper is mainly restricted to studies in human fetuses in which simultaneous recordings of fetal behavioral states by ultrasound techniques and abdominal fetal ECG recordings are made.

It is, however, difficult to reach unanimous conclusions from these studies because of several factors:

- Definitions of fetal behavioral states are not uniform
- Periods during which fetal breathing or no fetal breathing, gross fetal trunk movements, or fetal limb movements are present are probably not always exactly defined or excluded in the results presented

- Definition and properties of the quantitative processing methods for fetal heart rate parameters are not uniform in all studies
- The epochs under study are different in the studies cited.

Nevertheless some phenomena described have more or less consistently been found by different research groups.

Dawes et al. (1981) found a lower heart frequency during fetal breathing with an increase in beat-to-beat variability compared with periods of no fetal breathing. Although not in all fetuses there was a strict and highly significant correlation between the basal heart frequency and short-term variability during periods of fetal breathing as well as during periods without fetal breathing.

In the case of fetal trunk movements basal heart frequency increased with a significant reduction in beat-to-beat variability.

Wheeler et al. (1980) found the change in the basal heart frequency unpredictable when fetal breathing occurred, but variability increased during fetal breathing in their experiments. Moreover, they found a sinus arrhythmia during fetal breathing in all recordings.

Campogrande et al. (1982) using the same quantitative processing methods as Wheeler et al. (1980) found an increase in both the short- and long-term variability during fetal breathing compared with periods without breathing. The changes in basal heart rate were unpredictable. This increase in variability is probably mainly caused by changes in venous umbilical blood flow during fetal breathing as shown by Hasaart and de Haan (1982, 1983) (Fig. 6) and Reuss et al. (1983) in chronically instrumented fetal lambs by electromagnetic flow measurements as well as in men during pregnancy by means of ultrasound techniques (Trudinger and Cook 1982).

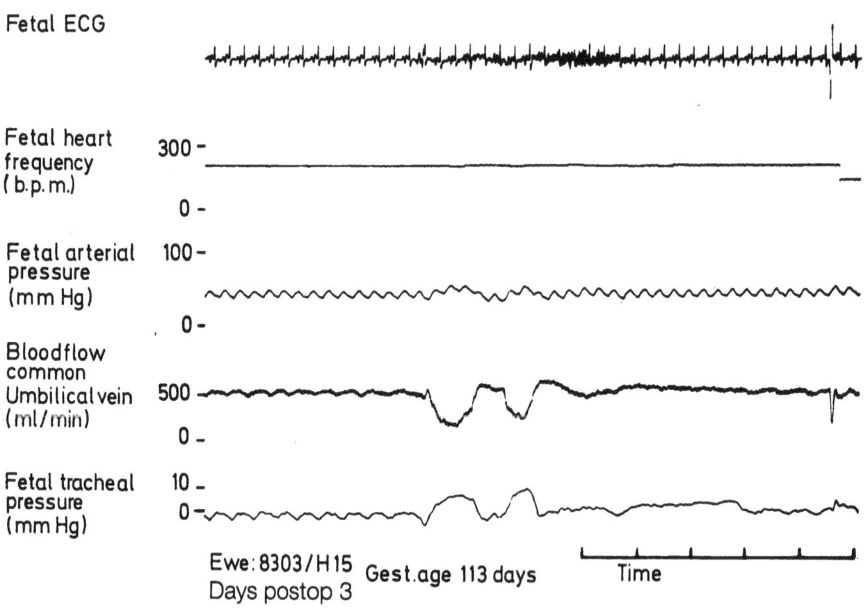

Fig. 6. Changes in umbilical venous blood flow and fetal tracheal pressure

Bots et al. (1978), however, found no statistical difference in mean heart rate and short- and long-term variability between periods of fetal breathing and no fetal breathing.

In regard to fetal behavioral states more problems arise:

Nijhuis et al. (1982) tried to define fetal activity states in utero. From 36 weeks onwards well-organized behavioral states are recognizable. In state 1F (quiet sleep) long-term variability, assessed as band width, is lower than in a fetal behavioral state which is more or less equal to neonatal behavioral state 2 (REM sleep).

Junge (1979a, b) found a lower basal heart frequency in quiet sleep (state 1) than in REM sleep state in fetuses and neonates, as van Geyn et al. (1980a) determined only in neonates. Long-term variability in the neonate was lower in state 1 than in state 2 in the studies by van Geyn et al. (1980a). In contrast short-term variability was higher in state 1 than in state 2. Junge (1979b) differentiated between the amplitude and frequency of the macrofluctuations. These two aspects of this parameter also changed in different directions when the fetal behavioral state changed. In this way Junge (1979b) found a lower amplitude of fluctuations during non-REM sleep than in REM sleep whereas the frequency of the macrofluctuations showed the reverse pattern.

3. For obvious reasons it is impossible to subject the human fetus to standardized degrees of hypoxemia under experimental conditions. Nevertheless from clinical experience during fetal monitoring, important conclusions can be drawn regarding the relation between fetal heart rate variability and basal heart frequency and hypoxemia and/or acidemia.

Hammacher et al. (1968), in the early days of fetal electronic monitoring, found an increase in the amplitude of the bandwidth of the fetal heart rate pattern (saltatory pattern) in cases of umbilical cord complications and with Apgar scores below 7.

Krebs et al. (1979) underlined this point by also finding an increased oscillation amplitude in the case of low Apgar scores.

Roemer et al. (1979) found an increase in oscillation frequency and oscillation amplitude in fetal heart rate patterns during the last 30 min in fetuses which were born with an umbilical artery pH between 7.20 and 7.25. Those born with an umbilical artery pH below 7.15 showed a significant decrease in oscillation frequency and amplitude.

At first glance this seems not in line with the findings in chronically distressed fetuses showing a silent heart rate pattern. More insight into this obvious discrepancy can be obtained in animal experiments during which more or less standardized hypoxemic and/or acidemic conditions can be realized.

In chronic fetal sheep experiments we occluded intermittently the maternal common internal iliac artery, simulating the pathophysiological mechanisms causing late decelerations (de Haan et al. 1979). The first reaction of the fetus to hypoxemia was a decrease in basal heart frequency, with an increase in short-term variability concomitant with an increase in fetal arterial blood pressure. Variability (especially short-term variability) remained present until the fetus became severely acidemic (Fig. 7). This phenomenon was also found in fetal lambs by Dalton et al. (1977), Parer et al. (1980), and Martin et al. (1974) in fetal monkeys.

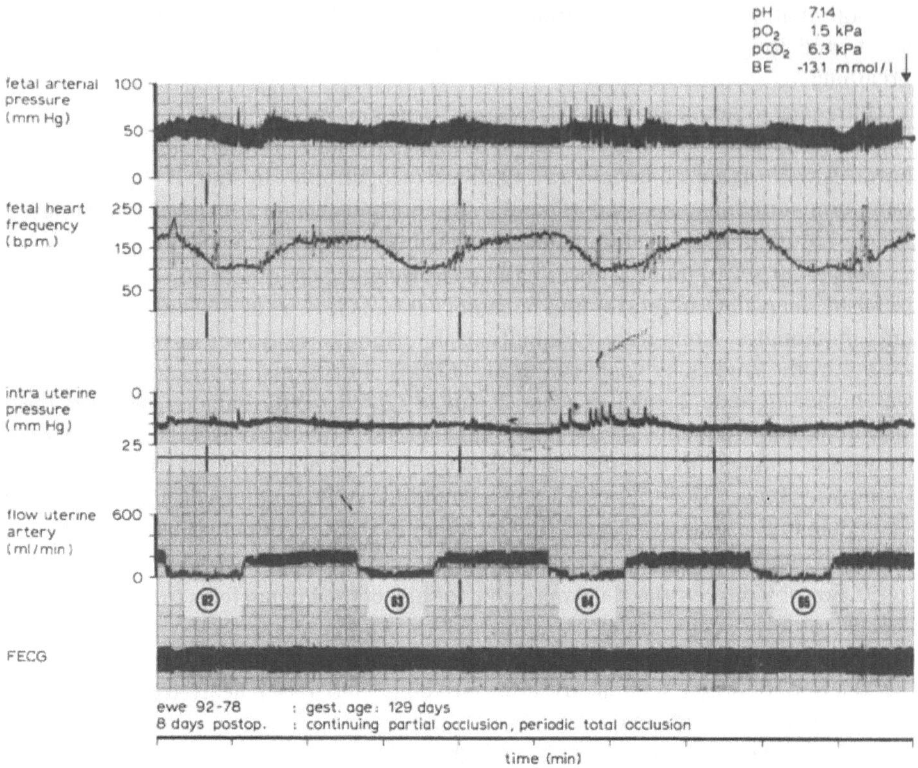

Fig. 7. Fetal response to continuing partial occlusion and intermittent total occlusions *(numbers)* of the maternal common internal iliac artery simulating late decelerations. Note the wide decelerations and the presence of short-term variability during fetal hypoxemia judged by the fetal arterial acid base balance

During severe hypoxemia and acidemia the basal heart rate tended to increase again but was still significantly lower in Parer's experiments than in the control period (probably caused by an increase in vagal oscillating activity or an increase in alpha-adrenergic activity).

The differences in phenomena in the case of fetal hypoxemia (increase in variability on one hand and the silent pattern on the other hand) can probably be explained by the differences in the mechanisms of fetal hypoxemia: in animal experiments hypoxemia experiments are rather acute accidents whereas the chronic fetal distress with a silent pattern has a much longer time constant. A substantial decrease in short- and long-term variability resulting in a silent fetal heart rate pattern was also observed in chronic distress with a long time constant (days) in rhesus monkeys by Martin et al. (1974).

Conclusions

Within the fetal heart rate pattern oscillations are present with different time constants. As a consequence studies concerning the basal heart frequency and variability within the fetal heart rate pattern must account for this fact, by defining accurately the time during which the studies were performed. Moreover, due to the effects of fetal breathing, gross fetal trunk movements, fetal behavioral state, and fetal limb movements the epochs studied must be performed during one and the same activity state. Within one activity state a clear relation seems to be present between short-term variability and basal heart rate frequency. Long-term variability behaves less consistently in this respect. The definition and properties of the quantitative indices to describe the short- and long-term variability can, however, influence the results of the experiments substantially.

Comparison of short-term variability between different parts of a fetal heart rate tracing or between different fetuses must take into account basal heart rate frequency. The quantitative methods used for quantitating the short- and long-term variability should not be interdependent.

References

Boddy K, Dawes GS, Fisher R, Pinter S, Robinson IS (1974) Foetal respiratory movements, electrocortical and cardiovascular responses to hypoxemia and hypercapnia in sheep. J Physiol (Lond) 243:599

Bots RSG, Jongsma HW, Braat AJHM, Martin CB, De Haan J (1978) Human fetal breathing movements and heart rate variability. In: Proceedings of the 5th conference on fetal breathing. Catholic University, Nijmegen, The Netherlands, p 45

Campogrande M, Alemanno MG, Viora E, Bussolino S (1982) FHR short and long term variability associated with fetal breathing. J Perinat Med 10:203

Dalton KJ, Dawes GS, Patrick JE (1977) Diurnal, respiratory and other rhythms of fetal heart rate in lambs. Am J Obstet Gynecol 127:414

Dawes GS, Visser GHA, Goodman JDS, Levine DH (1981) Numerical analysis of the human fetal heart rate: modulation by breathing and movement. Am J Obstet Gynecol 140:535

de Haan J (1971) The short term irregularity in the foetal heart rate pattern (in Dutch). Thesis, Free University, Amsterdam

de Haan J (1973a) Fetal monitoring by physical methods. I. Technical questions. Eur J Obstet Gynecol Reprod Biol 3:57

de Haan J (1973b) Fetal monitoring by physical methods. II. Interpretation of phenomena. Eur J Obstet Gynecol Reprod Biol 3:95

de Haan J, Van Bemmel JH (1970) Proceeding methods for fetal R-R intervals. Scientific exhibition, 6th world congress of gynaecology and obstetrics, New York, Sandoz, Basel, p 2

de Haan J, van Bemmel JH, Versteeg B, Veth AFL, Stolte LAM, Janssens J, Eskes TKAB (1971a) Quantitative evaluation of fetal heart rate patterns. I. Processing methods. Eur J Obstet Gynecol Reprod Biol 3:95

de Haan J, van Bemmel JH, Stolte LAM, Janssens J, Eskes TKAB, Versteeg B, Veth AFL, Braaksma JT (1971b) Quantitative evaluation of fetal heart rate patterns. II. The significance of the fixed heart rate during pregnancy and labor. Eur J Obstet Gynecol Reprod Biol 3:103

de Haan J, Stolte LAM, Veth AFL, Van Bemmel JH, Janssens J, Eskes TKAB (1973) The significance of short term irregularity in the fetal heart rate pattern. In: Dudenhausen JW, Saling E (eds) Perinatale Medizin. Thieme, Stuttgart, p 398

de Haan J, Martin CB, Evers JLH, Jongsma HW (1979) Pathophysiological mechanisms underlying fetal heart rate patterns. In: Thalhammer O, Baumgarten K, Pollak A (eds) Perinatale Medizin. Thieme, Stuttgart, p 200

Detweiler JS, Jarisch W, Caritis SN (1980) Statistical fluctuations in heart rate variability indices. Am J Obstet Gynecol 136:243

Hammacher K, Huter KA, Bokelmann J, Werners PH (1968) Foetal heart frequency and perinatal condition of the fetus and newborn. Gynaecologia 166:349

Hammacher K, Brun Del Re, Gaudenz R, DeGrandi P, Richter R (1974) Kardiotokographischer Nachweis einer fetalen Gefährdung mit einem CTG-score. Gynakol Rundsch [Suppl 1] 14:61
Hasaart THM, deHaan J (1982) Reflections of fetal thoracal movements in the blood flow measurements of the common umbilical vein in the chronic sheep preparation. Proceedings of the 9th international symposium on fetal breathing and other measurements. University of Western Ontario, London, Canada, p 43
Hasaart THM, deHaan J (1983) Blood flow patterns in the common umbilical vein in fetal sheep. Abstracts of the 10th conference on fetal breathing movements and other fetal measurements. Malmö, Sweden, p 39
Ibarro Polo AA, Guiloff E, Gomez-Rogers C (1972) Fetal heart rate throughout pregnancy. Am J Obstet Gynecol 113:814
Jongsma HW, deHaan J, Martin CB (1978a) Review of heart rate variability parameters in perinatology. In: Proceedings of the 5th conference on fetal breathing. Catholic University, Nijmegen, The Netherlands
Jongsma HW, van Geyn HP, deHaan J (1978b) The analysis of heart rate variability in the perinatal period. In: Krause W (ed) Computerdiagnostik in der Geburtsmedizin. Friedrich Schiller Universität, Jena, p 249
Junge HD (1979a) Behavioral states and state related heart rate and motor activity patterns in the newborn infant and the fetus antepartum. A comparative study. I. Technique, illustration of recordings and general results. J Perinat Med 7:85
Junge HD (1979b) Behavioral states and state related heart rate and motor activity patterns in the newborn infant and the fetus ante partum. A comparative study. II. Computer analysis of state related heart rate baseline and macrofluctuations patterns. J Perinat Med 7:134
Krebs HB, Peters RE, Dunn LJ (1979) Intrapartum fetal heart rate monitoring. I. Classification and prognosis of fetal heart rate patterns. Am J Obstet Gynecol 133:762
Laros RK, Wong WS, Heilbron DC, Parer JT, Shnider SM, Naylor H, Butler J (1977) A comparison of methods for quantitating fetal heart rate variability. Am J Obstet Gynecol 128:381
Martin CB, Murata Y, Petrie RH, Parer JT (1974) Respiratory movements in fetal rhesus monkeys. Am J Obstet Gynecol 119:939
Nijhuis JG, Prechtl HFR, Martin CB, Bots RSGM (1982) Are there behavioural states in the human fetus? Early Hum Dev 6:177
Organ LW, Hawrylyshyn PA, Goodwin JW, Milligram JE, Bernstein A (1978) Quantitative indices of short and long term heart rate variability. Am J Obstet Gynecol 130:20
Parer JT, Dijkstra HR, Vredebregt PPM, Harris JL, Krueger TR, Reuss ML (1980) Increased fetal heart rate variability with acute hypoxia in chronically instrumented sheep. Eur J Obstet Gynecol Reprod Biol 10:393
Parer WJ, Holbrook H, Parer JT, Block BSB (1984) Validity of mathematical indices of fetal heart rate variability. Proceedings of the 31st annual meeting of the society for gynecologic investigations, San Francisco, p 212
Reuss ML, Rudolph AM, Dae MW (1983) Phasic blood flow patterns in the superior and inferior venae cavae and umbilical vein of fetal sheep. Am J Obstet Gynecol 145:70
Roemer VM, Holzhauser B, Heinzl S (1979) The evaluation and significance of intrapartum FHR oscillation patterns. J Perinat Med 7:46
Trudinger BJ, Cook CM (1982) Quantification of human fetal breath cycle. Proceedings of the 9th international symposium on fetal breathing and other measurements. University of Western Ontario, London, Canada, p 59
van Geyn HP, Jongsma HW, deHaan J, Eskes TKAB, Prechtl HFR (1980a) Heart rate as an indicator of the behavioural state. Studies in the newborn and prospects for fetal heart rate monitoring. Am J Obstet Gynecol 136:1061
van Geyn HP, Jongsma HW, deHaan J, Eskes TKBS (1980b) Analysis of heart rate and beat to beat variability: the interval difference index (ID index). Am J Obstet Gynecol 138:246
Wheeler T, Cooke E, Murrills A (1979) Computer analysis of fetal heart rate variation during normal pregnancy. Br J Obstet Gynaecol 86:186
Wheeler T, Gennser G, Lindvall R, Murrils AJ (1980) Changes in the fetal heart rate associated with fetal breathing and fetal movement. Br J Obstet Gynaecol 87:1068
Wladimiroff JW, Seelen JC (1972) Fetal heart rate action in early pregnancy. Developments of fetal vagal function. Eur J Obstet Gynecol Reprod Biol 2:55

Long-Term Observation of Fetal Heart Rate Irregularities

H. D. Junge[1]

Numerous proposals for antepartum assessment of fetal well-being have been published in recent years. Undoubtedly the nonstress test (NST) plays a major role as a screening method for detecting the fetus at risk of chronic hypoxia.

According to various recommendations the NST is performed once a week to several times a day, each test lasting 15–30 min. FHR is evaluated by mere eyeballing or according to various semiquantitative scores. Items for scoring are baseline, variability, and deviations from baseline, i.e., accelerations and decelerations.

It has been shown that this clinically well-accepted routine of surveillance lowered antepartum death from chronic hypoxia substantially but not totally. On the other hand it has been shown that in the healthy fetus seemingly suspicious FHR pattern due to decreased variability and missing accelerations: nonreactive patterns occur in about 10%–20% of all NSTs and induce unnecessary further measures.

Most probably our present understanding of FHR regulation in the healthy and in the hypoxic fetus throughout gestation is still incomplete and it is likely that present recommendations for routine antepartum FHR monitoring are not well adapted to the latest findings in this field.

Looking at our present management of surveillance with the NST from the standpoint of information theory, it would be taking short signal samples from a signal continuum at more or less irregular and distant intervals in order to detect changes in signal properties.

This pattern of signal sampling would only be justified and effective if discontinuous and short signal samples were representative of the signal continuum. In other words the undisturbed signal must be stationary and its measures of location and dispersion must be invariant to random time transposition, whereas signal disturbances must have a slow and monotonous trend.

The latest findings in long-term observations of FHR indicate that there is little doubt that neither is FHR an absolutely stationary signal in the healthy undisturbed fetus nor do FHR alterations from chronic hypoxia progress in an absolutely slow and monotonous fashion.

In continuous and long-lasting FHR recordings of healthy term fetuses (Fig. 1) cyclic changes of FHR pattern can be seen. These cyclic changes may be somewhat obscured, when short or even long strip charts of 10 mm/min time base are evaluated by eyeballing, but they can be easily detected in compressed records of 1 mm/min time base.

In one of these alternating FHR patterns, let us call it pattern B, the baseline is generally less stable; variability, or to be precise macrofluctuation amplitude and frequency, is in the normal range; and accelerations occur at more or less regular

[1] Univ.-Frauenklinik, Josef-Schneider-Str. 4, D-8700 Würzburg

Fetal Heart Rate Monitoring
Ed. by W. Künzel

intervals. The alternative pattern, let us call it pattern A, is characterized by a baseline that is more stable, by a decreased macrofluctuation amplitude, and by the fact that accelerations are rare or missing. If present, accelerations are generally of decreased amplitude and short duration, frequently somewhat biphasic.

In 16 mature fetuses with 8 h of recording each and a total of 62 complete cycles of FHR pattern A + B, the mean duration of these cycles was 77 min, range 25–134 min; the mean duration of periods of FHR pattern A was 20 min, range 8–

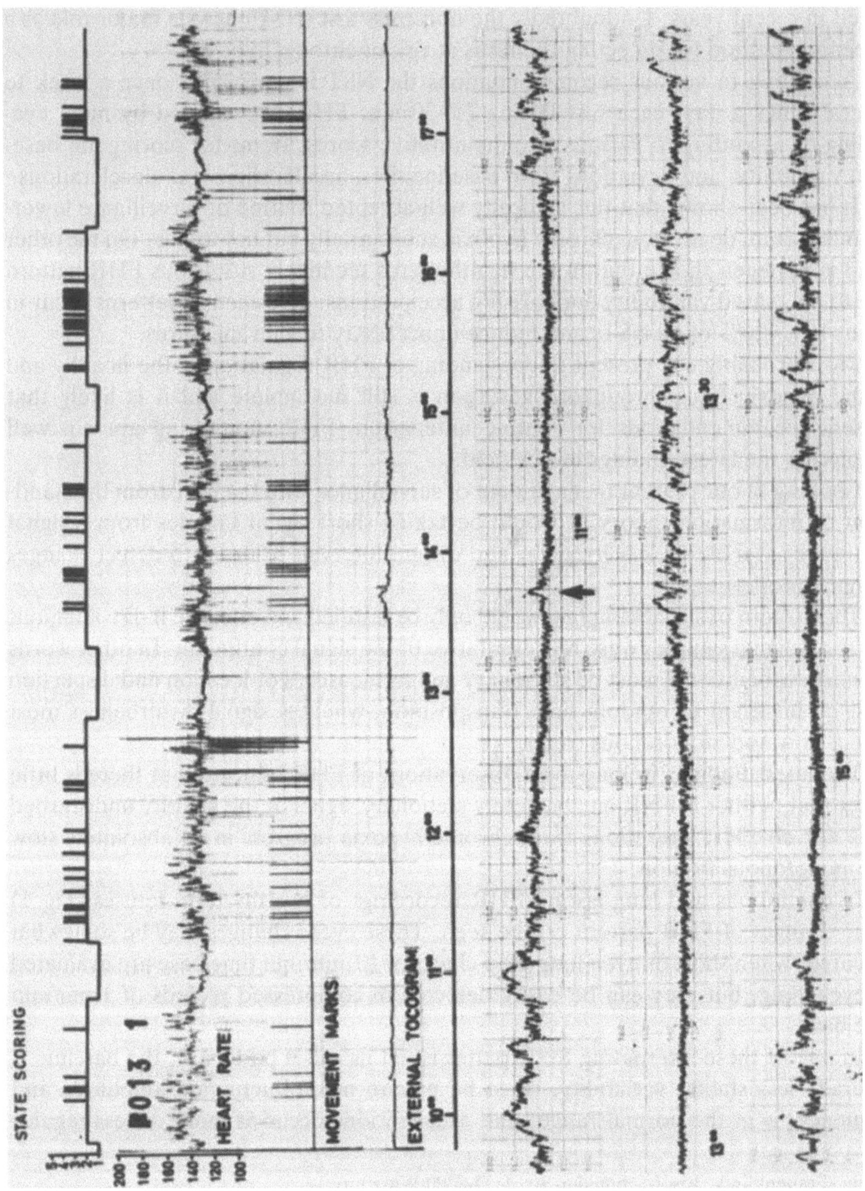

Fig. 1

37 min; and the mean duration of periods of FHR pattern B was 56 min, range 15–119 min (Fig. 2) (Junge 1979).

In addition, we saw another FHR pattern in some of the recordings (Fig. 3). It is characterized by accelerations of large amplitude, repetitive and often merging so that heart rate rises abruptly and the high level can often be taken as a sequence of peaks of these repetitive and merging accelerations with their interspersed downward and upward slopes. In between a marked and more or less straight-lined tachycardia may be present. Let us call this pattern D.

FHR pattern D could be seen in 7 out of 16 FHR recordings. When present, it generally persisted for prolonged periods.

The relative distribution of FHR patterns A, B, and D for total recording time, i.e., 16 × 8 h, was 24.5%, 65.0%, and 8.8% respectively. These data are in a good agreement with data in the literature.

After separating FHR patterns A and B by eyeballing, computerized quantitation of these patterns according to methods developed by the author gave the following results:

Baseline, the statistical mean of 1-min heart rate segments after exclusion of accelerations, is more stable during pattern A than during pattern B (Fig. 4).

Macrofluctuation is defined as the variation of heart rate around the baseline after elimination of its high-frequency component, called microfluctuation, by a short moving average window, and of course after elimination of accelerations. As quantitative measures mean macrofluctuation amplitude for 1-min segments and mean frequency for 1-min segments were calculated. Figure 5 shows histograms of macrofluctuation amplitude and frequency and a scattergram of amplitude versus frequency for FHR patterns A and B.

A highly significant difference in respect to location and dispersion of macrofluctuation amplitude can be seen and there is a shift in frequency to lower values with a change from FHR pattern A to pattern B. From the scattergram of amplitude versus frequency a negative correlation can be seen.

During FHR pattern A, decile range of macrofluctuation amplitude is from 3 to 7.6 beats/min and during FHR pattern B from 6.5 to 21.8 beats/min. Macrofluctuation frequency differs less. It tends to be higher during FHR pattern A (Table 1).

As has been mentioned the difference in macrofluctuation is not the only one comparing FHR patterns A and B. The difference is enhanced by the uneven distribution of accelerations. These accelerations occur synchronously with fetal body movements, as can be seen from the simultaneous recording of the tick marks for fetal movements felt by the mother (see Fig. 1).

Fig. 1. Compressed writeout of 8 h' recording of FHR, movement marks, and external tocogram together with state scoring. In the FHR recording a regular change in macrofluctuation pattern can be seen clearly. The low-amplitude macrofluctuation pattern corresponds to a heart rate pattern seen in the newborn infant during state 1 (FHR pattern A), and the FHR pattern with higher amplitude and accelerations corresponds to a heart rate pattern seen in the newborn in state 2 (FHR pattern B). Movement marks are state related, they are seen in state 2 and are absent or rare in state 1. *Bottom:* three segments 45 min in duration of original FHR writeout (Hewlett-Packard machine at 10 mm/min time base). FHR pattern A during state 1F *(middle part of upper segment, left side of middle segment, middle part of lower segment)* and FHR pattern B during state 2F are demonstrated. Accelerations during state 2F are synchronous with movement marks

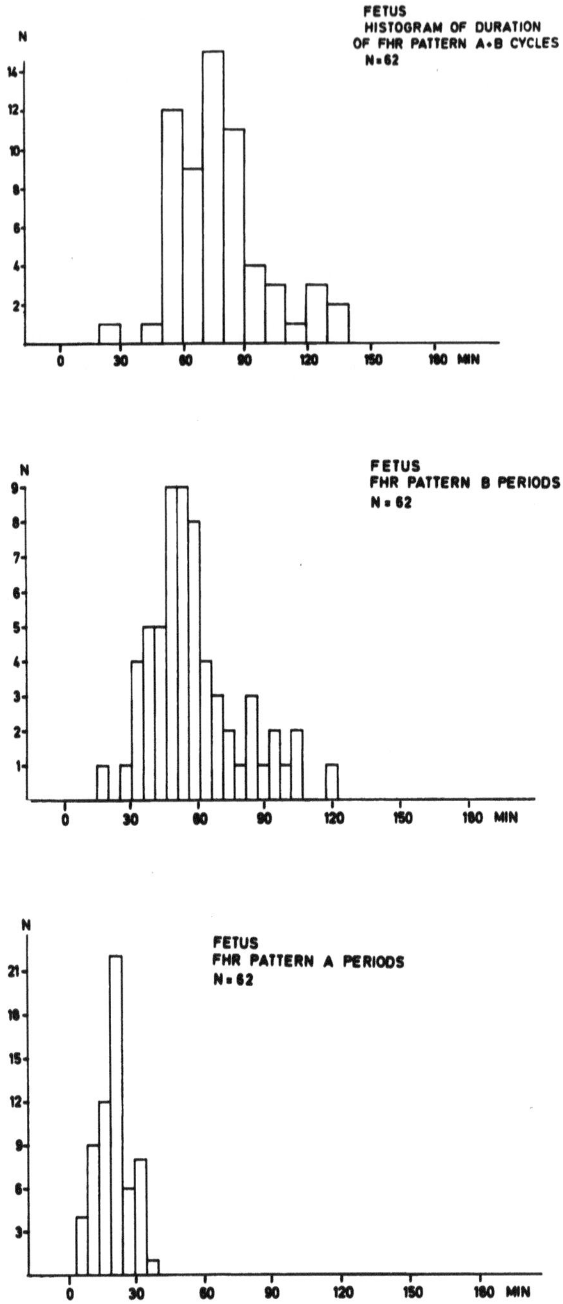

Fig. 2. Histograms of duration of FHR pattern A + B *(top)*, FHR pattern B periods *(center)*, and FHR pattern A periods *(bottom)* from 16 × 8 h of FHR recording

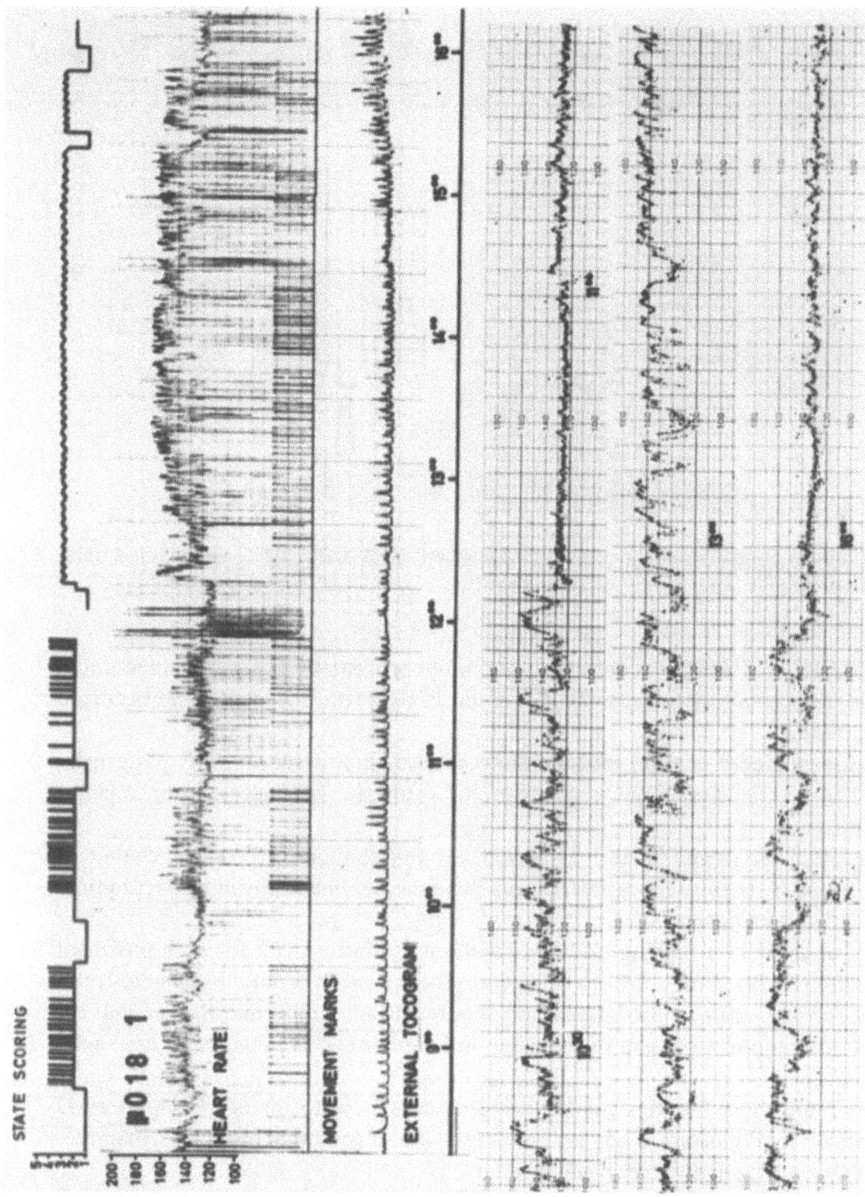

Fig. 3. *Top:* compressed writeout of 8 h' recording of FHR, movement marks, and external tocogram together with state scoring. Besides a regular change in FHR macrofluctuation as in Fig. 1, a long-lasting period of FHR pattern D, identical to the newborn heart rate pattern during wakefulness, is seen (marked by ∼∼∼ in the state scoring). Movement marks are much more frequent during this period. *Bottom:* three segments 45 min in duration of original FHR writeout (Hewlett-Packard machine at 10 mm/min time base). *Middle tracing and left side of lower tracing:* FHR pattern D

In other words: the occurrence of repetitive accelerations reflects the clustering of fetal movements during an FHR pattern B period within the cycles of patterns A + B.

The uneven distribution of motor activity is demonstrated in Fig. 6. The total number of fetal movements for the periods of FHR patterns A and B is plotted. In nearly 50% of all periods of pattern A no movements occurred and in 80% of all these periods the total number did not exceed two movements. In contrast in all

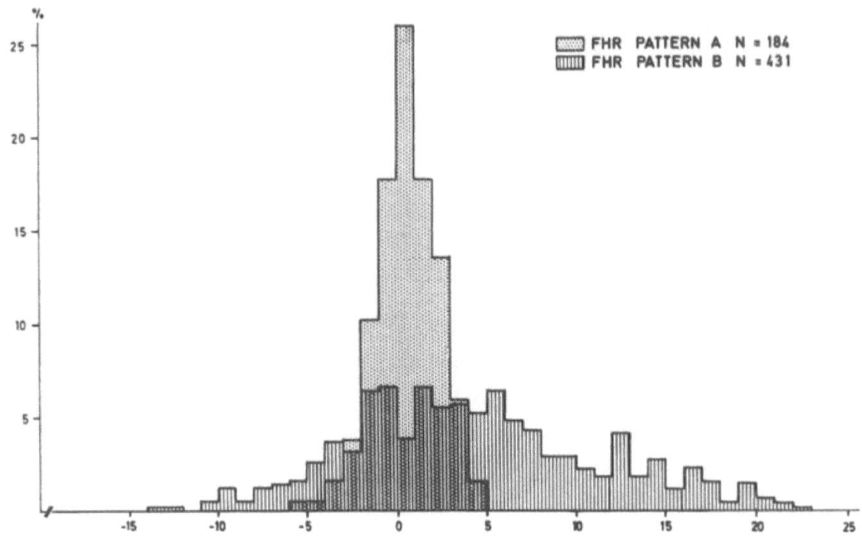

Fig. 4. Histograms of relative baseline values for FHR patterns A and B. The baseline is less stable during pattern B

periods of FHR pattern B except 1 the total number exceeded two movements. On the whole 90% of all motor activity during an FHR pattern A + B cycle occurred during pattern B.

A further increase of fetal motor activity is associated with an FHR pattern D, which is characterized by large, repetitive, and often merging accelerations, as has been mentioned.

These often prolonged pattern D periods are not related to the cyclic change of patterns A and B. In our recordings, during day time, no clustering in respect to time of the day could be detected.

Visser et al. (1982) making 24-h observations, found a peak for high-pass root mean square (RMS), a measure that calculates the variation around basal heart rate, i.e., accelerations, around the late evening hours and midnight; and Patrick and coworkers (1982) found a peak in the number and percentage of movements at exactly the same time.

To my mind these findings can be interpreted as a clustering of FHR pattern D and enhanced fetal motor activity in the early hours of the night and this is in agreement with what pregnant women often tell us.

Longitudinal studies have revealed that FHR patterns change in the course of pregnancy.

In early and mid-pregnancy, FHR pattern is characterized by a mild tachycardia and variability in respect to amplitude, and frequency is substantially reduced. Deviations from baseline are rare and slim decelerations prevail. According to general standards this immature pattern would be suspected of being pathologic. In part FHR pattern is uncharacteristic but not suspect. As gestation advances basal heart rate decreases, variability increases, and accelerations increasingly prevail. Successively distinct FHR patterns A, B, and D emerge. At last duration of pattern

a
b
c
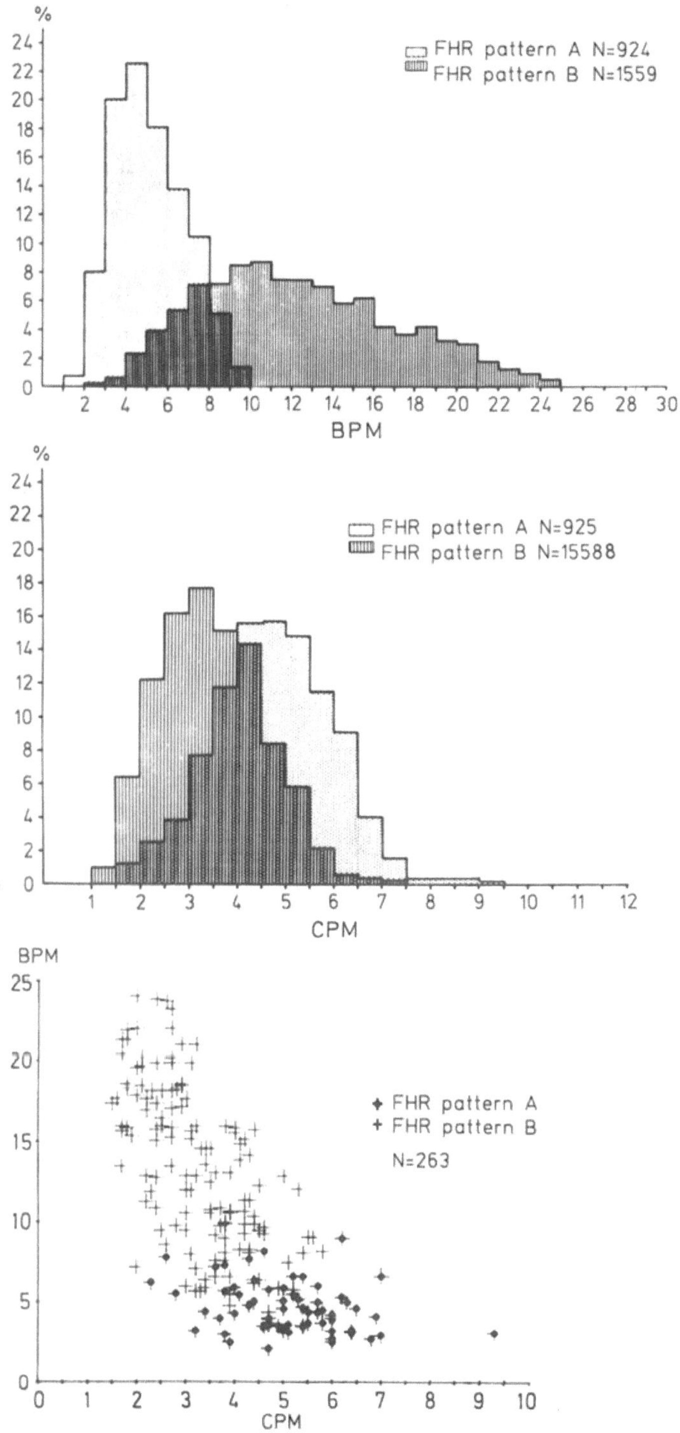

Fig. 5a–c. Histograms of macrofluctuation amplitude (**a**), macrofluctuation frequency (**b**), and scattergram of amplitude versus frequency (**c**) for FHR patterns A and B

Table 1. Order statistics of amplitude and frequency of macrofluctuation for FHR patterns A and B

	Amplitude							Frequency						
	N	Range	D_1	Q_1	Median	Q_3	D_9	N	Median	D_1	Q_1	Range	Q_3	D_9
FHR pattern A	924	9	3.0	3.8	4.9	6.4	7.6	925	8.0	3.1	3.9	4.7	5.5	6.3
FHR pattern B (accelerations excluded)	1559	23	6.5	8.7	11.8	17.2	21.8	1558	6.5	2.1	2.6	3.4	4.2	4.9

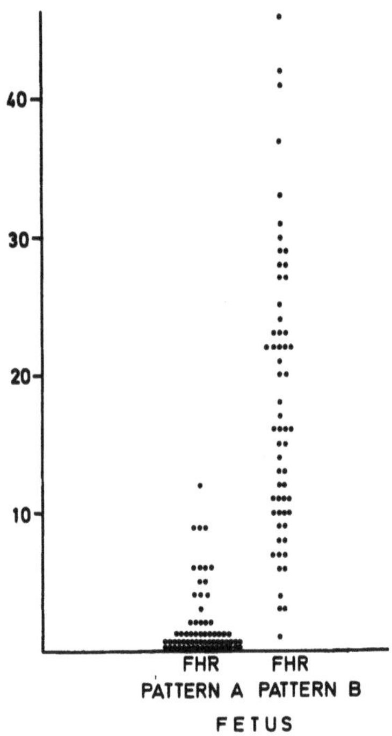

Fig. 6. State-related fetal motor activity. The total number of movements per state period is plotted for periods of FHR pattern A ($N=65$) and FHR pattern B ($N=60$)

A periods increases, giving the relative distribution of patterns mentioned above, in the last 2 or 3 weeks of pregnancy.

Consideration of long-term observation of FHR patterns would be incomplete without discussion of results in the context of fetal state behavior. The existence of "sleep" and "wakefulness" or "rest and activity cycles" in the fetus has been postulated for some time and recently several investigators and myself have argued

Table 2. Definition of states in the newborn infant by visual observation according to Prechtl (1974)

State 1:	eyes closed, regular respiration, no movements
State 2:	eyes closed, irregular respiration, small movements
State 3:	eyes open, no movements
State 4:	eyes open, gross movements
State 5:	crying (vocalization)

that the regular changes in FHR and motor activity patterns are correlates of distinct fetal state behavior identical to that in the newborn infant.

The concept of state behavior in the newborn infant is well accepted in developmental neurology and pediatrics and this concept has been used fruitfully for a descriptive categorization of newborn behavioral patterns and for a theory of brain function in respect to central nervous coordination of vital body functions.

A behavioral state is a centrally coordinated mode of neural activity characterized by a set of biological phenomena: state variables, the criteria of which form a stable combination for the time of a state period and change simultaneously at the onset and end of each period. State concomitants are events or phenomena which occur only during particular states. According to Prechtl (1974), five states can be defined in the newborn infant by mere visual observation (Table 2).

From the truth table for states and their state variables (Table 3) it can be seen that state criteria are not state specific but each set of state variables is mutually exclusive.

These and additional state variables, i.e., eye movements, electroencephalogram, and electromyogram, can be recorded electronically to give a polygraphic recording of state behavior.

Using these methods we investigated the same population, whose data have been demonstrated at the beginning of this presentation, postnatally and after full adaptation to extrauterine life. The results were strikingly similar in respect to FHR and motor activity patterns as well as duration and relative distribution of periods, when analyzed with our methods as described above.

Based on these results I postulated that in the mature fetus in the last weeks of gestation a regular change in central nervous coordination, i.e., state behavior comparable to state behavior in the newborn infant, does exist and that fetal states can be identified by adequate polygraphic recording of a set of state variables.

Table 3. Truth table for state variables of newborn states (Prechtl 1974)

	Eyes open	Respiration regular	Gross movements	Vocalization
State 1	−1	+1	−1	−1
State 2	−1	−1	−1	−1
State 3	+1	+1	−1	−1
State 4	+1	−1	+1	−1
State 5	0	−1	+1	+1

Table 4. Definition of states in the fetus (Nijhuis et al. 1982)

State 1F (Fig. 2):	quiescence, which can be regularly interrupted by brief gross body movements, mostly startles Eye movements absent Heart rate stable, with a small oscillation bandwidth. Isolated accelerations occur. These are strictly related to movements. This heart rate pattern is called FHRPA
State 2F (Fig. 2):	frequent and periodic gross body movements—mainly stretches and retroflexions—and movements of the extremities Eye movements continually present (REMs and SEMs) Heart rate (called FHRPB) with a wider oscillation bandwidth than FHRPA and frequent accelerations during movements
State 3F (Fig. 3):	gross body movements absent Eye movements continually present Heart rate (called FHRPC) stable, but with a wider oscillation bandwidth than FHRPA and no accelerations
State 4F (Fig. 3):	vigorous, continual activity including many trunk rotations Eye movements continually present (when observable) Heart rate (called FHRPD) unstable, with large and long-lasting accelerations, frequently fused into a sustained tachycardia

Table 5. Truth table for state variables of fetal states (Nijhuis et al. 1982)

	State 1F	State 2F	State 3F	State 4F
Body movements	Incidental	Periodic	Absent	Continuous
Eye movements	Absent	Present	Present	Present
Heart rate pattern	A	B	C	D

The concept of state behavior and especially state identification in the fetus has received some criticism, in part for general considerations, in part for particular shortcomings of the investigations.

The argument that fetal states comparable to states of wakefulness in the newborn infant with eyes open or even crying is beyond our imagination is not a good argument to my mind against the concept of fetal state behavior. Central nervous control of vital functions during a fetal state of wakefulness will be adapted to the special needs of the fetus and to its environment and there may be no need for the fetus to scan its environment with open eyes during fetal state 3 and there is definitely no need to call for the mother by crying. Criticism in regard to inadequate investigations has to be accepted insofar as simultaneous recordings of FHR and fetal motor activity alone may be insufficient for safe discrimination of fetal states and—in the earlier weeks of gestation—insufficient as evidence of coordinated central nervous activity and true state behavior at all.

This has been documented by the latest publication of Nijhuis et al. (1982). Besides recording of breathing movements they added recording of eye movements and mouthing movements as additional state variables or concomitants via US-B-scan. Based on their recordings they first of all defined four distinct fetal behavioral states (states 1F–4F) (Tables 4, 5) and their state criteria and I emphasize the fact that they defined an FHR pattern C typical for state 3F.

Nijhuis et al. (1982) also demonstrated that central nervous coordination of state variables, i.e., the establishment of coherent states with synchronous changes of coherent state criteria can only be seen from 36 to 38 weeks of gestation onward. In the earlier weeks of pregnancy, from 30 to 32 weeks onward, state variables alternate in an uncoordinated manner and because of the length of alternating periods particular state criteria may coincide randomly. This coincidence of state criteria by chance is not proof of true central nervous coordination, i.e., state behavior.

To my mind the following conclusions for clinical routine may be derived from the long-term observations of FHR described above.

Application of the nonstress test as a routine method for fetal surveillance must be based on knowledge of the wide variety of normal as well as pathological FHR patterns and their components, their time course of changes due to gestational age, state behavior, development of distress, and with that their probability densities.

Because FHR in the healthy fetus is not stationary, because alterations in the hypoxic fetus do not develop in a slow and monotonous trend, short-lasting nonstress tests performed at longer intervals may fail in clinical routine.

No schedule when strictly applied will guarantee early and safe detection of the fetus at risk. It is just the principle: the higher the density of monitoring the better the success rate and density of monitoring can be increased by increasing duration and frequency of nonstress tests, making long-term observations for several hours, and adding a stress test. Of course this principle cannot be maximized; it should be optimized according to the estimated risk and previous monitoring results.

Last but not least, the question of whether and how polygraphic observations of the fetus will improve results of fetal monitoring in clinical routine awaits further investigation.

References

Junge HD (1979) Behavioral states and state related heart rate and motor activity patterns in the newborn infant and the fetus ante partum—a comparative study. I. Technique, illustration of recordings, and general results. J Perinat Med 7:85

Junge HD (1979) Behavioral states and state related heart rate and motor activity patterns in the newborn infant and the fetus ante partum—a comparative study. II. Computer analysis of state related heart rate baseline and macrofluctuation patterns. J Perinat Med 7:134

Junge HD (1980) Behavioral states and state releated heart rate and motor activity patterns in the newborn infant and the fetus ante partum—a comparative study. III. Analysis of sleep state related motor activity patterns. Eur J Obstet Gynecol Reprod Biol 10(4):239

Nijhuis JG, Prechtl HFR, Martin CB Jr, Bots RSGM (1982) Are there behavioral states in the human fetus? Early Hum Dev 6:177

Patrick J, Campbell K, Carmichael L, Natale R, Richardson B (1982) Pattern of gross fetal body movements over 24-h observation intervals during the last 10 weeks of pregnancy. Am J Obstet Gynecol 142:363

Prechtl HFR (1974) The behavioral states in the newborn infant (a review). Brain Res 76:185

Visser GHA, Goodman JDS, Levine DH, Dawes GS (1982) Diurnal and other cyclic variations in human fetal heart rate near term. Am J Obstet Gynecol 142:535

Fetal Heart Rate Patterns in Experimental Intrauterine Growth Retardation*

J. F. Clapp, III[1], N. S. Peress, P. M. Catalano, and L. I. Mann

This report details our experience with fetal heart rate patterns in experimental intrauterine growth retardation (IUGR) using a chronically instrumented fetal lamb model. The data obtained indicate that increased variability, a relative baseline tachycardia, and magnified autonomic responses are characteristics of the fetal heart rate pattern in this IUGR model. Furthermore, when accentuated, this heart rate pattern is accompanied by functional and morphologic evidence of central nervous system damage. Preliminary retrospective data suggest that the former patterns may be present in the human IUGR fetus prior to the clinically emphasized patterns of diminished baseline variability; depressed or absent acceleration with fetal motion; and delayed decelerations in response to uterine contractions.

Since the introduction of electronic fetal heart rate monitoring by Hon (1959) interpretation has focused on these patterns as indicators of fetal compromise because they crudely correlate with the incidence of fetal acidosis and perinatal outcome (Kubli et al. 1969; Paul 1972; Lavery 1982; Collea and Holls 1982; Braly and Freeman 1977; Fox et al. 1976; Freeman and Garite 1981). In suspected IUGR, these depressed patterns are utilized as indicators for obstetrical intervention. However, several reports (Odendall 1976; Lin et al. 1981; Cetrulo and Freeman 1977; Tejani and Mann 1977) indicate that these fetal heart rate patterns occur late in the course of IUGR and are associated with significant perinatal morbidity and mortality. Furthermore, antenatal diagnostic accuracy of IUGR is poor (Tejani and Mann 1977; Lin et al. 1980) and many of these fetuses escape early detection. To date, little attention has been paid to the significance of early stress patterns as indicators of either this disorder or potential fetal compromise. This report emphasizes their potential value.

The Animal Model Utilized and Morphologic Outcome

The instrumentation employed in our IUGR model is illustrated in Fig. 1. The details of surgical preparation are detailed elsewhere (Clapp et al. 1980). Briefly, between 100 and 120 days' gestation electromagnetic flow transducers are placed on the main uterine and common umbilical arteries and polyvinyl catheters are placed in the distal maternal and fetal aorta, common umbilical vein, and main uterine vein. Solder ball electrodes are placed extradurally over the fetal temporoparietal cortex. An additional catheter is positioned in the main uterine artery for embolizing the

* Supported by NIH grant R01 HD 11122

[1] University of Vermont, Medical Center Hospital, Dept. of Obstetrics and Gynecology, Burlington, VT 05405, USA

Fetal Heart Rate Monitoring
Ed. by W. Künzel

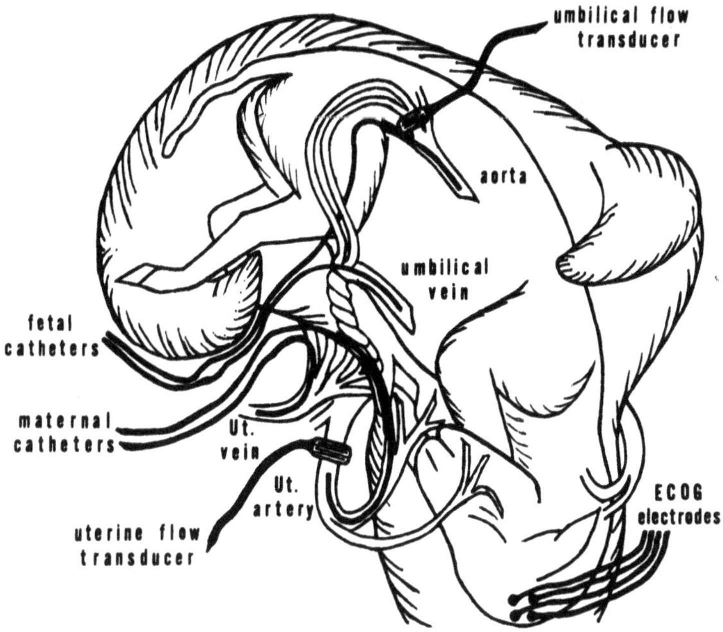

Fig. 1. The chronic animal model

uterine circulation with 15-μm microspheres which, by gradual occlusion of the placental vasculature, mimics progressive uteroplacental insufficiency with resultant IUGR. This instrumentation allows us to monitor electrocortical activity longitudinally in conjunction with numerous metabolic and cardiovascular parameters over the last 30 days of gestation. In this model fetal heart rate is obtained from the arterial pressure wave using a cardiotachometer coupler.

Immediately after surgical preparation functional parameters are monitored for 6 h and then daily for at least 60 min. Longitudinal data collection is begun on the fourth postoperative day; embolization is instituted on the eighth postoperative day and stopped when umbilical blood flow has returned to the level recorded on the fourth postoperative day. This report presents data obtained from 20 growth-retarded fetuses and 15 identically instrumented nonembolized, control animals, some of whom entered preterm labor.

As detailed in Table 1, the embolization produced clear morphometric evidence of growth retardation in both those animals who were killed near term (138th day) and those who entered preterm labor (129th day). At the time of death the fetal central nervous system was fixed in situ by perfusion to minimize artifact (Mann et al. 1978) and evaluated in detail by a neuropathologist who had no knowledge of antecedent events. The technical details and methodology employed are discussed elsewhere (Clapp et al. 1981a). As shown in Table 1, neuropathologic findings were confined to the cerebral white matter and the incidence was similar in the control, normally grown and embolized, IUGR fetal lambs. In all save one animal, the lesions were multifocal and located in the peripheral tongues of cerebral white matter just beneath the mantle of gray matter which was entirely spared. The lesions

Table 1. Morphologic data

	Morphologic data		
	Control	Embolized	Significance
Growth parameters			
1. Term (138 days)	$n = 10$	$n = 12$	
Body weight (kg)	3.77 ± 0.19	2.42 ± 0.15	0.001
Brain weight (g)	51.5 ± 1.7	44.9 ± 0.9	0.001
Hepatic weight (g)	156 ± 10	91 ± 6	0.001
2. Preterm (129 days)	$n = 5$	$n = 8$	
Body weight (kg)	2.54 ± 0.14	1.96 ± 0.11	0.001
Brain weight (g)	41.8 ± 3.2	38.6 ± 1.9	NS
Hepatic weight (g)	108 ± 6	87 ± 4	0.01
3. Ponderal index	4.08 ± 0.11	3.05 ± 0.07	0.001
CNS pathology	$n = 15$	$n = 20$	
Cortical gray	0	0	NS
Cortical white	5	5	NS
Fresh cellular	2	4	NS
Old cavitary	3	2	NS
Other	0	0	NS

were clearly separable into two age groups, the first being characterized by intense hypercellularity, the second by cavitation and glial scarring. In the fetal lamb the former occurs between the 4th and 7th day after injury while the latter does not occur for at least 35 days (Clapp et al. 1981a). As the older cavitary lesions antedated the fetal surgery they were excluded from statistical analysis.

Fetal Heart Rate Pattern Associated with Abnormal Brain Function and Neuropathology

Correlations between antecedent events and the presence (*n*, 6) or absence (*n*, 29) of fresh neuropathologic lesions were sought. Significant hypotension, a traditional etiologic factor in brain damage, was not observed in any animal. Likewise, metabolic abnormalities commonly associated with central nervous system damage (acidosis, hypoxia, hypoglycemia) were infrequent, marginal, and did not correlate with neuropathologic outcome. These data are reported in detail elsewhere (Clapp et al. 1981a).

As shown in Table 2, fetal electrocortical activity was an excellent predictor of neuropathologic outcome. In four of the six fetuses with neuropathology, delta wave voltage was reduced with a partial loss of the superimposed faster frequencies for 2 or more days and then returned to normal. This is illustrated for a single fetus in Fig. 2 with segments of recordings obtained over a 4-day interval. In two fetuses, electrocortical activity was normal but neuropathology was present. In one of these

Table 2. Correlations: ECOG vs fresh lesions

	Fresh lesions present	Fresh lesions absent
ECOG normal or transient abnormality	2	29
ECOG persistently abnormal	4	0

$P<0.001$ by Fisher's test of exact probability

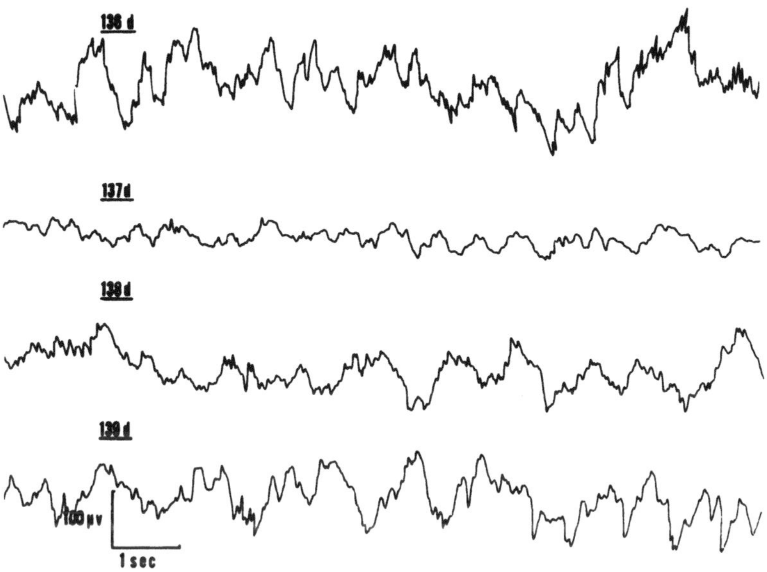

Fig. 2. Serial tracings of electrocortical activity during high voltage from a fetus with fresh hypercellular cortical white matter lesions—days 136 and 139 are normal. Note the reduction in voltage of the large delta waves on days 137 and 138 with marked suppression of the superimposed low-voltage high frequency on day 137

only a single fresh lesion was seen and electrode malfunction occurred 10 days prior to death in the other. No persistent abnormalities in electrocortical activity were observed in any fetus whose central nervous system was histologically normal.

As shown in Table 3 a similar relationship was present between antecedent cardiovascular parameters and neuropathologic outcome. In five of the six fetuses with neuropathology, evidence of recurrent cardiovascular instability, characterized by tachycardia and a marked increase in baseline variability exceeding 40 beats/min, was present. This heart rate pattern was episodic in nature and perhaps represented periodic changes due to its wide oscillatory nature and its association with inverse oscillatory changes in arterial pressure and umbilical blood flow. Representative heart rate tracings from three of the five fetuses are shown in Fig. 3 and the interrelationships between this heart rate pattern, arterial pressure, and umbilical flow are shown for a single fetus in Fig. 4. In one fetus, cardiovascular parameters were

Table 3. Correlations: cardiovascular instability vs fresh lesions

	Fresh lesions present	Fresh lesions absent
Recurrent cardiovascular instability absent	1	29
Recurrent cardiovascular instability present	5	0

$P < 0.001$ by Fisher's test of exact probability

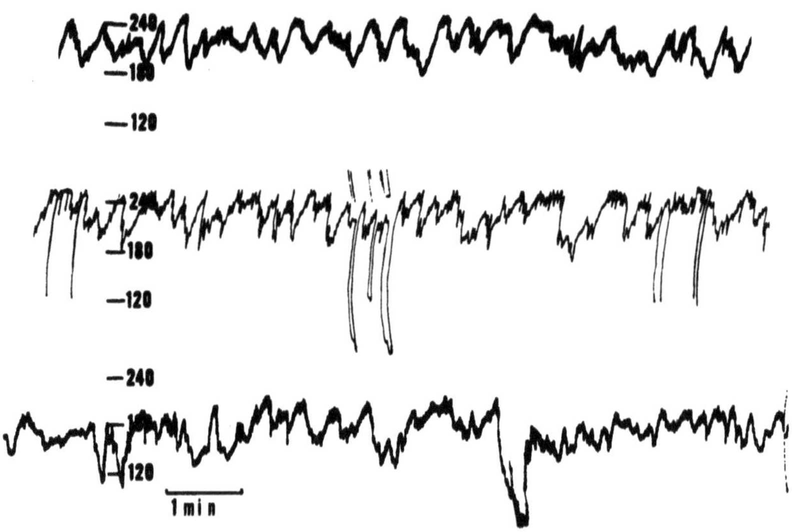

Fig. 3. Fetal heart rate recordings from three animals during episodes of cardiovascular instability. Note their wide oscillatory nature and their high baseline rate

entirely normal yet neuropathology was present. This was the fetus with a single fresh lesion. The aberrant heart rate pattern was not seen in fetuses with normal central nervous system histology.

Thus, in five of six fetuses with histologic evidence of neuropathologic damage a characteristic heart rate pattern suggesting intermittent partial occlusion of the umbilical circulation with increased sympathetic tone was seen and, in all fetuses with functioning electrodes, this was associated with abnormal electrocortical activity. This occurred in the absence of hypotension and without evidence of systemic hypoxia, hypoglycemia, or acidosis using intermittent sampling techniques. As shown in Figs. 3 and 4, the heart rate pattern is quite characteristic of an accentuated early stress response. From a physiologic point of view it is characteristic of a perturbed system attempting to regain equilibrium. The combined data support the conclusions of Duffy et al. (1982) that cerebral white matter is selectively vulnerable to injury during marginal systemic stress due to a local imbalance between metabolism and perfusion. Furthermore, the correlation between neuropathology

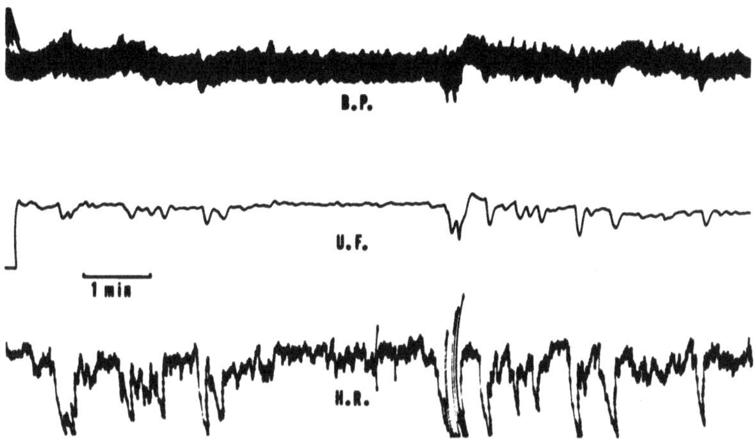

Fig. 4. A simultaneous recording of fetal arterial pressure, mean umbilical blood flow, and heart rate during an episode of cardiovascular instability. Note the inverse relationship between heart rate and arterial pressure and the instability of umbilical blood flow. During this episode blood gases drawn from the distal aorta were pH, 7.41; PO_2, 23; and PCO_2, 43

and a specific heart rate pattern provides a potential noninvasive marker which should be evaluated in the human.

Longitudinal Fetal Heart Rate Pattern in Experimental IUGR

The fetal heart rate recordings of the eight control, normally grown and nine embolized IUGR term fetuses without evidence of central nervous injury were visually reviewed to determine whether or not the longitudinal fetal heart rate pattern was different in the embolized group. Unfortunately, as we were dealing with a slow speed paper record, the data was difficult to quantitate but three distinct characteristics were identified.

Average Fetal Heart Rate for Gestational Age

Prior to the onset of embolization average daily heart rates were similar in the two groups. Following the initiation of embolization the average daily heart rate for gestational age was consistently higher in the embolized group. During embolization it averaged 15–35 beats/min higher and remained 10–25 beats/min higher in the postembolization period. Between the 135th day and the time of killing, mean values ($\pm$ SEM) were significantly ($P<0.01$) different in the control (142 ± 5) and embolized (160 ± 6) groups. As illustrated in Fig. 5 the longitudinal pattern was quite different. In the control animals there was a progressive gradual decrease with advancing gestational age. In the embolized animals average heart rate either remained in the same range or rose during embolization and changed erratically from day to day. Postembolization, the average daily heart rate fell but remained elevated for gestational age. The pattern observed in a single embolized normally grown fetus (lower left panel, Fig. 5), studied as we were developing the model,

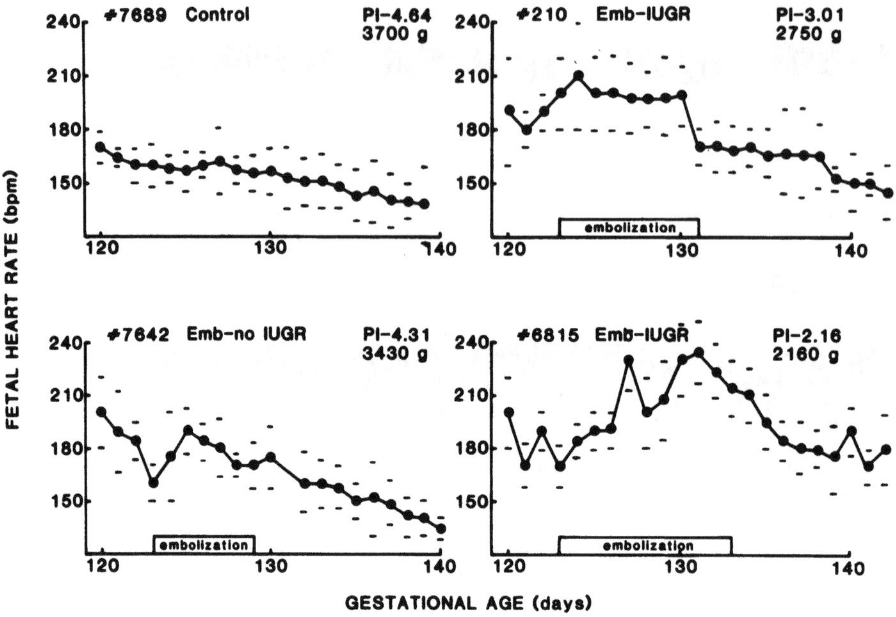

Fig. 5. Average daily heart rate over a 20-day interval in four chronically instrumented fetal lambs. In each graph the mean (●) and range for the day are shown. Note the difference in the longitudinal pattern between the embolized IUGR animals *(right panel)* and the control animal *(upper left panel)*. The embolized normally grown fetus *(lower left panel)* demonstrates an intermediate pattern

suggests that the differences in daily heart rate patterns represent a fetal sympathetic response to the repetitive placental damage rather than a response to the cessation of growth.

Variability

As illustrated in Figs. 5–7, the daily range and variability of the fetal heart rate was increased in the embolized, IUGR group. Unfortunately, this data is largely impressionistic as it was not stored in a form which allowed calculations of indices of short- and long-term variability as initially described by DeHaan (1971). Nonetheless, the visual impression of an increase in variability following the onset of embolization was consistently present. Although not recorded, it is unlikely that this was due to fetal breathing movements as the increased variability was most pronounced during high-voltage and indeterminate or transitional electrocortical activity, suggesting a relationship with complex fetal motion (Van der Wilt 1982) and/or changing autonomic tone.

Heart Rate Responsiveness

As illustrated by the tracings shown in Figs. 6 and 7, accelerations of the fetal heart rate were greater in magnitude, irregular, and in general more prolonged in the embolized IUGR group. Presumably these accelerations, accompanied by increases

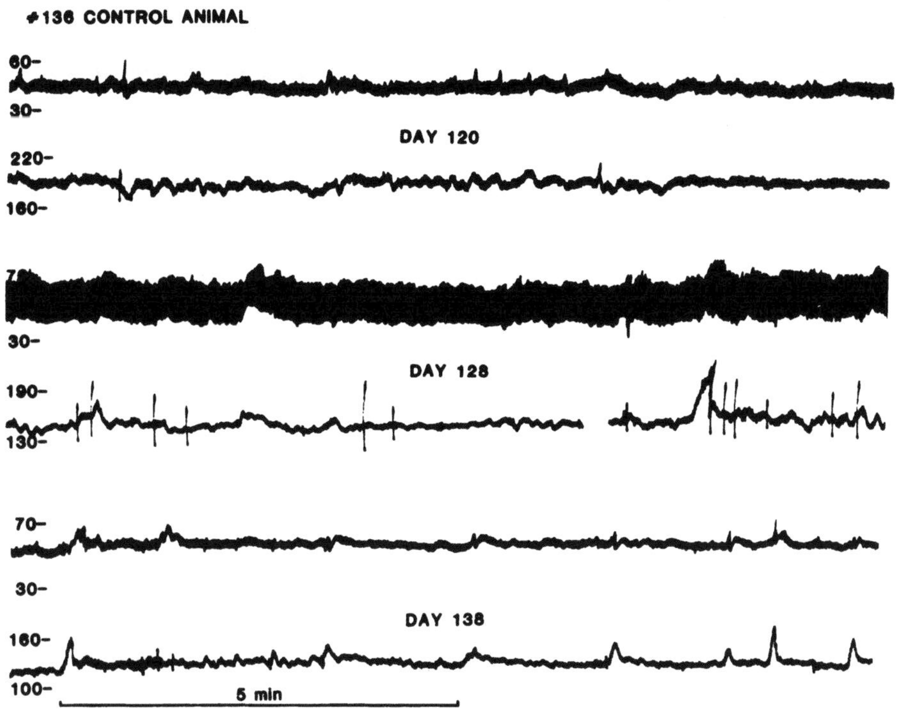

Fig. 6. Serial recordings of blood pressure and heart rate from a control animal. On each occasion the fetus moved from low-voltage fast-frequency electrocortical activity through intermediate or transitional activity to a high-voltage pattern as the recording progresses from left to right. Note the decrease in baseline heart rate and appearance of more defined accelerations with advancing gestation and the apparent decrease in baroreceptor activity

in arterial pressure, occurred in association with fetal motion, which we were unable to document accurately with the instrumentation available. As there is no reason to suspect that the growth-retarded fetus is more vigorous in its activity, the difference in the magnitude of the heart rate response suggests heightened sympathetic tone. Likewise, postacceleration and basal slowings of the heart rate in response to changes in arterial pressure were more frequent and pronounced in the embolized group, again suggesting an increase in autonomic tone producing a magnified heart rate response to baroreceptor stimulation.

Thus, serial fetal heart rate recordings revealed visually different longitudinal heart rate patterns in the embolized IUGR group characterized by an increase in the average daily heart rate for gestational age, a visually apparent increase in variability, and a magnified heart rate responsiveness. All suggest an increase in fetal autonomic tone which is consistent with the changes in the distribution of cardiac output (Creasy et al. 1973) and the rise in fetal cortisol levels (Clapp et al. 1982). However, this appears not to be accompanied by changes in mean arterial pressure (Clapp et al. 1980, 1981b; Creasy et al. 1973) and the heart rate patterns which suggest this etiology have not been appreciated in previous studies (Clapp et al. 1980, 1981a, b, 1982; Creasy et al. 1973) using this model.

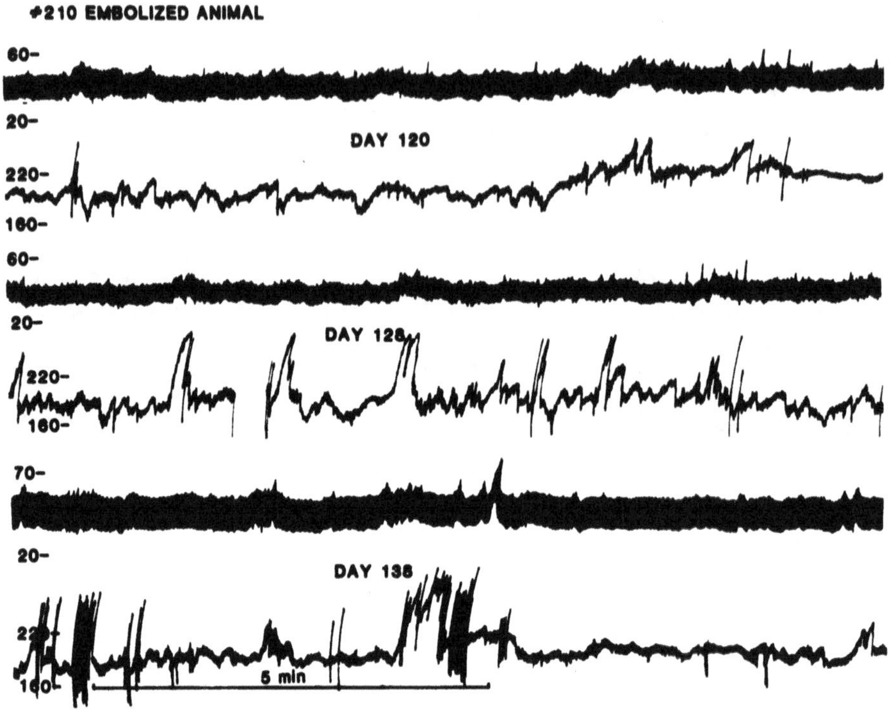

Fig. 7. Serial recordings of blood pressure and heart rate from an embolized animal at the same gestational age and during similar electrocortical patterns as the fetus in Fig. 6. The top recording was obtained prior to, the middle during, and the bottom tracing after the period of embolization. Note that baseline heart rate remains high and the baroreceptor effects on heart rate persist with advancing gestation. Note the contrast in heart rate variability and acceleration patterns in this fetus when compared with that shown in Fig. 6

Preliminary Retrospective Analysis of Heart Rate Patterns in the IUGR Human Fetus

In view of the heart rate patterns identified in our IUGR model, we designed a small retrospective study to see if similar longitudinal patterns could be identified in the growth-retarded human fetus. To obtain these data, the antepartum recordings obtained in the course of nonstress and contraction stress tests on the last 30 cases referred for evaluation of suspected IUGR were reviewed separately by two individuals who, save for estimated gestational age, were unaware of the clinical course and outcome. Three cases were rejected because there were less than three serial recordings made. In the remaining 27 cases between three and eight serial tracings obtained either weekly or twice weekly between the 35th and 42nd week of gestation were available for review. In each instance, the fetal heart rate was monitored using a wide-angle ultrasound transducer and recorded in standard fashion on a Hewitt-Packard 8030A. Each case was independently evaluated for: an increased baseline heart rate for gestational age (> 140 after 38 weeks, > 150 between the 35th and 38th week); increased variability (> 20 beats/min); and the impression of increased responsiveness of the heart rate to fetal motion with frequent lambda (Aladjem et al. 1977) accel/decel patterns and an increase in baseline heart rate with the onset of uterine activity. If two of these three criteria were met on two consecutive tracings the case was classified as IUGR; if not, it was classified as normal. Scoring was uniform between observers save for one case which therefore was classified as normal.

Then, birthweight, crown-rump length, and gestational age at delivery were abstracted from the record and ponderal indices calculated. Based on the birthweight gestational age centiles in our populace and the ponderal index values reported by Miller and Merritt (1979), each infant was classified as normally grown (>10th centile and a ponderal index >2.33), asymmetrically small for gestational age (<10th centile, ponderal index <2.33), or symmetrically small for gestational age (<10th centile, ponderal index >2.33).

The predicted pattern of growth from analysis of the heart rate recordings was then plotted against the morphometric outcome obtained from chart review. These data are presented in Table 4. Using only the referral diagnosis, gestational age, and analysis of serial heart rate recordings, the intrauterine growth profile was correctly predicted in 20 of the 27 instances with a 14% false + diagnosis of IUGR and a false negative rate of 38%. The two false positives were infants who weighed in the 11th and 18th percentile for gestational age and had low normal ponderal indices of 2.35 and 2.42. Of the five false negatives, one was the product of a toxemic pregnancy with poor variability on all recordings, three were symmetrically growth retarded and may simply have been genetically small, and one was a clear misprediction. Currently we plan a prospective study to evaluate this in greater detail but the retrospective data appear promising in terms of improving the accuracy of antenatal diagnosis.

Summary

In summary, in both our IUGR animal model and in a preliminary retrospective clinical study, we find evidence that early in the course of IUGR fetal heart rate patterns are characterized by an increase in rate, variability, and responsiveness,

Table 4. Human fetal heart rate patterns and morphometric outcome

Heart rate pattern	Morphometric outcome			
	Normal growth	Asymmetric SGA	Symmetric SGA	Total
Prediction				
Normal	8	2	3	13
IUGR	2	9	3	14
Total	10	11	6	27

False positive rate, 14%; false negative rate, 38%
SGA, small for gestational age

suggesting increased fetal autonomic tone. This fetal heart rate pattern suggests an early stress response that may be of value in clinical diagnosis. In addition accentuation of this pattern, when recurrent, is an accurate predictor of cortical white matter injury in the animal model.

References

Aladjem S, Feria A, Rest J, Stojanovic J (1977) Fetal heart rate responses to fetal movements. Br J Obstet Gynaecol 84:487

Braly P, Freeman RK (1977) The significance of fetal heart rate reactivity with a positive oxytocin challenge test. Obstet Gynecol 50:689

Cetrulo CL, Freeman RK (1977) Bioelectric evaluation in intrauterine growth retardation. Clin Obstet Gynecol 20:979

Clapp JF, Szeto HH, Larrow R, Hewitt J, Mann LI (1980) Umbilical blood flow response to embolization of the uterine circulation. Am J Obstet 138:60

Clapp JF, Mann LI, Peress NS, Szeto HH (1981a) Neuropathology in the chronic fetal lamb preparation: structure-function correlates under different environmental conditions. Am J Obstet Gynecol 141:973

Clapp JF, Szeto HH, Larrow R, Hewitt J, Mann LI (1981b) Fetal metabolic response to experimental placental vascular damage. Am J Obstet Gynecol 140:446

Clapp JF, Auletta FJ, Farnham J, Larrow RW, Mann LI (1982) The ovine fetoplacental endocrine response to placental damage. Am J Obstet Gynecol 4:47

Collea JV, Holls WM (1982) The contraction stress test. Clin Obstet Gynecol 25:707

Creasy RK, DeSwiet M, Kahanpaa KV, Young WP, Rudolph AM (1973) Pathophysiological changes in the foetal lamb with growth retardation. In: Comline KS, Cross KW, Dawes GS, Nathanielsz PO (eds) Foetal and neonatal physiology. Cambridge University Press, Cambridge, UK, p 398

DeHaan J (1971) The short-term irregularity in the foetal heart rate pattern (in Dutch). Academic Thesis, Free University, Amsterdam

Duffy TE, Cavazzuti M, Cruz NF, Sokoloff L (1982) Local cerebral glucose metabolism in newborn dogs: effects of hypoxia and halothane anesthesia. Ann Neurol 11:233

Fox HE, Steinbrecher M, Ripton B (1976) Antepartum fetal heart rate and uterine activity studies. Am J Obstet Gynecol 126:61

Freeman RK, Garite TJ (1981) Fetal heart rate monitoring. Williams and Wilkins, Baltimore

Hon EH (1959) Observations on pathologic fetal bradycardia. Am J Obstet Gynecol 77:1084

Kubli FW, Hon EH, Khazin AF, Takemura H (1969) Observations of heart rate and pH in the human fetus during labor. Am J Obstet Gynecol 104:1190

Lavery JP (1982) Nonstress fetal heart rate testing. Clin Obstet Gynecol 25:689

Lin C, Moawad AH, Rowenow PJ, River P (1980) The acid base characteristics of fetuses with intrauterine growth retardation during labor and delivery. Am J Obstet Gynecol 137:553

Lin C, Devoe LD, River P, Moawad AH (1981) Oxytocin challenge test and intrauterine growth retardation. Am J Obstet Gynecol 140:282

Mann LI, Bhaktharathsalan A, Peress N, Szeto H, Lin M (1978) Fetal brain function, metabolism and neuropathology following acute hypoxia. In: Longo LD, Reneau DD (eds) Fetal and newborn cardiovascular physiology, vol 2. Garland, New York, pp 313–335

Miller HC, Merritt TA (1979) Fetal growth in humans. Yearbook Medical, Chicago, p 180

Odendall H (1976) Fetal heart rate patterns in patients with intrauterine growth retardation. Obstet Gynecol 48:187

Paul R (1972) Clinical fetal monitoring, experience on a large clinical service. Am J Obstet Gynecol 113:573

Tejani N, Mann LI (1977) Diagnosis and management of the small-for-gestational age fetus. Clin Obstet Gynecol 20:943

Van der Wilt B (1982) Heart rate, breathing movements and brain activity in fetal lambs. Academic thesis, University of Nijmegen, Nijmegen

Chemoreceptor and Baroreceptor Function with Respect to Fetal Heart Rate Variability

H. Acker[1]

The variability of the baseline heart rate has been accepted as a measurement of the fetal oxygen supply and thus fetal health. It has been found that late deceleration, tachycardia, and the loss of beat-to-beat variability produce an unstable heart rate pattern prior to fetal death. Late decelerations have been found to occur up to four times more often in hypoxic fetuses than in normal fetuses taking into account that late decelerations may be the result of both vagal stimulation and a direct myocardial response to hypoxemia (Hon 1968; Hon and Quilligan 1967; Willcourt et al. 1981).

To obtain more information about the variability of the fetal heart rate (FHR) in dependence on the oxygen supply of the fetus, in several studies the relationship between the fetal heart rate and transcutaneous (tc) PO_2 or arterial O_2 saturation was determined.

According to Huch et al. (1977), the relation between basal FHR and fetal $tcPO_2$ of human fetuses seems to be complex. In their studies there appeared to be no relation between basal FHR and fetal $tcPO_2$, except when the heart rate was below 100 or above 180 beats/min, in which case the fetal $tcPO_2$ was low. This demonstrates that the basal heart rate may vary due to factors which are not related to the oxygen level. The diagnosis of hypoxemia cannot be made from temporary changes in the heart rate variability. There seems to be a correlation between heart rate variability and low fetal $tcPO_2$. From the results of Huch et al. (1977), it appears that if $tcPO_2$ is higher than 15 mmHg there is no risk of fetal distress, whereas a fetal $tcPO_2$ level below 15 mmHg may suggest insufficient oxygen supply to the fetus.

Willecourt et al. (1981) could show that late decelerations were always associated with a declining fetal $tcPO_2$, although the magnitude of the FHR deceleration often did not reflect the extent of the decline in the fetal $tcPO_2$. The presence or absence of FHR variability did not reflect the baseline levels of fetal oxygenation, since maternal positioning or oxygen administration or both increased the fetal $tcPO_2$ and decreased the FHR variability. Künzel et al. (1981) could not establish a relationship between the oxygen saturation at control and the fetal heart rate and the blood pressure response. The duration and the fall of the fetal heart rate was not a good measure for estimating the severity of fetal hypoxia in their experiments. To elucidate this problem the complexity between the arterial PO_2 and the tissue PO_2 of different organs or, in other words, oxygen supply of the fetus should be discussed. According to the diffusion laws the PO_2 decrease in tissue, $\Delta PO_{2\,[t]}$, can be calculated. Hereby the dimension of the PO_2 gradient depends on the following:

1. Diffusion properties of tissue
2. Size of spatial distribution and oxygen uptake
3. Capillary distance and structure

[1] Max-Planck-Institut für Systemphysiologie, Rheinlanddamm 201, D-4600 Dortmund 1

Fetal Heart Rate Monitoring
Ed. by W. Künzel

This can be expressed by the following equations:

$$\Delta PO_{2\,[t]} = \frac{A\,[O_2]}{2\alpha \cdot D}\, g\,(r_t, r_c, r_z) \qquad \text{(Krogh-Erlang law) (1)}$$

$$\text{with } A\,[O_2] = [a\,[O_2] - v\,[O_2]] \cdot F \qquad \text{(Fick's law) (2)}$$

$$\text{and } g\,(r_t, r_c, r_z) = r_z^2 \ln\left(\frac{r_t}{r_z}\right) - (r_c^2 - r_t^2) \qquad (3)$$

where $a[O_2]$, arterial O_2 content; $v[O_2]$, venous O_2 content; F, blood flow; $A\,[O_2]$, oxygen uptake; $2\alpha \cdot D$, O_2 solubility coefficient and oxygen diffusion coefficient; r_c, radius of capillary; r_t, distance of PO_2 measuring point from capillary center; and r_z, radius of tissue cylinder.

Eq. (1) shows that the oxygen consumption is linearly related to the oxygen pressure difference ΔPO_2, which is necessary to transport oxygen into the tissue and that the geometry enters approximately as a squared function. The actual tissue PO_2, PtO_2, depends on the arterial PO_2, PaO_2, on the PO_2 decrease along the capillary, $\Delta PO_{2\,[cap]}$, and on the PO_2 decrease within the tissue $\Delta PO_{2\,[t]}$.

$$PtO_2 = PaO_2 - \Delta PO_{2\,[t]} - \Delta PO_{2\,[cap]} \qquad (4)$$

From Eqs. (1, 2, 4) one can recognize that the tissue PO_2 is a function of the blood flow and the actual hemoglobin dissociation curve when PaO_2, $A\,[O_2]$, $\alpha \cdot D$, and $g\,(r_t, r_c, r_z)$ are constant (Lübbers and Leniger-Follert 1978; Thews 1960).

To characterize the oxygen supply under normal and hypoxic conditions, we performed PO_2 measurements in different organs of the fetal and newborn lamb. Results of this experimental model should be discussed with cautiousness, since exteriorization causes (1) a fall of up to 50% in fetal cardiac output without changing the arterial gas tension and pH (Comline and Silver 1974), (2) a large increase in circulating catecholamines, and (3) profound effects on the sleep and waking pattern (Dawes et al. 1972). We measured the tissue PO_2 with surface electrodes as described by Lübbers and Leniger-Follert (1978). With these electrodes it is possible to measure the PO_2 on four different tissue spots as shown in Fig. 1. Clamping the umbilical cord, the surface PO_2 of the kidney decreases without reaching zero. After putting the fetus on the respiratory pump, simulating delivery, the tissue PO_2 increases to values known from adult animals. It is very interesting to observe that hypoxia, caused by an apnea, only causes a very small PO_2 decrease. In a 10-day-old lamb the same tissue PO_2 values of the kidney can be observed under normoxia. Now, an apnea causes a very drastic PO_2 decrease, a behavior of the tissue PO_2 which we know from the adult cat (Fig. 2). In the fetal state the skeletal muscle of the hind limb (Fig. 3) has low PO_2 values and, under hypoxic conditions, almost reaches a PO_2 of zero. After birth, the muscle PO_2 increases slowly and, after ½ h, reaches high values of up to 30 torr. These values are high in comparison to adult animals. An apnea always causes a marked PO_2 decrease. In the 10-day-old lamb the muscle PO_2 has values of between 10 and 20 torr, which are comparable with those in adult animals. We have to confirm these PO_2 measurements in further experiments and we

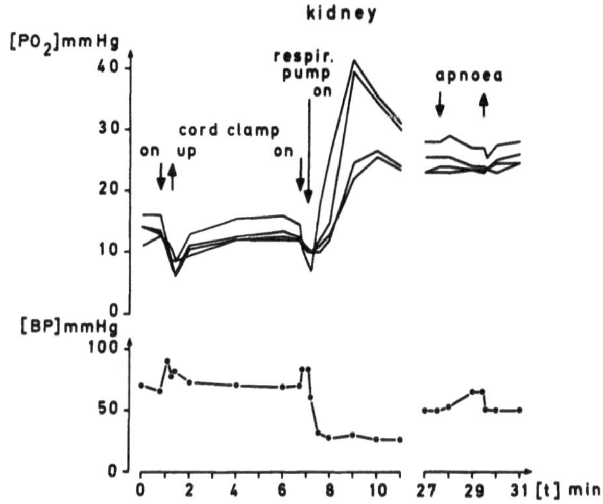

Fig. 1. Surface tissue PO_2 measured at four spots on the kidney and its behavior in the fetal lamb under cord clamp conditions, respiring conditions of the fetus, and the newborn lamb under apnea conditions. Mean arterial blood pressure under these circumstances is shown. *PO_2*, surface oxygen pressure; *BP*, mean arterial blood pressure; *t*, time

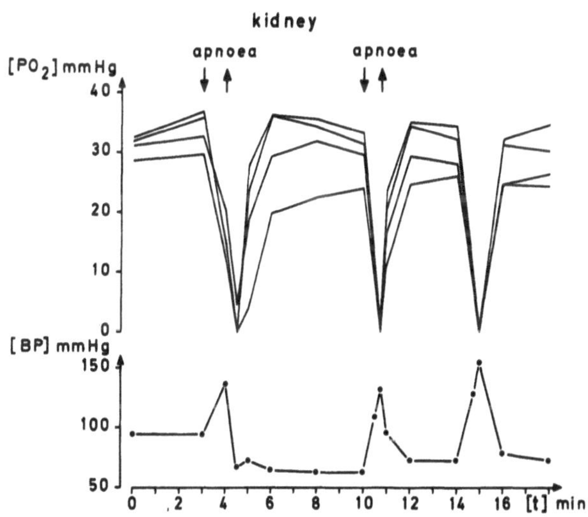

Fig. 2. Surface tissue PO_2 measured at four spots on the kidney of a 10-day-old lamb. Apnea is caused by cessation of the respirating pump. The behavior of the mean arterial blood pressure can be seen at the bottom. *PO_2*, surface oxygen pressure; *BP*, mean arterial blood pressure; *t*, time

must compare them with flow measurements in different fetal organs as described in the literature (Mott 1971; Reuss and Rudolph 1980; Robillard et al. 1981; Rudolph and Heymann 1973; Toubas et al. 1981).

For the fetal brain, a first attempt in this direction was made by Giulbeau and Reneau (1976). According to our measurements, fetal organs seem to possess

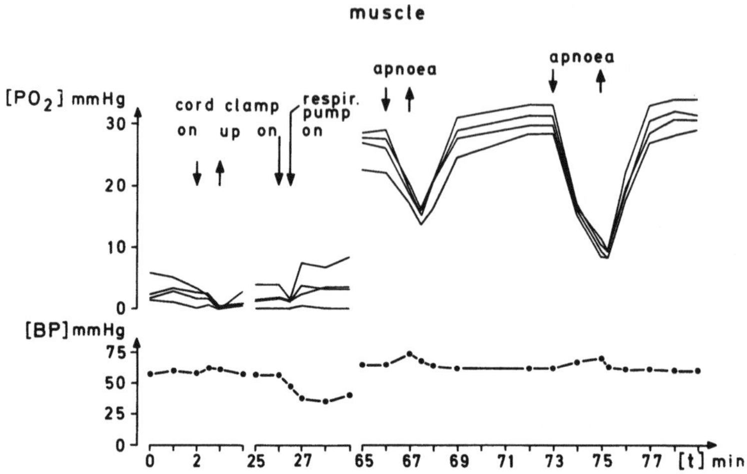

Fig. 3. Surface tissue PO_2 measured at four spots on the skeletal muscle of the hind limb and its behavior in the fetal lamb under cord clamp conditions, respiring conditions of the fetus, and the newborn lamb under apnea conditions. The mean arterial blood pressure under these circumstances is shown. *PO_2,* surface oxygen pressure; *BP,* mean arterial blood pressure; *t,* time

regulatory processes which compensate arterial hypoxemia. The left-shifted O_2 hemoglobin dissociation curve, a change in the general oxygen uptake (Rudolph and Heymann 1973) with a mitochondrial respiratory capacity different from the newborn and adult mitochondria (Goodwin et al. 1976), and special fetal local flow regulatory processes could be involved in the protection mechanism counterbalancing fetal arterial PO_2 decrease. Chemoreceptors and baroreceptors are certainly involved in regulating local flow. The four major baroreceptor nerves originate from the carotid sinus and the aortic arch baroreceptors. The effect of the baroreceptor reflex on the cardiovascular system depends on the anesthetic level of the animal. In conscious dogs carotid sinus hypotension induces heart rate changes characterized by a short-time constant together with transient changes in cardiac output (by about 15% of control). These heart-rate-dependent changes in cardiac output seem to be particularly suited for immediate adjustment of blood pressure. Under these conditions, a reflex sympathetic vasoconstriction has only been presented for the skeletal muscle resistance vessels. The changes observed in the renal and mesenteric vascular beds, which together comprise about 45% of the total peripheral resistance, seem to be solely due to autoregulation. In the anesthetized dogs carotid sinus hypotension induces a reflex tachycardia characterized by a low time constant and predominantly caused by sympathetic activation. This higher sympathetic tone also induces a vasoconstriction in the skeletal muscle, kidney, mesentery, and skin vasculature; there are several studies suggesting that the coronary vessels are also involved. Anesthesia probably blocks the influence of baroreceptor afferents, especially the effect on those central neurons responsible for cardiac vagal efferent activity. This might explain, at least in part, the low parasympathetic tone in the anesthetized dog (Kirchheim 1976). Dawes et al. (1980) were able to show a threshold at 60–65 mmHg for the heart period response to raising the arterial pressure in the

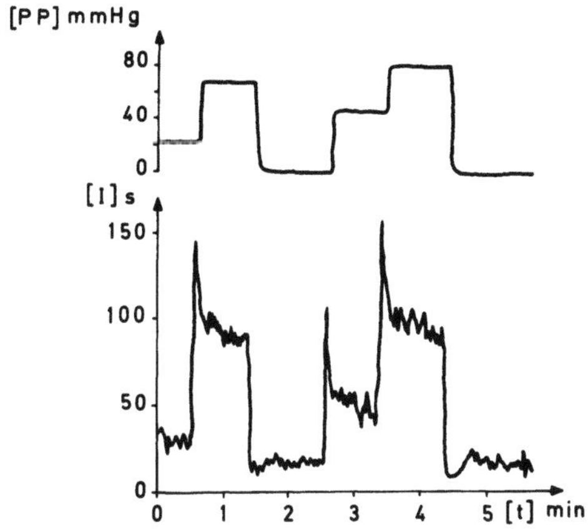

Fig. 4. Reaction of a few fiber baroreceptor preparations of the carotid sinus nerve to pressure changes in the isolated carotis sinus segment. *PP,* perfusion pressure; *I,* counted impulses of the nervous baroreceptor activity per time; *t,* time

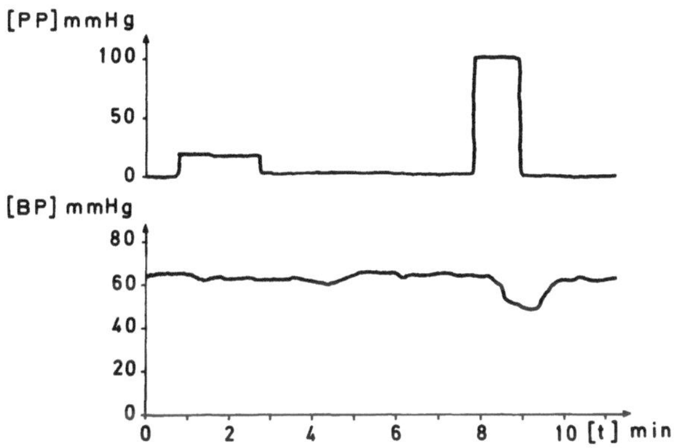

Fig. 5. Reaction of the blood pressure in the fetal lamb to changes in the perfusion pressure of the isolated carotic sinus segment. *PP,* perfusion pressure; *BP,* mean arterial blood pressure; *t,* minute

fetal lamb. The baroreflex control of heart rate does not operate at resting arterial pressures in a normal fetus in vitro. There is an increase in sensitivity of the reflex and an increase in the range over which the heart periods are changed when comparing the adult with the lamb (Dawes et al. 1980).

Figure 4 demonstrates the response of the baroreceptor activity in the carotid sinus nerve to pressure changes in the isolated carotid sinus segment of the fetal lamb. It can be seen that the baroreceptor activity adapts after a rapid pressure change. The blood pressure itself changes, too, if the pressure is changed in the isolated carotid sinus segment. The next two figures demonstrate this for the mature fetal (Fig. 5) and the newborn lamb (Fig. 6). A decrease in blood pressure during elevation of the carotid sinus pressure could always be observed.

The involvement of the chemoreceptors in the fetal cardiovascular changes to hypoxia has to be discussed in respect to the carotid and aortic bodies characteristics.

The elevation of arterial pressure under hypoxia is predominantly due to an increase in total peripheral resistance (De Burg Daly 1983; O'Regan and Majcherczyk

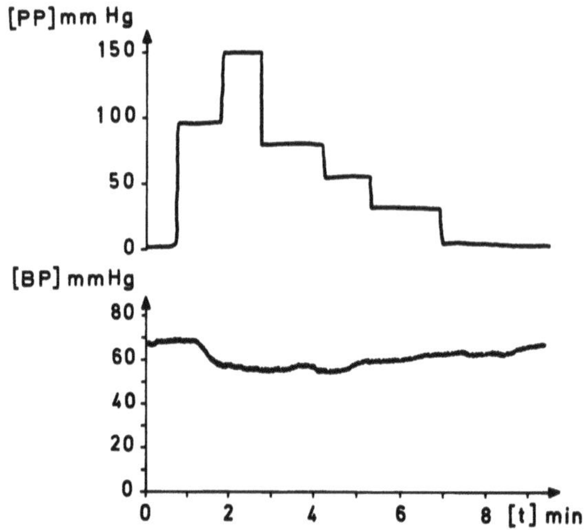

Fig. 6. Reaction of blood pressure in the newborn lamb to changes in perfusion pressure of the isolated carotis sinus segment. *PP*, perfusion pressure; *BP*, mean arterial blood pressure; *t*, minute

1982). Both groups of chemoreceptor carotid and aortic bodies reflexly cause this increase, the size of the primary response being on average the same. Vasoconstriction occurs in skeletal muscle, intestine, and kidney. The primary reflex effects on the heart by carotid chemoreceptors are bradycardia and variable effects on contractility, whereas stimulation of aortic chemoreceptors induces tachycardia and positive ionotropic effects. In the mature fetal lamb, hypoxemia causes tachycardia and hypertension and with a further fall of PO_2, bradycardia, and further hypertension. These responses are accompanied by femoral vasoconstriction, an increase in cardiac output and an increase in umbilical blood flow (Dawes et al. 1969a, b). The physiological importance of these changes is expressed in a reduction of the somatic oxygen consumption, a maximized oxygen uptake at the placenta, and an enhancement of the delivery of oxygen, in particular to the myocardium (Cohn et al. 1974; Reuss and Rudolph 1980). These cardiovascular responses depend on the integrity of the aortic nerves, whereas the carotid sinus nerve can be cut without abolishing the blood pressure response to hypoxia in the fetal lamb. These findings support reports from the literature (Blanco et al. 1982; Dawes et al. 1969a, b; Jansen and Chemick 1983; Purves 1974), indicating that the carotid body is discharging at a lower rate than in the adult at the same arterial PO_2. The aortic bodies, however, play a part in fetal blood gas homeostasis by their control of the circulation, since the maintenance of arterial pressure is essential to the maintenance of an adequate umbilical blood flow. The primary reflex effects on heart and blood vessels due to carotid chemoreceptor stimulation can be antagonized or potentiated by influences occurring simultaneously. Increases in vagal activity from pulmonary stretch receptors which are active in the sheep fetus (Ponte and Purves 1973), for instance, in the adult in association with hypocapnia and enhanced activity of respiratory neurons in the medulla, produce a reduction or even a reversal of the chemoreceptor-mediated hypertension, peripheral vasoconstriction, and bradycardia. Excitation of upper airway receptors (apnea) or stimulation of trigeminal receptors on the skin of the face enhance the primary influences due to chemoreceptor stimulation (O'Regan and Majcherczyk 1982). Cardiovascular response during carotid chemoreceptor stimulation can be modified by concomitant changes in baroreceptor afferent activity, so that hypotension potentiates these responses (Heistad et al. 1975). In our own experiments (Althoff and Acker, unpublished observations), we could observe that the baroreceptor reflex is diminished under isolated hypoxic stimulation conditions of the carotid sinus segment. Hypoxemia exerts influences on the autonomic nervous system, on the heart and blood vessels attenuating cardiovascular adjustments, which are mediated by peripheral chemoreceptors (Heistad and Abboud 1980).

The activation mechanism of the carotid body under or after birth is still unclear. Although the sympathetic nerve, which is activated with occlusion of the umbilical cord (Acker et al. 1980), contributes to the activation of the chemoreceptor, it cannot be the only mechanism, since an activation of the chemoreceptor occurs also in superfused preparation being free of efferent influences (Jansen et al. 1980).

We have tried to bring some light into the fetal carotid body physiology by comparative carotid body tissue PO_2 measurements in the fetal and newborn state (Acker et al. 1980). In the fetal state, the PO_2 difference between tissue PO_2 of the carotid body and the arterial blood is small and becomes very pronounced in the newborn state. It was supposed that this enhanced PO_2 difference could induce metabolic processes which would activate the chemoreceptor mechanism. In continuation of these experiments we performed measurements of the extracellular ion activity changes under hypoxia in the fetal and newborn carotid body of the lamb.

Figure 7 shows a simultaneous measurement of tissue PO_2 and extracellular potassium activity with a three-barrel microelectrode in the fetal carotid body. The potassium activity increases with the declining tissue PO_2 due to cord clamp. The

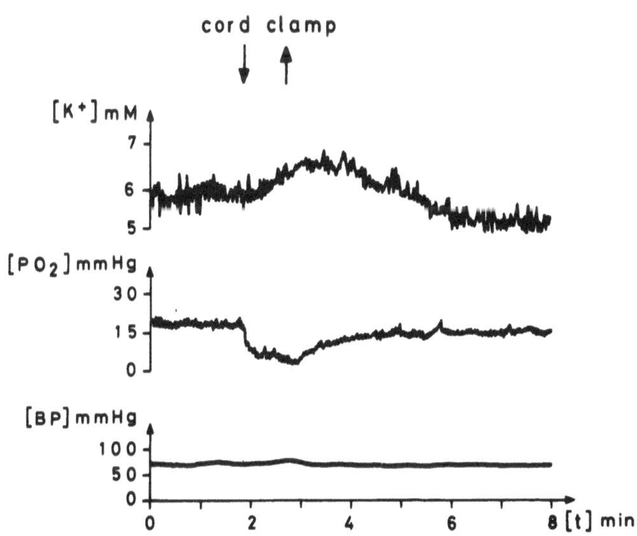

Fig. 7. Changes of extracellular potassium activity and tissue PO_2 in the fetal lamb carotid body under cord clamp conditions. *[K^+]*, extracellular potassium activity; *PO_2*, tissue PO_2; *BP*, blood pressure; *t*, time

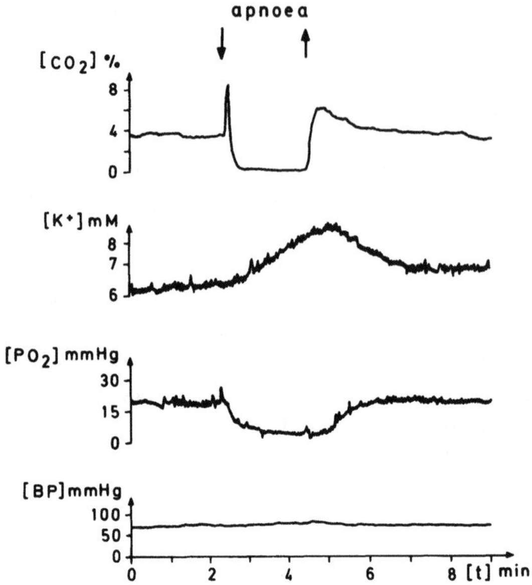

Fig. 8. Changes of extracellular potassium activity and tissue PO_2 in the newborn lamb carotid body under apnea conditions. Apnea was produced by cessation of the respiratory pump. *CO_2*, peak values of the endexpiratory CO_2; *$[K^+]$*, extracellular potassium activity; *PO_2*, tissue PO_2; *BP*, blood pressure; *t*, time

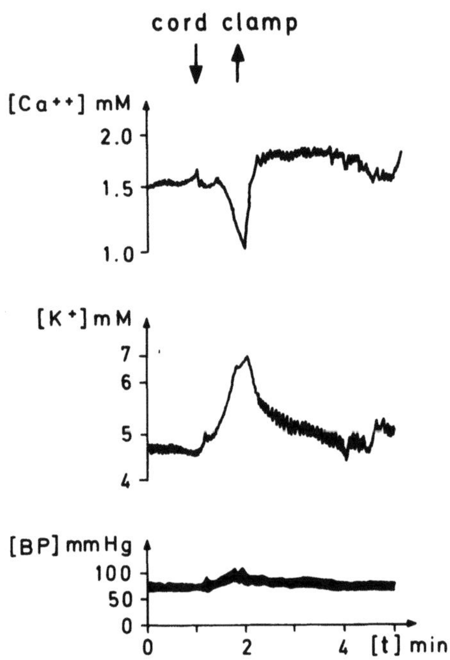

Fig. 9. Changes of extracellular potassium and calcium activities in the fetal lamb carotid body under cord clamp conditions. *$[Ca^{++}]$*, extracellular calcium activity; *$[K^+]$*, extracellular potassium activity; *BP*, blood pressure; *t*, time

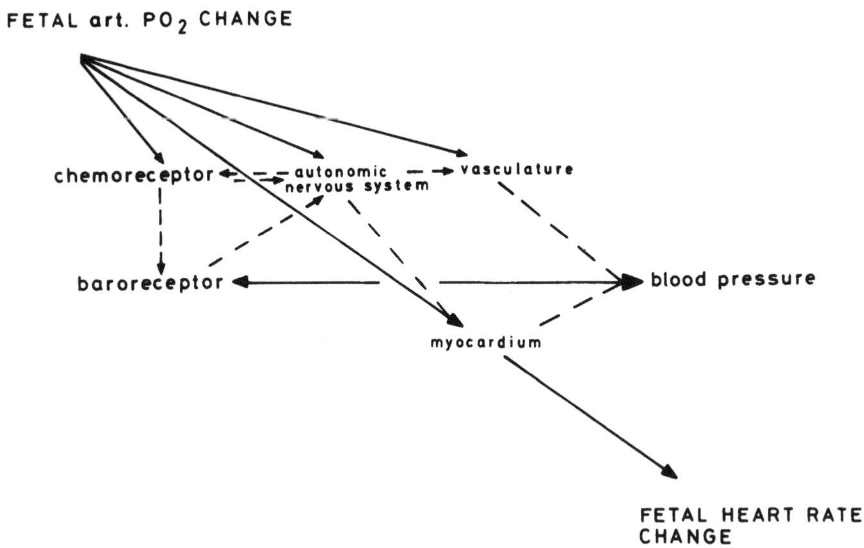

Fig. 10. Schematic drawing of the interaction between PO_2 changes and different compartments of the fetal lamb resulting in a change in the fetal heart rate

same behavior of potassium activity and tissue PO_2 could be observed in the newborn lamb carotid body under apnea as to be seen from Fig. 8. Concomitant with the potassium increase a decrease of the extracellular calcium activity is to be observed under cord clamp conditions in the fetus as shown in Fig. 9. Extracellular potassium and calcium activities in the carotid body were measured simultaneously with microelectrodes as described by Dufau et al. (1982). We can interpret these results in analogy to the results of the cat carotid body (Acker 1980) that hypoxia induces a calcium influx into cells to release transmitter and a concomitant potassium efflux. To explain the lower chemoreceptive nervous activity of the fetal carotid body we would like to follow in further experiments the idea that the amount of released transmitters is too low for a normal excitation. Highly active cytosolic calcium activity controller could be responsible for this.

The complicated relationship between the fall in fetal arterial PO_2 and the change in fetal heart rate is demonstrated in Fig. 10. Hypoxemia exerts its influence separately on chemoreceptors, autonomic nervous system, vasculature, and the myocardium. Via the autonomic system the chemoreceptors themselves control the heart dynamics and the vasculature. Chemoreceptors and autonomic nervous system are interconnected. The changes in blood pressure excite the baroreceptors, which again have their efferent output in the autonomic nervous system. Chemoreceptors and baroreceptors antagonize their afferent input to the medulla. Except the very severe hypoxemia, changes in the fetal arterial PO_2 can hardly have predictable changes in the fetal heart rate due to the magnitude of influences. In further experiments, we would like to investigate whether the relationship between fetal heart rate changes and tissue PO_2 changes in different organs under hypoxemia gives better criteria to judge the fetal oxygen supply situation.

References

Acker H (1980) The meaning of tissue pO_2 and local blood flow for the chemoreceptive process of the carotid body. Fed Proc 39:2641–2647

Acker H, Lübbers DW, Purves MJ, Tan ED (1980) Measurements of the partial pressure of oxygen in the carotid body of fetal sheep and newborn lambs. J Dev Physiol 2:323–338

Biscoe TJ, Purves MJ, Sampson SR (1969) Types of nervous activity which may be recorded from the carotid sinus nerve in the sheep foetus. J Physiol 202:1–23

Blanco CE, Dawes GS, Hanson MA, McCooke HB (1982) The arterial chemoreceptors in fetal sheep and newborn lambs. J Physiol 330:38

Cohn HE, Sacks EJ, Heymann MA, Rudolph AM (1974) Cardiovascular responses to hypoxemia and acidemia in fetal lambs. Am J Obstet Gynecol 120:817–824

Comline RS, Silver M (1974) Recent observations on the undisturbed foetus in utero and its delivery. In: Linden RJ (ed) Recent advances in physiology. Churchill, Edinburgh, pp 406–454

Dawes GS, Duncan SLB, Lewis BV, Merlet CL, Owen-Thomas JB, Reeves JT (1969a) Hypoxaemia and aortic chemoreceptor function in foetal lambs. J Physiol 201:105–116

Dawes GS, Duncan SLB, Lewis BV, Merlet CL, Owen-Thomas JB, Reeves JT (1969b) Cyanide stimulation of the systemic arterial chemoreceptors in foetal lambs. J Physiol 201:117–128

Dawes GS, Fox HE, Leduc BM, Liggins GC, Richards RT (1972) Respiratory movements and rapid eye movement sleep in the foetal lamb. J Physiol 220:119–143

Dawes GS, Johnston BM, Walker DW (1980) Relationship of arterial pressure and heart rate in fetal, newborn and adult sheep. J Physiol 309:405–417

De Burg Daly M (1983) Peripheral arterial chemoreceptors and the cardiovascular system. In: Acker H, O'Regan R (eds) Physiology of the peripheral arterial chemoreceptors. Elsevier/North Holland, Amsterdam

Dufau E, Acker H, Sylvester D (1982) Triple-barrelled ion-sensitive microelectrode for simultaneous measurements of two extracellular ion activities. Med Progr Technol 9:33–38

Giulbeau EJ, Reneau DD (1976) Experimental and theoretical analysis of oxygen transport in fetal brain. In: Grote J, Reneau D, Thews G (eds) Oxygen transport to tissue II. Plenum, New York, pp 721–730 (Advances in experimental medicine and biology, vol 75)

Goodwin CW, Mela L, Deutsch C, Forster RE, Miller LD, Delivoria-Papadopoulus M (1976) Development and adaptation of heart mitochondrial respiratory chain function in fetus and in newborn. In: Grote J, Reneau D, Thews G (eds) Oxygen transport to tissue II. Plenum, New York, pp 713–720 (Advances in experimental medicine and biology, vol 75)

Heistad DD, Abboud FM (1980) Circulatory adjustments to hypoxia. Circulation 61:463–470

Heistad DD, Abboud FM, Mark AL, Schmid PG (1975) Modulation of the chemoreceptor reflex by changes in baroreceptor activity. In: Purves MJ (ed) The peripheral arterial chemoreceptor. Cambridge University Press, Cambridge

Heymann MA, Rudolph AM (1967) Effect of exteriorization of the sheep fetus on its cardiovascular function. Circ Res 21:741–745

Hon EH (1968) An atlas of fetal heart rate patterns. Harty, New Haven

Hon EH, Quilligan EJ (1967) The classification of fetal heart rate. Conn Med 31:779

Huch A, Huch R, Schneider H, Rooth G (1977) Continuous transcutaneous monitoring of fetal oxygen tension during labour. Br J Obstet Gynaecol [Suppl 1] 84:1–39

Jansen AH, Chemick V (1983) Development of respiratory control. Physiol Rev 63(2):437–483

Jansen AH, Purves MJ, Tan ED (1980) The role of sympathetic nerves in the activation of the carotid chemoreceptors at birth in the sheep. J Dev Physiol 2:305–321

Kirchheim HR (1976) Systemic arterial baroreceptor reflexes. Physiol Rev 56:100–176

Künzel W, Kurz CS, Kastendieck E (1981) Die Variabilität der fetalen Herzfrequenzreaktion auf die Reduktion der uterinen Durchblutung. Z Geburtshilfe Perinatol 185:343–350

Lübbers DW, Leniger-Follert E (1978) Capillary flow in the brain cortex during changes in oxygen supply and state of activation. In: Cerebral vascular smooth muscle and its control. Ciba Found Symp 56:21–47

Moll W, Herberger J (1976) Oxygen uptake of the guinea pig at decreased and increased maternal placental blood flow. In: Grote J, Reneau D, Thews G (eds) Oxygen transport to tissue II. Plenum, New York, pp 705–712 (Advances in experimental medicine and biology, vol 75)

Mott JC (1971) Baro- and chemoreceptor mechanisms in hemorrhage. In: Kovach AGB, Stoner HB, Spitzer JJ (eds) Neurohumoral and metabolic aspects of injury. Plenum, NewYork, pp 415–461
O'Regan RGO, Majcherczyk ADS (1982) Role of peripheral chemoreceptors and central chemosensitivity in the regulation of respiration and circulation. J Exp Biol 100: 23–40
Ponte J, Purves MJ (1973) Types of afferent nervous activity which may be measured in the vagus nerve of the sheep foetus. J Physiol 229: 51–76
Purves MJ (1974) Onset of respiration at birth. Arch Dis Child 49: 333–343
Reuss ML, Rudolph AM (1980) Distribution and recirculation of umbilical and systemic venous blood flow in fetal lambs during hypoxia. J Dev Physiol 2: 71–84
Robillard JE, Weitzman RE, Burmeister L, Smith FG (1981) Developmental aspects of the renal response to hypoxemia in the lamb fetus. Circ Res 48(1): 128–138
Rudolph AM, Heymann N (1973) Control of the foetal circulation. In: Comline RS, Cross KW, Dawes GS, Nathanielsz PW (eds) Foetal and neonatal physiology. Cambridge University Press, London
Rurak DW (1978) Plasma vasopressin levels during hypoxaemia: the cardiovascular effects of exogenous vasopressin in foetal adult sheep. J Physiol (Lond) 277: 341–457
Thews G (1960) Die Sauerstoffdiffusion im Gehirn. Pflügers Arch 271: 197–226
Toubas PL, Silverman NH, Heymann MA, Rudolph AM (1981) Cardiovascular effects of acute hemorrhage in fetal lambs. Am J Physiol 240(1): H45–H48
Willcourt RJ, King JC, Indyk L, Queenan JT (1981) The relationship of fetal heart rate patterns to the fetal transcutaneous PO_2. Am J Obstet Gynecol 140(7): 760–769

Blood Flow Measurements in the Human Fetus

J. W. WLADIMIROFF[1], H. M. TONGE, and P. C. STRUIJK

Introduction

Recently, noninvasive methods using 2D real-time and continuous-wave or pulsed-wave Doppler ultrasound have been used to record blood flow velocity waveforms in the human fetus. In 1977 Fitzgerald and Drumm reported on the measurement of blood flow velocity in the umbilical cord by means of continuous-wave Doppler ultrasound. McCallum et al. (1978) recorded blood flow velocity waveforms from the umbilical artery. Measurements on blood flow in the fetal descending aorta and umbilical vein using Doppler ultrasound were first described by Gill and Kossoff (1979) and by Eik-Nes et al. (1980a).

Methodology

The system which will be described in this paper was introduced by Eik-Nes et al. (1980a, b). First the fetal descending aorta was located by means of a 2D dynamically focused linear array transducer (Fig. 1). The sound velocity was calibrated at 1540 m/s. The transducer frequency was 3.5 MHz, and the axial and lateral resolutions

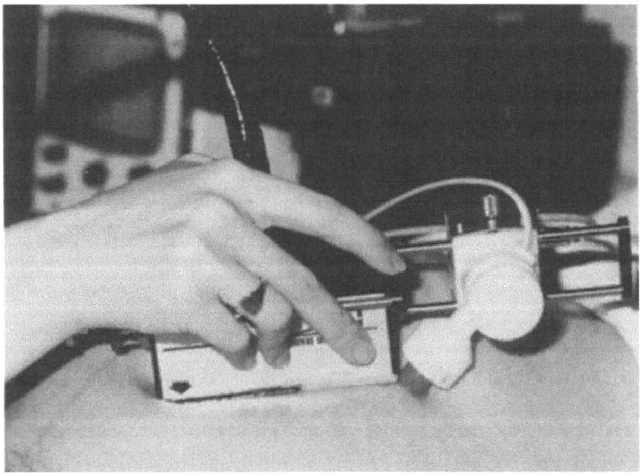

Fig. 1. Combined 2D linear array real-time and pulsed Doppler system

[1] Dept. of Obstetrics and Gynaecology, Academic Hospital Dijkzigt – Rotterdam, Erasmus University Rotterdam, Dr. Molewaterplein 40, NL-3015 GD Rotterdam

Fetal Heart Rate Monitoring
Ed. by W. Künzel

were 1 and 3 mm respectively. A 2-MHz pulsed Doppler transducer with a diameter of 12 mm was used for measurement of the blood flow velocity. The ultrasound pulses were emitted with a duration of 10 ms each at a repetition frequency of 6.5 or 9.75 kHz, which allows measurements of velocities up to 1.7 m/s to a depth of 8.5 cm and velocities up to 1 m/s to a depth of 11.0 cm.

The Doppler probe was attached to the linear array real-time transducer so that the Doppler beam intersected the fetal descending aorta at a fixed angle of 45° (Fig. 1). The beam direction with the sample gate position (electronic marker) could be displayed on the real-time screen.

The Doppler shift (f_d) is given by the equation:

$$f_d = \frac{2 f_o v \cos \alpha}{c}$$

where f_o is the ultrasound frequency, v is the velocity of the erythrocytes, c is the sound velocity in soft tissues (1540 m/s), and α is the angle between the ultrasound beam and the direction of erythrocyte movement. The frequency shift of the reflected ultrasound will be increased in proportion to v. The reflected Doppler signals were fed into estimators of maximum and mean Doppler shifts, which produced analogue output voltages.

Due to unacceptable interference, which results from simultaneous emission of ultrasound pulses from 2D real-time and Doppler pulses, we introduced an interface system. This reduces the image representation from 50 to 1 image/s by switching off the real-time for a period of 980 ms. During this period flow velocity in the fetal descending aorta can be measured. During the remaining 20 ms the pulsed Doppler probe is switched off and the real time-scanner builds up an image; the last measured flow velocity is then contained by means of "hold circuits." This system thus allows instantaneous resetting of the sample volume relative to the vessel lumen, resulting in more accurate flow velocity measurements over a longer period.

Blood flow *(Q)* is calculated according to the equation:

$$Q = \frac{v \pi^2}{\cos \alpha}$$

where v is blood flow velocity and r is vessel diameter.

Following location and determination of vessel orientation, the following measurements are essential in the calculation of volume blood flow: the flow velocity within the vessel and the vessel size.

The first step was positioning of the real-time transducer parallel to the aorta, ensuring maximum display of the vessel length on the real-time screen. An electronic marker representing the sample gate was subsequently moved along the path toward the intersection of the vessel above the diaphragm (descending thoracic aorta). The marker was then placed in the center of the vessel and audio signals were used to ensure that the sample gate was covering the whole lumen of the vessel. A recording of the mean flow velocity was subsequently made.

Aortic diameter measurements have been carried out from 2D real-time images (Eik-Nes et al. 1980a, b; Wladimiroff et al. 1981a, b; Griffin et al. 1983; Jouppila et al. 1983), *M*-mode (Eik-Nes et al. 1982a, b), and time distance recordings (TD) (Eik-Nes et al. 1984). Whereas the first method only provides fractional information on vessel size, the latter method allows continuous monitoring of the pulsatile aortic wall movements and calculation of instantaneous flow in the cardiac cycle using the pulsatile velocity and diameter profile (Tonge et al. 1983).

Clinical Data

Normal Pregnancy

Blood flow in the fetal descending aorta has been studied during the third trimester of pregnancy. The mean blood flow velocity was measured at the lower thoracic level of the descending aorta. The pulsatile vessel diameter was registered at the same level using the dual-time distance recorder. Simultaneous recording of blood flow velocity pulsatile diameter is not possible due to the interference between the ultrasound signals from real-time and Doppler transducers. Instead, these profiles were compared in cardiac cycles of equal R-R intervals as obtained by an external fetal

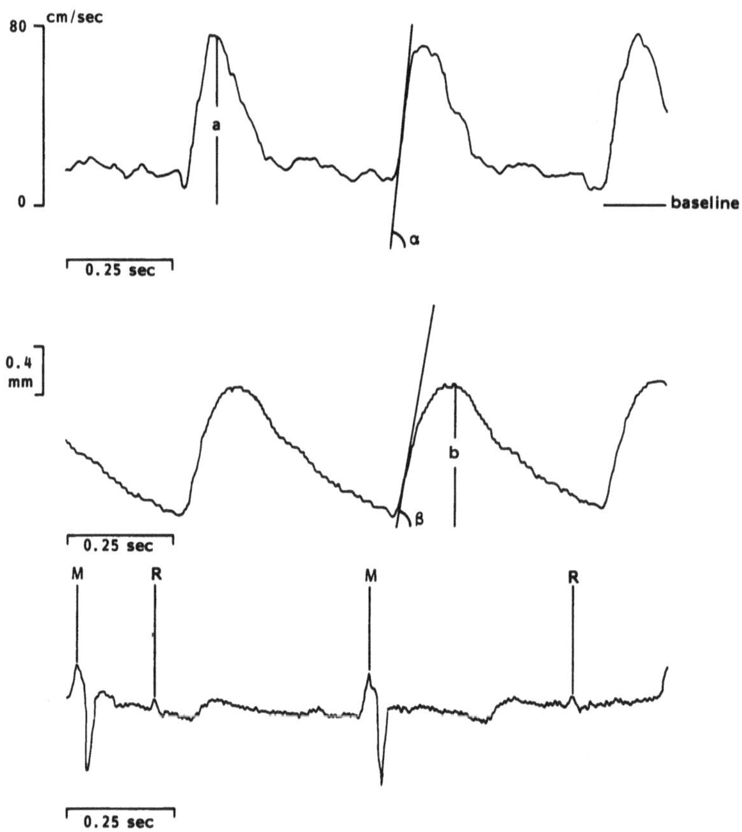

Fig. 2. Tracings of mean flow velocity and pulsatile diameter changes compared in cardiac cycles of equal R-R intervals. *a*, peak mean velocity (cm/s); *b*, diameter change, α, acceleration of mean flow velocity (cm/s^2); β, rate of vessel wall expansion (cm/s); *R*, R-top fetal ECG; and, *M*, R-top maternal ECG

ECG (Fig. 2) (Tonge et al. 1983). Note that the blood flow velocity profile is elevated above the baseline throughout the cardiac cycle. For each of these cardiac cycles, the following parameters were established:

1. Mean blood flow velocity profile, i.e., peak mean velocity and time-averaged mean velocity (cm/s) and acceleration of mean flow velocity (cm/s^2).
2. Pulsatile diameter profile: diastolic diameter (mm), maximum diameter change, i.e., diameter change at peak height of pulse wave (%) and rate of vessel wall expansion (cm/s).
3. Pulsatile index (PI): trough to peak height divided by mean height over one cardiac cycle.
4. Combined flow velocity and pulsatile diameter profile: pulsatile flow integrated over one cardiac cycle, i.e., aortic stroke volume. During one cardiac cycle the flow velocity and pulsatile diameter profile was divided into equal periods. The blood flow velocity and vessel diameter were sampled at these periods and the flow velocity was subsequently calculated using the formula: $Q = 0.25 \times \pi \times d^2 \times v$, where Q is flow, d is diameter, and v is velocity.

From Fig. 2 it can be seen that the blood flow velocity profile is elevated above the baseline throughout the cardiac cycle. The actual data are presented as mean values ± SD in Table 1. Fetal heart, blood flow velocity profile, rate of vessel wall expansion, and maximum diameter change were not significantly different in the two groups. However, the diastolic diameter of the descending aorta, aortic stroke volume, and averaged mean blood flow showed a significant increase during the study period.

Comments

The advantage of pulsed wave over continuous wave Doppler is that the former is range selective. Each short pulse of ultrasound has to travel to the vessel and back.

Table 1. Flow data in the human fetal descending aorta during the third trimester of pregnancy

Gestational age (weeks)	Heart rate (bpm)	Mean blood flow velocity profile		Pulsatile diameter profile			Combined blood flow velocity profile and pulsatile diameter profile	
		Peak mean velocity (cm/s)	Acceleration of mean flow velocity (cm/s^2)	Diastolic diameter (mm)	Rate of vessel wall expansion (cm/s)	Maximum diameter change (%)	Averaged mean blood flow (ml/min)	Stroke volume (ml)
30–35	136.7	70.1	1855.9	5.1	1.4	14.6	390.2	2.8
(mean, 31)	±9.0	±7.9	±339.6	±0.5	±0.6	±3.9	±94.0	±0.7
36–41	142.1	70.4	1748.3	6.5	1.7	12.4	602.0	4.2
(mean, 37)	±8.9	±13.3	±518.2	±0.9	±0.5	±3.2	±142.0	±1.2
Statistical significance				$P<0.0005$			$P<0.0005$	$P<0.005$

It should be realized that there is a depth limitation determined by the pulse repetition frequency (PRF). Moreover, the highest Doppler frequency which can be picked without ambiguity is determined by the PRF. Therefore peak maximum velocities up to 1.4 m/s in the fetal descending aorta can only be accurately recorded up to a depth of 11 cm when insonation angles of 45°–50°, a PRF of 6.4 kHz, and Doppler ultrasound frequencies of 2–3 MHz are employed.

Mean flow velocity calculations are based upon the assumption that flow in major arterial vessels is laminar. Recently, Griffin et al. (1983) pointed out that in the fetal descending thoracic aorta blood flow depicts a plug profile during systolic acceleration and a parabolic profile during diastole. Measurement of mean blood flow velocity is subject to the following errors:

Incorrect Positioning of the Real-time Transducer Relative to the Longitudinal Cross-section of the Aorta. It has been established that when the angle (α) between real-time and pulsed Doppler transducer exceeds 60°, an error in flow velocity measurement of at least 20% can be expected (Griffin et al. 1983).

Incorrect Positioning of the Sample Gate. The sample gate should cover the entire lumen in order to make a correct measurement over the cross-sectional area of the vessel. In the present set-up this is feasible in vessels with diameters between 4 and 9 mm, which is the range usually encountered during the third trimester of pregnancy. Inappropriate positioning of the sample gate may result in erroneous information of flow velocity due to the inclusion of other major vessel structures within the sample gate.

Incorrect High-Pass Filters. High-pass filters are used to eliminate high-intensity, low-frequency Doppler signals originating from the pulsating aortic wall movements. Initially the cut-off point was set at 600 Hz, resulting in considerable loss of frequency information during diastole. Nowadays, a cut-off level at 150 Hz is generally accepted.

Since errors in vessel diameter measurement will be squared when calculating volume blood flow, one should have detailed knowledge of the possible problems which one may encounter in the vessel measurement.

Pulsatility of the Arterial Vessel Wall. The pulsatility in aortic diameter can be a major source of error in volume flow measurements. We found that blood flow calculations based on the maximum vessel diameter may lead to a volume flow overestimation of 9%, whereas blood flow calculations based on the minimum vessel diameter may result in a volume flow underestimation of 19%. In practice this means that if a vessel diameter measurement is carried out from one frozen 2D real-time image, the error in volume flow will vary between +9% and −19%, approaching an underestimation of 5% if ten randomly selected real-time images are taken. From *M*-mode recordings, in which usually the mean of the minimum and maximum diameter is taken, a volume flow underestimation of 5% can be expected.

Origin of the Vessel Wall Echoes. It is not known whether the echo-reflecting boundary of the fetal aortic wall is determined by the muscular layer or by the surrounding connective tissue. In nearly all studies the vessel diameter is measured between the leading edges of echoes from the proximal and distal vessel wall. We found an overestimate in volume blood flow of 8% when the muscular layer alone is taken into account, but an overestimate of 11.5% when both muscular and surrounding tissue are considered.

The blood flow velocity waveform is biphasic with a systolic peak and forward flow during diastole. The end-diastolic forward flow indicates continuous perfusion as a result of the low placental resistance. The relative constancy of the PI as a measure of placental flow resistance has also been reported by Griffin et al. (1983) and Lingman et al. (1983). The constancy of the mean blood flow velocity observed by us and others (Griffin et al. 1983; Marsál et al. 1984) indicates that the rise in volume blood flow in the fetal descending aorta during the third trimester of pregnancy is solely determined by the increase in cardiac ventricular and aortic vessel size. The large standard deviations of the mean blood flow values are not only determined by the grouping of data over several gestational weeks, but also by the limited accuracy of the Doppler technique as a result of the pitfalls described earlier.

References

Eik-Nes SH, Brubakk AO, Ulstein MK (1980a) Measurement of human fetal blood flow. Br Med J I:280–283

Eik-Nes SH, Marsál K, Brubakk AO, Ulstein MK (1980b) Ultrasonic measurements of human fetal blood flow in aorta and umbilical vein: influence of fetal breathing movements. In: Kurjak A (ed) Recent advances in ultrasonic diagnosis 2. Excerpta Medica, Amsterdam, pp 233–240

Eik-Nes SH, Marsál D, Brubakk AO, Kristoffersen K, Ulstein M (1982a) Ultrasonic measurement of human fetal blood flow. J Biomed Eng 4:28–36

Eik-Nes SH, Gröttum P, Anderson NJ (1982b) Estimation of fetal weight by ultrasound measurement. II. Clinical application of a new formula. Acta Obstet Gynecol Scand (1982b) 61:307–312

Eik-Nes SH, Marsál K, Kristoffersen K (1984) Methodology and basic problems related to blood flow studies in the human fetus. Ultrasound Med Biol (in press)

Fitzgerald DE, Drumm JF (1977) Non-invasive measurement of human fetal circulation using ultrasound: a new method. Br Med J 2:1450–1451

Gill RW, Kossoff G (1979) Pulsed Doppler combined with B-mode imaging for blood flow measurement. Contrib Gynecol Obstet 6:139–141

Griffin D, Cohen-Overbeek T, Campbell S (1983) Fetal and uteroplacental blood flow. In: Campbell S (ed) Clinics in obstetrics and gynecology. Saunders, London, pp 565–602

Jouppila P, Kirkinen P, Eik-Nes SH (1983) Acute affect of maternal smoking on the human fetal blood flow. Br J Obstet Gynecol 90:7–10

Lingman G, Laurin J, Marsál K (1983) Aortic blood flow in normal and growth retarded fetuses. In: Proceedings of the 10th conference on fetal breathing movements and other fetal measurements, Malmö, p 79

Marsál K, Lindblad A, Lingman G, Eik-Nes SH (1984) Blood flow in the fetal descending aorta. Intrinsic factors affecting fetal blood flow, i.e. fetal breathing movements and cardiac arrhythmia. Ultrasound Med Biol 10:339–349

McCallum WD, Williams CS, Napel S, Daigle RE (1978) Fetal blood velocity waveforms. Am J Obstet Gynecol 132:425–429

Tonge HM, Struyk P, Custers P, Wladimiroff JW (1983) Vascular dynamics in the descending aorta of the human fetus in normal late pregnancy. Early Hum Dev 9:21–26

Wladimiroff JW, McGhie J, Vosters R (1981a) Fetal cardiac activity. In: Rijstenborgh H (ed) Echocardiology. Martinus Nijhoff, The Hague, pp 417–423

Wladimiroff JW, McGhie J (1981b) M-mode ultrasonic assessment of fetal cardiovascular dynamics. Br J Obstet Gynaecol 88:1241–1245

Subject Index

Acceleration 13, 26, 76, 191, 201, 212, 219, 221, 223
Acetylcholine 172
Acid base 94, 100, 136, 156
Acidemia 147, 170, 197
  metabolic 84, 189
Acidosis 50, 120, 170, 212
  metabolic 94
  respiratory 105
Activity state 195
Adenylate cyclase 132
Adrenal gland 82, 127, 152
Adrenaline 127, 171
  infusion 171, 188
Adrenal-medullary activity 127
Adrenocorticotropic hormone 188
Adrenosympathetic system 97
Afterload 68
Alpha receptor 228
Alpha-adrenergic system
  activity 83
  blocker 83
  mechanism 171
  receptor 68
Amniotic fluid 115
Amplitude 197
  oscillation 197
  saltatory 197
  silent 197
Anaerobic glycolysis 102
Anaerobic metabolic rate 161
Anaerobic metabolism 82, 86
Anaesthesia 140, 226
  halothane 119
  ketamine 104
  sodium pentobarbital 104
Analgetics 193
Anoxia 164
Aortic diameter 235
Aortic occlusion 88, 89, 108, 144
  partial 108
Aortic stroke volume 237
Aortic wall movements 236
Apgar score 77, 146, 197
Apnea 224
Asphyxia 82, 86, 144, 150
  history 5
  mild 172
  phasic 176
ATP production 165
Atropine 89, 105, 106, 112, 171, 189
Auscultation 34
  history 3
Autocorrelation technique 55
  history 13
Autonomic blocking agents 170
Autonomic nervous system 170
Autonomic tone 218

Baroreceptor 89, 100, 106, 120, 129, 172, 187, 219, 226
  aortic arch 226
  carotid sinus 226
  reflex 226
Baroreflex 172
Basal heart rate frequency 191
Basal rate 73
Base deficit 162
Base excess 136, 142
Base line 104, 146, 201, 220
  level 13, 170
  variability 212, 215
Beat to beat
  alteration 146
  history 13
  interval difference 172
  variability 172, 196, 223
Behavioral state 195
Beta-adrenergic blockade 89, 171
Beta-adrenergic effect 171
Beta-endorphin 181
Beta-receptor 132
Biophysical profile 28
Birthweight 221
Blood flow 66, 150, 152, 156, 224, 234
  brain 153
  cerebellum 153
  cortex 153
  glands 152
  heart 152
  hemispheres 153
  interbrain 153
  kidneys 152
  liver 152

medulla oblongata 153
midbrain 153
myocardial 171
pons 153
skin 96, 146, 152
spleen 152
stem 153
thymus 152
thyroid 152
Blood flow ultrasound measurements
continuous-wave Doppler 234
2D real-time 234
pulse-wave Doppler 234
Blood flow velocity profile 237
Blood flow velocity wave forms
descending aorta 234
umbilical artery 234
umbilical cord 234
umbilical vein 234
Blood gas 100, 156
Blood pressure 118
arterial pressure 68, 84, 94, 97, 106, 156, 197, 215, 219, 223
diastolic 98
systolic 98, 140
Bradycardia 69, 73, 82, 86, 88, 134, 228
history 6
reflex 171
Brain 82, 104, 152, 225
activity state 170
function 214
Breathing 170
history 5
Buffer base 136

Calcium
activity 230
influx 230
Capillary
distance 223
structure 223
Carcase 83, 171
Cardiac cycle 237
Cardiac output 66, 68, 83, 85, 89, 98, 104, 132, 171, 172, 188, 219, 224, 228
Cardiotocography
history 12
score 48
Cardiovascular control 127
Carotid artery 161
Catecholamine 68, 127, 132, 144, 178, 188, 224
concentration 97
output 128
release 170
secretion 88, 108
Centralization 156
Central nervous coordination 211
Central nervous system 180, 213
damage 212
Cerebral blood flow 84
Cerebral circulation 86
Cerebral matter
gray 213
white 213
Cesarean section 77, 140
rate 19, 31, 48
Chemoreceptor 89, 100, 106, 107, 120, 129, 172, 223, 226
aortic 171, 187, 228
carotid 228
Chemoreflex 172
Chorioid plexus 160
Chromafin cells 129
Chronotropic 132, 172
CO_2 82, 105, 133
Computer 73
Contraction
history 5
uterine 88, 114, 131, 212
Cord
blood 168
complication 197
compression 90, 179
occlusion 104, 106, 114, 119, 164, 224
occlusion (partial) 106, 114, 216
prolapse 115
Cortisol 219
Crown-rump length 221

Deceleration 13, 76, 79, 88, 94, 97, 118, 144, 146, 156, 164, 191, 221
delayed 212
early deceleration 76, 90
late deceleration 23, 76, 89, 108, 197, 223
pattern 48
variable deceleration 76, 90, 106
Delivery
cesarean section 77, 136
forceps 80, 136
simulating 224
spontaneous 77
vaginal operation 77
Delta wave voltage 214
Diffusion property 223
Dip area 97, 136, 147

Electrocardiography
history 11
Electrocortical activity 214, 218
high voltage 180, 218
low voltage 180
Electrode 13, 26
spiral type electrode 54
Electroencephalogram 209

Electromyogram 209
Embolisation 213
Enkephalin 127
Epinephrine 147, 152
Erythrocyte movement 235

Fetal circulation 66
 pulmonary circulation 67
Fetal distress 77, 223
Fetal death 223
Fetal electrocorticogram 188
Fetal heart rate 68, 73, 78, 86, 94, 104, 118, 132, 136, 144, 156, 170, 189, 201, 212
Fetal heart rate alteration 114, 161
 history 4, 22
Fetal heart rate monitoring 34, 42, 50, 82, 212
 abdominal wall ECG 26, 55, 195
 autocorrelation technique 13, 55
 beat to beat measurement 54
 computer aided 58, 63
 direct 26, 54
 Doppler ultrasound 26, 55, 195
 history 3, 40
 indirect 26
 jitter
 phonocardiogram 26
Fetal heart rate variability 23, 64, 89, 97, 170, 172, 191, 212, 220, 223
 long term variability 23, 105, 191, 218
 low heart variation 64
 short term irregularity index 191
 short term variability 23, 105
Fetal movement 4, 26, 76, 203, 212, 218, 221
 breathing 180, 187, 195, 210, 218
 eye 187, 209, 210
 history 4
 limbs 187, 195
 mouthing 210
 neck 187
 trunk 187, 195
Fetal outcome 212
Fetal oxygen consumption 82
Fetal-placental unit 168
Fetal respiration 64
Fetal scalp blood 21, 145
 fetal scalp stimulation 31
Fetal state behaviour 209
Fever 4
 history 4
Flow measurements
 electromagnetic 196, 212
 ultrasound 196
Frequency shift 235
Frequent lambda 221

Gas tension
 arterial 224
Gestational age 188, 195, 217
Glucose homeostasis 127
Glykogen 132
Guinea pig 161
Gut 83, 171

Haemorrhage 128
Head compression 132
 history 6, 10
Heart 82
Hemoglobin dissociation curve 224
Hemoglobin saturation 105
High-pass filters 238
Home delivery 17
Hypercapnia 108, 128, 170, 189
Hypertension 228
 arterial 170, 178
Hypocapnia 228
Hypoglycaemia 128
Hypotension 171, 214
Hypoxemia 85, 96, 100, 104, 171, 195, 223, 228
Hypoxia 48, 77, 82, 104, 128, 133, 139, 161, 170, 189, 201, 223, 224
 hypercapnic 172
 isocapnic 172, 187, 189
Hypoxic stress 94, 170
Hysterotomy 104

Iliac artery
 occlusion 176, 197
Internal recording
 history 12
Intrauterine growth retardation 212
Ionotropic 133, 172
 effect 228
Isoprenaline 172

Kidney 83, 171, 224

Labor monitoring 46
 intrauterine catheter 46
Lactate 86, 94, 100, 142, 161
 concentration 161
 production 165
 removal 168
 transport 166
Lactic acid 161
 transfer 166
 utilization 166
Laparoscopy 104
Linear array transducer 234
Liver 83, 171
Long-term observation 201
Lung 171
 fluid 132

Macrofluctuation
 amplitude 197, 201

frequency 137
Mechanism of alteration
history 5
Medulla 127
adrenal 127, 170
Medullary centre 188
Metabolism
fetal 166
placental 166
Metarimonol 171
Microblood 18, 43, 145
Microfluctuation 208
Microsphere 151, 156, 213
Mitochondrial respiratory capacity 226
Multineuronal limb reflexes 181
Muscarinic cholinerg blockade 172
Myocardial contractility 68
Myocardial failure 89
Myocardial response 223
Myocardial rhythmicity 170

Naloxone 84, 181
Neurohumoral mechanism 171
Neuromuscular blockade 189
Neuropathologic outcome 214
Neuropathology 214
Noradrenaline 127, 171
infusion 133, 171
Norepinephrine 144, 152, 172
Normoxia 83, 105, 224

O_2-Concentration 161
O_2-Content 85
arterial 224
venous 224
Opioid 83
Oscillation 13, 73, 172
long term irregularity 172
O_2-Solubility coefficient 224
O_2-Uptake 85, 161
Oxygen 82
administration 223
supply 223
uptake 223
Oxygenation 66
Oxygen consumption 85, 118, 131, 224
Oxygen diffusion coefficient 224
Oxygen dissociation curve 85

Parasympathetic
stimulation 133
tone 226
PCO_2 84, 94, 106, 129, 142
transcutan 43
Perfusion pressure 116
Perinatal morbidity 17, 51, 212
Perinatal mortality 17, 31, 43, 51, 212

pH 85, 94, 100, 106, 129, 142, 152, 224
area 143
umbilical artery 78, 197
Phenoxy benzamine 83
Phentolamine 171, 189
Phonocardiography
history 7, 9
Placenta 66, 83
epitheliochorial 161
hemochorial 104, 161
Placental diffusional clearance 167
Placental transfer 165, 166
PO_2 82, 94, 104, 106, 129, 142, 170, 223, 224
difference 224
scalp blood 145
transcutan 43, 95, 97, 106, 144, 223
umbilical artery 85
umbilical venous 85
Posthypoxic period 161
Potassium
activity 229
Pre-ejection period 171
Preload 68
Pressoreceptor
history 6
Primate 104
Propanolol 84, 89, 171, 188
Proton 167
Pulmonary stretch receptors 228
Pulsatile diameter profile 237
Pulsatile index 237
Pulse pressure 99, 118
Pulse repetition frequency 238
Pyrogene 128

Radius
of capillary 224
of tissue cylinder 224
Real-time transducer 235
Reflex mechanism 171
Resistance
peripheral 226
vascular 83, 106, 114, 120
Respiratory neurons
medulla 228
Respiratory pump 224
Rhesus monkey 104, 164, 170, 197
Root mean square (RMS) 206
R-R Interval 191, 236
Rupture of membranes 115

Saturation kinetics 166
Sedatives 193
Sheep 94, 144
fetus 82, 104, 127, 170, 195, 212, 224
Shock 146
Sinoaortic denervation 171

Sinus arrhythmia 196
Skeletal muscle
hind limb 224
Skin blood flow 96, 146, 152
Skin perfusion 99, 108
Sleep
quiet 197
REM 197
SO_2 94, 116, 118, 142, 144, 152, 156, 161, 223
Somatic movements 170
Spatial distribution 223
Spleen 83, 171
Stress test 27
contraction stress test (CST) 27, 220
nonstress test (NST) 27, 201
oxytocin challenge test (OCT) 27
Stroke volume 99, 133
Suprapontine centre 188
Sympathectomy 171
Sympathetic innervation 127
myocardium 68
Sympathetic response 218
Sympathetic stimulation 133
Sympathetic system 127

Tachycardia 73, 88, 212, 215, 223, 228
history 6
Telemetric systems 46, 58
history 13, 26
Thermogenesis 132
Transducer frequency 234
Transection
brain stem 189
suprapontine 189
Trigeminal receptor 228

Ultrasonography
history 13
Umbilical artery 114
Umbilical blood flow 67, 85, 116, 118, 171, 215, 228
venous 196
Umbilical circulation 82, 114
Umbilical vein 106, 114
occlusion 115, 118
Uterine activity 221
Uterine blood flow 82, 85, 114, 128
reduction 83, 88, 94, 139, 161
Uteroplacental insufficiency 213

Vagal
activity 133, 172, 228
cardiodecelerator 172
origin 89
stimulation 223
Vagotomy 179, 187
Vagus nerve 106
Vascular bed
mesenteric 226
renal 226
Vasoconstriction 83, 171
femoral 228
peripheral 97
sympathetic reflex 226
Vasodilatation 84
Vasopressin 83, 181, 188
Vessel diameter 236
Vessel wall echoe 238

MIX
Papier aus verantwortungsvollen Quellen
Paper from responsible sources
FSC® C105338

FSC
www.fsc.org

If you have any concerns about our products,
you can contact us on
ProductSafety@springernature.com

In case Publisher is established outside the EU,
the EU authorized representative is:
Springer Nature Customer Service Center GmbH
Europaplatz 3, 69115 Heidelberg, Germany

Printed by Libri Plureos GmbH
in Hamburg, Germany